MEASUREMENT OF
JOINT MOTION:
A Guide to Goniometry

MEASUREMENT OF JOINT MOTION:
A Guide to Goniometry

Second Edition

CYNTHIA C. NORKIN, EdD, PT
Associate Professor and Director
School of Physical Therapy
College of Health and Human Services
Ohio University
Athens, Ohio

D. JOYCE WHITE, DSc, PT
Assistant Professor of Physical Therapy
College of Health Professions
University of Massachusetts at Lowell
Lowell, Massachusetts

Photographs by Lucia Grochowska Littlefield

Illustrations by Jennifer Daniell
and Meredith Taylor Stelling

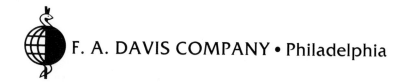
F. A. DAVIS COMPANY • Philadelphia

F. A. Davis Company
1915 Arch Street
Philadelphia, PA 19103

Printed in the United States of America

Last digit indicates print number: 10 9 8 7 6

Publisher, Allied Health: Jean-François Vilain
Senior Allied Health Developmental Editor: Ralph Zickgraf
Production Editor: Crystal S. McNichol
Cover Designer: Donald B. Freggens, Jr. and Steven R. Morrone

As new scientific information becomes available through basic and clinical research, recommended treatments and drug therapies undergo changes. The authors and publisher have done everything possible to make this book accurate, up to date, and in accord with accepted standards at the time of publication. The authors, editors, and publisher are not responsible for errors or omissions or for consequences from application of the book, and make no warranty, expressed or implied, in regard to the contents of the book. Any practice described in this book should be applied by the reader in accordance with professional standards of care used in regard to the unique circumstances that may apply in each situation. The reader is advised always to check product information (package inserts) for changes and new information regarding dose and contraindications before administering any drug. Caution is especially urged when using new or infrequently ordered drugs.

Library of Congress Cataloging-in-Publication Data

Norkin, Cynthia C.
    Measurement of joint motion : a guide to goniometry/Cynthia
Claire Norkin, D. Joyce White ; photographs by Lucia Grochowska
Littlefield ; illustrations by Jennifer Daniell and Meredith Taylor
Stelling.—2nd ed.
      p. cm.
    Includes bibliographical references and index.
    ISBN 0-8036-6579-2 (pbk. : alk. paper)
    1. Joints—Range of motion—Measurement. I. White, D. Joyce.
II. Title.
    [DNLM: 1. Joints—physiology. 2. Movement. 3. Physical
Examination—methods. WE 300 N841m 1995]
RD734.N67 1995
612.7′5—dc20
DNLM/DLC
for Library of Congress

94-29823
CIP

To Carolyn, Alexandra, and Jonathan
Without their support and encouragement this book would not have been possible.

Preface

The measurement of joint motion is an important component of a comprehensive physical examination of the extremities and spine, one which enables health professionals to accurately assess dysfunction and rehabilitative progress. Many educational programs spend considerable time teaching goniometric evaluation. The lack of an appropriate text on goniometry has forced instructors to expend a great deal of effort not only in preparing their own teaching material but also in demonstrating testing positions, stabilization techniques, and goniometer alignments. Students often have difficulty remembering specific aspects of the instructor's demonstration and may not have adequate resources available for study purposes.

Measurement of Joint Motion: A Guide to Goniometry evolved from teaching materials on goniometry originally prepared in 1974 for physical therapy students at Boston University. Over the years, our teaching experience in goniometry made increasingly evident the need for a comprehensive, well-illustrated goniometry text that went beyond a compendium with line sketches. In the early 1980s, we decided to undertake a major revision and expansion of the original teaching materials for the purpose of publication. The first edition of the book that resulted has been well received. It is used as an instructional text in a wide variety of educational programs for health professionals and as a reference guide in many clinical settings.

Since 1985, when the first edition was published, members of the physical therapy profession and other health professions that use goniometry have made significant contributions to the research literature on the measurement of joint motion. Many research studies have been published on the reliability and validity of goniometric measurement, and a few studies have been conducted to examine the effects of age and gender on range of motion.

Our intent in preparing the second edition was not only to enhance the text by adding information on the structure, osteokinematics, arthrokinematics, and capsular pattern of limitation of each joint but also to incorporate some of the research results on goniometric measurement. Our purpose in making these additions was to provide students, faculty, and clinicians with more comprehensive information about each joint, including normal range-of-motion values, joint motion needed for functional activities, effects of age and gender on motion, and the reliability and validity of measurements. We hope that the additional information will help with interpreting the results of goniometric evaluations. Much of the new information is found in Chapter 3 and in well-identified sections within each chapter on specific joints. For readers wishing to focus on measurement techniques, that information is still readily available.

The book presents goniometry logically and clearly. Chapter 1 discusses basic concepts, including the use of goniometry in patient evaluation, arthrokinematic and osteokinematic motions, age and gender effects on motion, and elements of active and passive range of motion. The inclusion of end-feels and capsular and noncapsular patterns of joint limitation introduces readers to current concepts in orthopedic manual therapy and encourages them to consider joint structure while measuring joint motion.

Chapter 2 takes the reader through a step-by-step process to master the techniques of goniometric evaluation. Positioning, stabilization, instruments used for measurement, goniometer alignment, and the recording of results are all addressed. The chapter includes exercises that help develop necessary psychomotor skills and demonstrate direct application of theoretical concepts. In the second edition, we have expanded this chapter to include other devices, in addition to universal goniometers, that may be used to measure joint motion. We also have clarified the documentation process and introduced the sagittal-frontal-transverse-rotation (SFTR) recording method and the AMA *Guides to the Evaluation of Permanent Impairment.*

Chapter 3 discusses the validity and reliability of measurement. The results of validity and reliability studies on the measurement of joint motion are summarized to help the reader focus on ways of improving and interpreting goniometric measurements. Mathematical methods of evaluating reliability are presented along with examples and exercises so that the reader can assess his or her reliability in taking measurements.

Chapters 4 to 12 present detailed information on goniometric testing procedures for the upper and lower extremities, spine, and temporomandibular joint. The text presents the testing position, stabilization, normal end-feel, and goniometer alignment for each joint and motion; this format reinforces a consistent approach to evaluation. The extensive use of photographs and captions should eliminate the need for repeated demonstrations by the instructor. The photographs provide the reader with a permanent reference for visualizing the procedures. The opened book lies flat on a table and therefore can be used easily in a laboratory and in a clinical setting. New to the second edition is the inclusion of information on joint structure, osteokinematic and arthrokinematic motion, and capsular patterns of limitation. A review of current literature regarding normal range-of-motion values, range of motion needed for functional tasks, the effects of age and gender on motion, and reliability and validity also has been added.

We hope this book will make the teaching and learning of goniometry easier and improve the standardization and thus the reliability of this evaluative tool. We believe that the second edition provides a more comprehensive coverage of the measurement of joint motion and hope that the additions will promote new research and use of research results in evaluation.

CCN
DJW

Acknowledgments

We wish to express our appreciation to the following people for their invaluable assistance in the preparation of this book.

To photographer Lucia Grochowska Littlefield we owe a special debt of gratitude. Her patience, good humor, and friendship helped to carry us through the many picture-taking sessions necessary to illustrate each measurement. Lucia's good-natured willingness to pursue excellence combined with her talents is responsible for the high quality of the photographs that are such an important feature of the book. We also extend our thanks to Claudia Van Bibber, who was a subject for some of the photographs.

We are also grateful to Jennifer Daniell and Meredith Taylor Stelling for the various line drawings to which they gave their talents and knowledge.

We are grateful to the many dedicated professionals at F. A. Davis, whose hard work helped make the first edition a success, and those, in particular Allied Health Publisher Jean-François Vilain, who encouraged and aided us in preparing the second edition. We also are indebted to the following rehabilitation educators and clinicians, for carefully reading and fruitfully criticizing the manuscript of the second edition: Mark Westover Cornwall, PhD, PT, Northern Arizona University; Leonard Elbaum, MM, PT, Florida International University; Edmund M. Kosmahl, EdD, PT, University of Scranton; David A. Rohe, MPH, PT, Medical College of Georgia; and R. Scott Ward, PhD, PT, University of Utah.

Contents

PART 1: INTRODUCTION TO GONIOMETRY   1

1 BASIC CONCEPTS   3
   GONIOMETRY   3
   JOINT MOTION   4
      Arthrokinematics and Osteokinematics   4
      Planes and Axes   4
   RANGE OF MOTION   6
   FACTORS AFFECTING RANGE OF MOTION   6
      Age   7
      Gender   7
      Active Range of Motion   8
      Passive Range of Motion   8
   END-FEEL   9
   CAPSULAR PATTERNS OF RANGE-OF-MOTION LIMITATION   10
   NONCAPSULAR PATTERNS OF RANGE-OF-MOTION LIMITATION   10

2 PROCEDURES   13
   POSITIONING   13
   STABILIZATION   14
      *Exercise 1. Determining the end of the
      range of motion and end-feel.*   15
   MEASUREMENT INSTRUMENTS   16
      Universal Goniometer   16
      Gravity-Dependent Goniometers   18
      Electrogoniometers   20
      Visual Estimation   21
      Exercise 2. The universal goniometer   21
   ALIGNMENT   22
      Exercise 3. Goniometer alignment for elbow flexion   25
   RECORDING   26
      Numerical Tables   28
      Pictorial Charts   28

Sagittal-Frontal-Transverse-Rotation Method 28
American Medical Association
Guide to Evaluation Method. 30
PROCEDURES. 30
Explanation Procedure 30
Exercise 4. Explanation of goniometry 31
Testing Procedure 31
Exercise 5. Testing procedure for goniometric
evaluation of elbow flexion. 32

3 VALIDITY AND RELIABILITY 35
VALIDITY. 35
RELIABILITY 36
Summary of Goniometric Reliability Studies 36
Mathematical Methods of Evaluating Measurement Reliability. . . 37
EXERCISES TO EVALUATE RELIABILITY 41
Exercise 6. Intratester reliability 42
Exercise 7. Intertester reliability 44

PART 2: UPPER-EXTREMITY TESTING 47

4 THE SHOULDER. 49
GLENOHUMERAL JOINT. 49
Structure. 49
Osteokinematics 49
Arthrokinematics 49
Capsular Pattern 49
STERNOCLAVICULAR JOINT 49
Structure. 49
Osteokinematics 50
Arthrokinematics 50
ACROMIOCLAVICULAR JOINT 50
Structure. 50
Osteokinematics 50
Arthrokinematics 50
SCAPULOTHORACIC JOINT. 50
Structure. 50
Osteokinematics 50
Arthrokinematics 50
RANGE OF MOTION 50
Functional Range of Motion 50
Effects of Age and Gender 50
Reliability and Validity 52
TESTING PROCEDURES 53
Flexion 54
Extension 56
Abduction 58
Adduction 61
Medial (Internal) Rotation. 62
Lateral (External) Rotation 64

5 THE ELBOW AND FOREARM 67
HUMEROULNAR AND HUMERORADIAL JOINTS 67
Structure. 67

Osteokinematics 67
Arthrokinematics 67
Capsular Pattern 67
SUPERIOR AND INFERIOR RADIOULNAR JOINTS 67
    Structure 67
    Osteokinematics 68
    Arthrokinematics 68
    Capsular Pattern 68
RANGE OF MOTION 68
    Functional Range of Motion 69
    Effects of Age and Gender 70
    Reliability and Validity 70
TESTING PROCEDURES 72
    Flexion 72
    Extension 72
    Pronation 74
    Supination 76

6   THE WRIST AND HAND 79
RADIOCARPAL AND MIDCARPAL JOINTS 79
    Structure 79
    Osteokinematics 79
    Arthrokinematics 79
    Capsular Pattern 79
WRIST RANGE OF MOTION 80
    Functional Range of Motion 80
    Effects of Age and Gender 81
    Reliability and Validity 82
TESTING PROCEDURES: THE WRIST 84
    Flexion 84
    Extension (Dorsal Flexion) 86
    Radial Deviation (Radial Flexion) 88
    Ulnar Deviation (Ulnar Flexion) 90
METACARPOPHALANGEAL JOINTS (FINGERS) 92
    Structure 92
    Osteokinematics 92
    Arthrokinematics 92
    Capsular Pattern 92
PROXIMAL INTERPHALANGEAL AND DISTAL
INTERPHALANGEAL JOINTS (FINGERS) 92
    Structure 92
    Osteokinematics 92
    Arthrokinematics 92
    Capsular Pattern 92
FINGER RANGE OF MOTION 92
    Functional Range of Motion 92
    Effects of Age and Gender 93
    Reliability and Validity 93
TESTING PROCEDURES: METACARPOPHALANGEAL
JOINTS (FINGERS) 94
    Flexion 94
    Extension 96
    Abduction 98
    Adduction 98

TESTING PROCEDURES: PROXIMAL
INTERPHALANGEAL JOINTS (FINGERS) 100
    Flexion 100
    Extension 100
TESTING PROCEDURES: DISTAL
INTERPHALANGEAL JOINTS (FINGERS) 102
    Flexion 102
    Extension 102
CARPOMETACARPAL JOINT (THUMB) 102
    Structure 102
    Osteokinematics 102
    Arthrokinematics 102
    Capsular Pattern 103
    Carpometacarpal Range of Motion 103
METACARPOPHALANGEAL AND INTERPHALANGEAL JOINTS (THUMB) 103
    Structure 103
    Osteokinematics 103
    Arthrokinematics 103
    Capsular Pattern 103
    Metacarpophalangeal and Interphalangeal Range of Motion 103
TESTING PROCEDURES: CARPOMETACARPAL JOINT (THUMB) 104
    Flexion 104
    Extension 106
    Abduction 108
    Adduction 108
    Opposition 110
TESTING PROCEDURES: METACARPOPHALANGEAL JOINT (THUMB) 112
    Flexion 112
    Extension 112
TESTING PROCEDURES: INTERPHALANGEAL JOINT (THUMB) 114
    Flexion 114
    Extension 116

PART 3: LOWER-EXTREMITY TESTING 117

7 THE HIP 119
STRUCTURE 119
OSTEOKINEMATICS 119
ARTHROKINEMATICS 119
CAPSULAR PATTERN 119
RANGE OF MOTION 119
    Functional Range of Motion 120
    Effects of Age and Gender 121
    Reliability and Validity 123
TESTING PROCEDURES 124
    Flexion 124
    Extension 126
    Abduction 128
    Adduction 130
    Medial (Internal) Rotation 132
    Lateral (External) Rotation 134

8 THE KNEE 137
STRUCTURE 137
OSTEOKINEMATICS 137
ARTHROKINEMATICS 138

CAPSULAR PATTERN 138
RANGE OF MOTION 138
    Functional Range of Motion 138
    Effects of Age and Gender 139
    Reliability and Validity 140
TESTING PROCEDURES 142
    Flexion 142
    Extension 144

9   THE ANKLE AND FOOT. 147
PROXIMAL AND DISTAL TIBIOFIBULAR AND TALOCRURAL JOINTS 147
    Structure. 147
    Osteokinematics 147
    Arthrokinematics 147
    Capsular Pattern 148
SUBTALAR JOINT 148
    Structure. 148
    Osteokinematics 148
    Arthrokinematics 148
    Capsular Pattern 148
TRANSVERSE TARSAL (MIDTARSAL) JOINT 148
    Structure. 148
    Osteokinematics 148
    Arthrokinematics 148
TARSOMETATARSAL JOINTS 148
    Structure. 148
    Osteokinematics 149
    Arthrokinematics 149
METATARSOPHALANGEAL JOINTS 149
    Structure. 149
    Osteokinematics 149
    Arthrokinematics 149
    Capsular Pattern 149
INTERPHALANGEAL JOINTS 149
    Structure. 149
    Osteokinematics 149
    Arthrokinematics 149
RANGE OF MOTION 149
    Functional Range of Motion 149
    Effects of Age and Gender 150
    Reliability and Validity 151
TESTING PROCEDURES: TALOCRURAL JOINT 154
    Dorsiflexion 154
    Plantar Flexion 156
TESTING PROCEDURES: TARSAL JOINTS 158
    Inversion 158
    Eversion 160
TESTING PROCEDURES: SUBTALAR JOINT (HINDFOOT) 162
    Inversion 162
    Eversion 164
TESTING PROCEDURES: TRANSVERSE TARSAL JOINT 166
    Inversion 166
    Eversion 168
TESTING PROCEDURES: METATARSOPHALANGEAL JOINT 170
    Flexion 170
    Extension 172

Abduction	. . . .	174
Adduction	. . . .	174
TESTING PROCEDURES: PROXIMAL INTERPHALANGEAL JOINT	. . . .	176
Flexion	. . . .	176
Extension	. . . .	176
TESTING PROCEDURES: DISTAL INTERPHALANGEAL JOINT	. . . .	176
Flexion	. . . .	176
Extension	. . . .	177

PART 4: TESTING OF THE SPINE AND TEMPOROMANDIBULAR JOINT 179

10	**THE CERVICAL SPINE**	**181**
	ATLANTO-OCCIPITAL AND ATLANTOAXIAL JOINTS	181
	Structure.	181
	Osteokinematics	181
	Capsular Pattern	181
	INTERVERTEBRAL AND ZYGAPOPHYSIAL JOINTS	181
	Structure.	181
	Osteokinematics and Arthrokinematics	181
	Capsular Pattern	182
	RANGE OF MOTION	182
	Effects of Age and Gender	182
	Reliability and Validity	185
	TESTING PROCEDURES	188
	Flexion	188
	Extension	190
	Lateral Flexion	192
	Rotation	196
11	**THE THORACIC AND LUMBAR SPINE**	**199**
	THORACIC SPINE: INTERVERTEBRAL, ZYGAPOPHYSIAL,	
	COSTOVERTEBRAL, AND COSTOTRANSVERSE JOINTS	199
	Structure.	199
	Osteokinematics	199
	Capsular Pattern	199
	LUMBAR SPINE: INTERVERTEBRAL AND ZYGAPOPHYSIAL JOINTS	200
	Structure.	200
	Osteokinematics	200
	Capsular Pattern	200
	RANGE OF MOTION	200
	Effects of Age and Gender	200
	Reliability and Validity	203
	TESTING PROCEDURES	206
	Flexion	206
	Extension	208
	Lateral Extension	210
	Rotation	212
12	**THE TEMPOROMANDIBULAR JOINT**	**215**
	STRUCTURE	215
	OSTEOKINEMATICS AND ARTHROKINEMATICS.	215
	CAPSULAR PATTERN	215
	RANGE OF MOTION	215
	Effects of Age and Gender	215

Reliability and Validity 215
TESTING PROCEDURES 216
    Depression of the Lower Jaw (Opening Mouth) 216
    Anterior Protrusion of the Lower Jaw. 218
    Lateral Deviation of the Lower Jaw 219

APPENDIX A: AVERAGE RANGES OF MOTION 221

APPENDIX B: JOINT MEASUREMENTS BY
               BODY POSITION 225

APPENDIX C: SAMPLE NUMERICAL RECORDING FORM . . . 227

INDEX 237

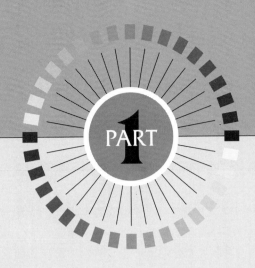

PART 1

Introduction to Goniometry

OBJECTIVES

On completion of Part 1 the reader will be able to:

1. Define:
   goniometry
   planes and axes
   range of motion
   end-feel
   reliability
   validity

2. Identify the appropriate planes and axes for each of the following motions:
   flexion-extension, abduction-adduction, and rotation

3. Compare:
   active and passive ranges of motion
   arthrokinematic and osteokinematic motions
   soft, firm, and hard normal end-feels
   capsular and noncapsular patterns of limitation
   reliability and validity
   intratester and intertester reliability

4. Explain the importance of:
   recommended testing positions
   stabilization
   clinical estimates of range of motion
   recording starting and ending positions

5. Describe the parts of universal, fluid, and pendulum goniometers

6. List:
   the six-step explanation sequence
   the 12-step testing sequence
   the 10 items included in recording

7. Perform a goniometric evaluation of the elbow joint including:
   a clear explanation of the procedure
   positioning of a subject in the recommended testing position
   adequate stabilization of the proximal joint component
   a correct determination of the end of the range of motion
   a correct identification of the end-feel
   palpation of the correct bony landmarks
   accurate alignment of the goniometer
   correct reading of the goniometer and recording of the measurement

8. Perform and interpret intratester and intertester reliability tests

Basic Concepts

This book is designed to serve as a guide to learning the technique of human joint measurement called goniometry. Background information on principles and procedures necessary for an understanding of goniometry is found in Part 1. Practice exercises are included at appropriate intervals to help the examiner apply this information and develop the psychomotor skills necessary for competency in goniometry. Procedures for the goniometric evaluation of joints of the upper extremity, lower extremity, spine, and temporomandibular joint are presented in Parts 2, 3, and 4, respectively.

GONIOMETRY

The term **goniometry** is derived from two Greek words, *gonia*, meaning angle, and *metron*, meaning measure. Therefore, goniometry refers to the measurement of angles, in particular the measurement of angles created at human joints by the bones of the body. When using a universal goniometer, the examiner obtains these measurements by placing the parts of the measuring instrument along the bones immediately proximal and distal to the joint being evaluated. Goniometry may be used to determine both a particular joint position and the total amount of motion available at a joint.

> **Example:** The elbow joint is evaluated by placing the parts of the measuring instrument on the humerus (proximal segment) and the forearm (distal segment) and measuring either a specific joint position or the total arc of motion (Fig. 1–1).

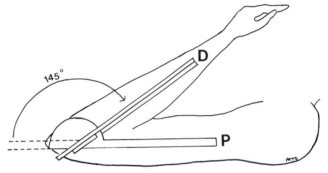

FIGURE 1 – 1. This figure shows the upper left extremity of a subject in the supine position. The humerus (proximal component) is designated by the letter P. The forearm (distal component) is designated by the letter D. The parts of the measuring instrument have been placed along the proximal and distal components and centered over the axis of the elbow joint. When the distal component has been moved toward the proximal component (elbow flexion), a measurement of the arc of motion can be obtained.

Goniometry is an important part of a comprehensive evaluation of joints and surrounding soft tissue. A comprehensive evaluation typically begins by interviewing the subject and reviewing records to obtain an accurate description of current symptoms, functional abilities, occupational and recreational activities, and past medical history. Observation of the body to assess soft tissue contour and skin condition usually follows the interview. Gentle palpation is used to determine skin temperature and the quality of soft tissue deformities and to locate pain symptoms in relation to anatomical structures. Anthropometric measurements such as leg length, circumference, and body volume may be indicated.

The performance of active joint motions by the subject during the evaluation allows the examiner to screen for abnormal movements and gain information about the subject's willingness to move. If abnormal active motions are found, the examiner performs passive joint motions in an attempt to determine reasons for joint limitation and joint end-feels. Goniometry is used to measure and document the amount of available active and passive joint motion. Goniometry is also used to accurately describe abnormal fixed joint positions. Resisted isometric muscle contractions and special tests are used in conjunction with goniometry to help isolate the injured anatomical structures. Tests to assess muscle strength and neurological function are often included. Radiographs, scans, and laboratory tests may be required.

Goniometric data used in conjunction with other information can provide a basis for:

- Determining the presence or absence of dysfunction
- Establishing a diagnosis
- Developing treatment goals
- Evaluating progress or lack of progress toward rehabilitative goals
- Modifying treatment
- Motivating the subject
- Researching the effectiveness of specific therapeutic techniques or regimens, for example, exercises, medications, and surgical procedures
- Fabricating orthoses and adaptive equipment

JOINT MOTION

ARTHROKINEMATICS AND OSTEOKINEMATICS

Motion at a joint occurs as the result of movement of one joint surface in relation to another. **Arthrokinematics** is the term used to refer to the movement of joint surfaces. The movements of joint surfaces are described as slides (glides), spins, and rolls.[1] A slide (glide), which is a translatory motion, is the sliding of one joint surface over another, as when a braked wheel skids. A spin is a rotary (angular) motion, similar to a toy top spinning. All points on the moving joint surface rotate at a constant distance around a fixed axis of motion. A roll is a rotary motion similar to the bottom of a rocking chair rolling on the floor, or a tire rolling on the road. In the human body, glides, spins, and rolls usually occur in combination with each other and result in movement of the shafts of the bones.

Osteokinematics refers to the movement of the shafts of the bones, rather than the movement of joint surfaces. The movements of the shafts of bones are usually described in terms of the rotary motion produced, as if the movement occurs around a fixed axis of motion. Goniometry measures the angles created by the rotary motion of the shafts

of the bones. However, some translatory motion usually accompanies rotary motion and creates a slightly changing axis of motion during movement. Nevertheless, most clinicians find the description of osteokinematic movement in terms of rotary motion sufficiently accurate and use goniometry to measure osteokinematic movements.

PLANES AND AXES

Osteokinematic motions are classically described as taking place in one of the three cardinal **planes** of the body (sagittal, frontal, and transverse) around three corresponding **axes** (medial-lateral, anterior-posterior, and vertical). The three planes lie at right angles to one another, whereas the three axes lie at right angles both to one another and to their corresponding planes.

The sagittal plane proceeds from the anterior to the posterior aspect of the body. The median sagittal plane divides the body into right and left halves. The motions of flexion and extension occur in the sagittal plane. The axis around which the motions of flexion and extension occur may be envisioned as a line that is perpendicular to the sagittal plane and proceeds from one side of the body to the other. This axis is called a medial-lateral axis. All motions in the sagittal plane take place around a medial-lateral axis.

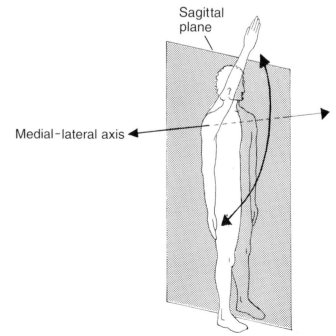

FIGURE 1 – 2. The shaded areas in the illustration indicate the sagittal plane. This plane extends from the anterior aspect of the body to the posterior aspect. Motions in this plane, such as flexion and extension of the upper and lower extremities, take place around a medial-lateral axis.

Example: Flexion and extension occur in the sagittal plane around a medial-lateral axis (Fig. 1–2).

The frontal plane proceeds from one side of the body to the other and divides the body into front and back halves. The motions that occur in the frontal plane are abduction and adduction. The axis around which the motions of abduction and adduction take place is an anterior-posterior axis. This axis lies at right angles to the frontal plane and proceeds from the anterior to the posterior aspect of the body. Therefore, the anterior-posterior axis lies in the sagittal plane.

Example: Abduction and adduction occur in the frontal plane around an anterior-posterior axis (Fig. 1–3).

The transverse plane is horizontal and divides the body into upper and lower portions. The motion of rotation occurs in the transverse plane around a vertical axis. The vertical axis lies at right angles to the transverse plane and proceeds in a cranial to caudal direction.

Example: Medial and lateral rotation occur in the transverse plane around a vertical axis when a person is in anatomical position (Fig. 1–4A and B).

The motions described in the examples above are considered to occur in a single plane around a single axis. Com-

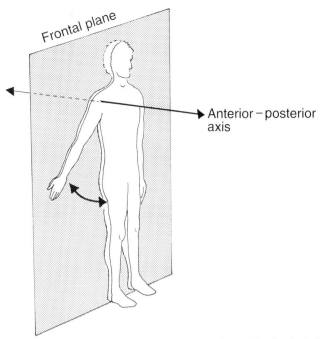

FIGURE 1–3. The frontal plane, which is indicated by the shaded area, extends from one side of the body to the other. Motions in this plane, such as abduction and adduction of the upper and lower extremities, take place around an anterior-posterior axis.

bination motions such as circumduction (flexion-abduction-extension-adduction) are possible at many joints, but because of the limitations imposed by the uniaxial design of the measuring instrument, only motions occurring in a single plane are measured in goniometry.

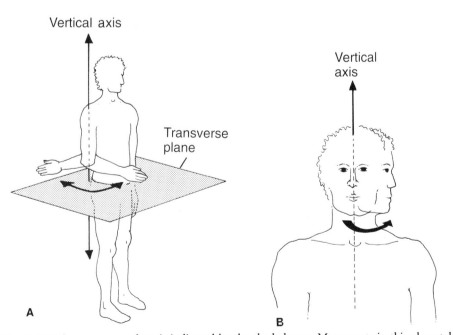

FIGURE 1–4. (A) The transverse plane is indicated by the shaded area. Movements in this plane take place around a vertical axis. These motions include rotation of the head (B), shoulder (A) and hip, as well as pronation and supination of the forearm.

The type of motion that is available at a joint varies according to the structure of the joint. Some joints, such as the interphalangeal joints of the digits, permit a large amount of motion in only one plane around a single axis: flexion and extension in the sagittal plane around a medial-lateral axis. A joint that allows motion in only one plane is described as having 1 **degree of freedom of motion**. The interphalangeal joints of the digits have 1 degree of freedom of motion. Other joints, such as the glenohumeral joint, permit motion in three planes around three axes: flexion and extension in the sagittal plane around a medial-lateral axis, abduction and adduction in the frontal plane around an anterior-posterior axis, and medial and lateral rotation in the transverse plane around a vertical axis. The glenohumeral joint has 3 degrees of freedom of motion.

The planes and axes for each joint and joint motion to be measured are presented for the examiner in Chapters 4 to 12.

RANGE OF MOTION

The amount of motion that is available at a joint is called the **range of motion (ROM)**. The starting position for measuring all ROM, except rotations in the transverse plane, is the anatomical position. Three notation systems have been used to define ROM: the 0- to 180-degree system, the 180- to 0-degree system, and the 360-degree system.

In the **0- to 180-degree notation system**, the upper and lower extremity joints are at 0 degrees for flexion-extension and abduction-adduction when the body is in anatomical position (Fig. 1–5A). A body position in which the extremity joints are halfway between medial (internal) and lateral (external) rotation is 0 degrees for the ROM in rotation (Fig. 1–5B). A ROM begins at 0 degrees and proceeds in an arc toward 180 degrees. This 0- to 180-degree system of notation is widely used throughout the world. First described by Silver[2] in 1923, its use has been supported by many authorities, including Cave and Roberts,[3] Moore,[4,5] the American Academy of Orthopaedic Surgeons,[6] and the American Medical Association.[7]

> **Example:** The range of motion for shoulder flexion, which begins with the shoulder in the anatomical position (0 degrees) and ends at full flexion, is expressed as 0 to 180 degrees.

In the preceding example, the portion of the extension ROM from full shoulder flexion back to the zero starting position does not need to be measured because this ROM represents the same arc of motion that was measured in flexion. However, the portion of the extension ROM that is available beyond the zero starting position must be measured (Fig. 1–6). Documentation of extension ROM usually incorporates only the extension that occurs beyond the

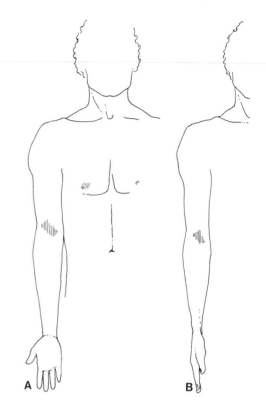

FIGURE 1–5. (*A*) In the anatomical position, the forearm is supinated so that the palms of the hands face anteriorly. (*B*) When the forearm is in a neutral position (with respect to rotation), the palm of the hand faces the side of the body.

zero starting position. The term **extension**, as it is used in this manual, refers to both the motion that is a return from full flexion to the zero starting position and the motion that normally occurs beyond the zero starting position. The term **hyperextension** is used to describe a greater than normal extension ROM.

Two other systems of notation have been described. The **180- to 0-degree notation system** defines anatomical position as 180 degrees.[8] A ROM begins at 180 degrees and proceeds in an arc toward 0 degrees. The **360-degree notation system** also defines anatomical position as 180 degrees.[9] The motions of flexion and abduction begin at 180 degrees and proceed in an arc toward 0 degrees. The motions of extension and adduction begin at 180 degrees and proceed in an arc toward 360 degrees. These two notation systems are more difficult to interpret than the 0- to 180-degree notation system and are rarely used. Therefore, we have not included them in this text.

FACTORS AFFECTING RANGE OF MOTION

Normal ROM varies among individuals and is influenced by factors such as age, gender, and whether the motion is performed actively or passively.

geons,[6] the American Medical Association,[7] and Boone and Azen.[14] Therefore, age-appropriate norms should be used whenever possible for newborns, infants, and young children up to 2 years of age.

Most investigators who have studied a wide range of age groups have found that older adult groups have somewhat less ROM of the extremities than younger adult groups. As in the findings of studies comparing newborns, infants, and young children with adults, these age-related changes in the ROM of older adults also are joint and motion specific but may affect males and females differently. Allander et al.[15] found that wrist flexion-extension, hip rotation, and shoulder rotation ROM decreased with increasing age, whereas flexion ROM in the metacarpophalangeal joint of the thumb showed no consistent loss of motion. Roach and Miles[16] generally found a small decrease (3 to 5 degrees) in mean active hip and knee motions between the youngest age group (25 to 39 years) and the oldest age group (60 to 74 years). Except for hip extension ROM, these decreases represented less than 15 percent of the arc of motion. Boone et al.[17] studied hip and knee motions, ankle plantar flexion, and subtalar inversion-eversion. Comparisons between a group of 20- to 21-year-olds and a group of 61- to 69-year-olds showed decreases, increases, and no changes in ROM with increasing age depending on the motion and gender.

As with the extremities, age-related effects on spinal ROM appear to be motion specific. Investigators have reached varying conclusions regarding how large a change in ROM occurs with increasing age. Moll and Wright[18] found an initial increase in thoracolumbar spinal mobility (flexion, extension, lateral flexion) from 15 to 24 years of age through 25 to 34 years of age followed by a progressive decrease with increasing age. These authors concluded that age alone may decrease spinal mobility 25 percent to 52 percent by the seventh decade, depending on the motion. Loebl[19] found that thoracolumbar spinal mobility (flexion-extension) decreases with age an average of 8 degrees per decade. Fitzgerald et al.[20] found a systematic decrease in lateral flexion and extension of the lumbar spine at 20-year intervals but no differences in rotation and forward flexion. Youdas et al.[21] concluded that with each decade both females and males lose approximately 5 degrees of active motion in neck extension and 3 degrees in lateral flexion and rotation.

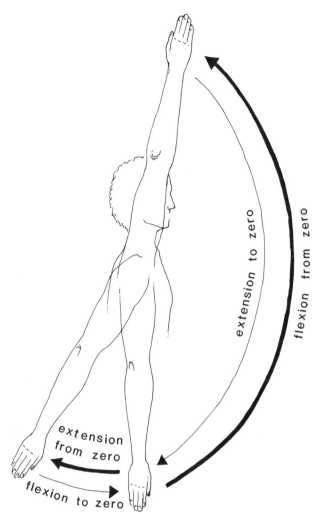

FIGURE 1–6. Shoulder flexion and extension. Flexion begins with the shoulder in anatomical position and the forearm in the neutral position. The ROM in flexion proceeds from the zero position through an arc of 180 degrees. The long, bold arrow shows the ROM in flexion, which is measured in goniometry. The short, bold arrow shows the ROM in extension, which is measured in goniometry.

AGE

Numerous studies have been conducted to determine the effects of age on ROM of the extremities and spine. General agreement exists among investigators regarding the age-related effects on the ROM of the extremity joints of newborns, infants, and young children up to about 2 years of age.[10–13] These effects are joint and motion specific but do not seem to be affected by gender. In comparison with adults, the youngest age groups have more hip flexion, hip abduction, hip lateral rotation, ankle dorsiflexion, and elbow motion. Limitations in hip extension, knee extension, and plantar flexion are considered to be normal for these age groups. Mean values for these age groups differ by more than two standard deviations from adult mean values published by the American Academy of Orthopaedic Sur-

GENDER

The effects of gender on the ROM of the extremities and spine also appear to be joint and motion specific. Boone et al.[17] found that females across an age range of 21 to 69 years have less hip extension, but more hip flexion, than males in the same age groups. Females in the age range of 1 to 29 years had less hip adduction and lateral rotation than males in the same age groups. Beighton et al.,[22] in a study of an African population, found that females between 0 and 80 years of age were more mobile than their male counterparts. Looking at the spine, Moll and Wright[18] found that female thoracolumbar left lateral flexion exceeded male left lateral flexion by 11 percent. On the other hand, male mobility exceeded female mobility in thoracolumbar flexion and extension. O'Driscoll and Thomenson[23] found that age accounted for 57 percent to 70 percent of the variation in ROM of the cervical spine in males but accounted for only 44 percent to 64 percent of the variation in females.

Ideally, to determine whether a ROM is impaired, the ROM of the joint under consideration should be compared with ROM values from people of the same age and gender and from studies that used the same method of measurement. Often such comparisons are not possible, because age- and gender-related norms have not been established for all groups. In such situations the ROM of the joint under consideration should be compared with the same joint of the individual's contralateral extremity. If the contralateral extremity is also impaired, the individual's ROM may be compared with average ROM values found in the handbook by the American Academy of Orthopedic Surgeons[6] and other standard texts.[7,24-31] However, in many of these texts, the populations from which the average values were derived are undefined or the specific testing positions and type of measuring instruments used are not identified.

To assist the examiner, in the beginning of Chapters 4 to 12 a brief review of studies that examine age and gender effects on the featured joint are included. Examiners are urged to refer to these studies for more detailed information. Also, average ROM values published in several standard texts and studies are summarized in tables at the beginning of the chapters and in Appendix A. The average ROM values presented in these tables should serve only as a general guide to identifying normal versus impaired ROM. Considerable differences in average ROM values are noted between the various references.

ACTIVE RANGE OF MOTION

Active range of motion (AROM) refers to the amount of joint motion attained by a subject during unassisted voluntary joint motion. Having a subject perform active ROM provides the examiner with information about the subject's willingness to move, coordination, muscle strength, and joint ROM. If pain occurs during active ROM, it may be due to contracting or stretching of "contractile" tissues, such as muscles, tendons, and their attachments to bone. Pain also may be due to stretching or pinching of noncontractile (inert) tissues, such as ligaments, joint capsules, and bursa. Testing active ROM is a good screening technique to help focus a physical examination. If a subject can complete active ROM easily and painlessly, then further testing of that motion probably is not needed. If, however, active ROM is limited, painful, or awkward, then the physical ex-

amination should include additional testing to clarify the problem.

PASSIVE RANGE OF MOTION

Passive range of motion (PROM) is the amount of motion attained by an examiner without assistance from the subject. The subject remains relaxed and plays no active role in producing the motion. Normally the passive ROM is slightly greater than the active ROM because each joint has a small amount of available motion that is not under voluntary control. The additional passive ROM that is available at the end of the normal active ROM helps to protect joint structures because it allows the joint to absorb extrinsic forces.

Testing passive ROM provides the examiner with information about the integrity of the articular surfaces and the extensibility of the joint capsule, associated ligaments, and muscles. To focus on these issues, passive rather than active ROM should be tested in goniometry. Unlike active ROM, passive ROM does not depend on the subject's muscle strength and coordination. Comparisons between the passive and active ROMs provide information about the amount of motion permitted by the joint structure (passive ROM) relative to the subject's ability to produce motion at a joint (active ROM). In cases of disability such as muscle weakness, the passive and active ROMs may vary considerably.

> **Example:** An examiner may find that a subject with a muscle paralysis has a full passive ROM but no active ROM at the same joint. In this instance, the joint surfaces and the extensibility of the joint capsule, ligaments, and muscles are sufficient to allow full passive ROM. The lack of muscle strength is preventing active motion at the joint.

The examiner should test passive ROM prior to performing a manual muscle test of muscle strength because the grading of manual muscle tests is based on completion of a joint ROM. An examiner must know the extent of the passive ROM before initiating a manual muscle test.

If pain occurs during passive ROM, it is often due to moving, stretching, or pinching of noncontractile (inert) structures. Pain occurring at the end of passive ROM may be due to stretching of contractile structures as well as noncontractile structures. Pain during passive ROM is not due to active shortening (contracting) of contractile tissues. By comparing which motions (active versus passive) cause pain and noting the location of the pain, the examiner can begin to determine which injured tissues are involved. Having the subject perform resisted isometric muscle contractions can help to isolate contractile structures. Having the examiner perform passive joint play tests and ligament

Table 1 – 1 **NORMAL (PHYSIOLOGICAL) END-FEELS**

End-feel	Structure	Example
Soft	Soft tissue approximation	Knee flexion (contact between soft tissue of posterior leg and posterior thigh)
Firm	Muscular stretch	Hip flexion with the knee straight (passive elastic tension of hamstring muscles)
	Capsular stretch	Extension of metacarpophalangeal joints of fingers (tension in the anterior capsule)
	Ligamentous stretch	Forearm supination (tension in the palmar radioulnar ligament of the inferior radioulnar joint, interosseous membrane, oblique cord)
Hard	Bone contacting bone	Elbow extension (contact between the olecranon process of the ulna and the olecranon fossa of the humerus)

stress tests on the subject can help determine which non-contractile structures are involved. Careful consideration of the end-feel during passive ROM also adds information about structures that are limiting ROM.

END-FEEL

The amount of passive ROM is determined by the unique structure of the joint being tested. Some joints are structured so that the joint capsules limit the end of the ROM in a particular direction, whereas other joints are structured so that ligaments limit the end of a particular ROM. Other normal limitations to motion include passive muscle tension, soft tissue approximation, and contact of joint surfaces.

The type of structure that limits a ROM has a character-istic feel, which may be detected by the examiner who is performing the passive ROM. This feeling, which is experienced by an examiner as a barrier to further motion at the end of a passive ROM, is called the **end-feel**. Developing the ability to determine the character of the end-feel requires practice and sensitivity. Determination of the end-feel must be carried out slowly and carefully to detect the end of the ROM and to distinguish among the various normal and abnormal end-feels. The ability to detect the end of the ROM is critical to the safe and accurate performance of goniometry. The ability to distinguish among the various end-feels helps the examiner identify the type of limiting structure. Cyriax,[32] Kaltenborn,[33] and Paris[34] have described a variety of normal (physiological) and abnormal (pathological) end-feels.[35] Table 1–1, which describes normal end-feels, and Table 1–2, which describes abnormal end-feels, have been adapted from the works of these authors.

Table 1 – 2 **ABNORMAL (PATHOLOGICAL) END-FEELS**

End-feel		Examples
Soft	Occurs sooner or later in the ROM than is usual, or in a joint that normally has a firm or hard end-feel. Feels boggy.	Soft tissue edema Synovitis
Firm	Occurs sooner or later in the ROM than is usual, or in a joint that normally has a soft or hard end-feel.	Increased muscular tonus Capsular, muscular, ligamentous shortening
Hard	Occurs sooner or later in the ROM than is usual, or in a joint that normally has a soft or firm end-feel. A bony grating or bony block is felt.	Chondromalacia Osteoarthritis Loose bodies in joint Myositis ossificans Fracture
Empty	No real end-feel because pain prevents reaching end of ROM. No resistance is felt except for patient's protective muscle splinting or muscle spasm.	Acute joint inflammation Bursitis Abscess Fracture Psychogenic disorder

In Chapters 4 to 12 we describe what we believe to be the normal end-feel and the structures that limit the ROM for each joint and motion. Because of the paucity of specific literature in this area, these descriptions are based on our experience in evaluating joint motion and on information obtained from established anatomy[36,37] and biomechanics texts.[26-28,38-41] In some parts of the body, such as the hand, there is considerable controversy among experts concerning the structures that limit the ROM. Also, normal individual variations in body structure may cause instances in which the end-feel differs from our description.

Examiners should practice trying to distinguish among the end-feels. In Chapter 2, Exercise 1 is included for this purpose. However, some additional topics regarding positioning and stabilization must be addressed before this exercise can be completed.

CAPSULAR PATTERNS OF RANGE-OF-MOTION LIMITATION

Cyriax[32] has proposed that pathological conditions involving the entire joint capsule cause a particular pattern of limitation involving all or most of the passive motions of the joint. This pattern of limitation is called a **capsular pattern**. The limitations do not involve a fixed number of degrees for each motion, but rather, a fixed proportion of one motion relative to another motion.

> **Example:** The capsular pattern for the elbow joint is a greater limitation of flexion than of extension. The elbow joint normally has a passive flexion ROM of 0 to 150 degrees. If the capsular involvement is mild, the subject might lose the last 15 degrees of flexion and the last 5 degrees of extension so that the passive flexion ROM is 5 to 135 degrees. If the capsular involvement is more severe, the subject might lose the last 30 degrees of flexion and the first 10 degrees of extension so that the passive flexion ROM is 10 to 120 degrees.

Capsular patterns vary from joint to joint. The capsular pattern for each joint, as presented by Cyriax,[32] is listed in the beginnings of Chapters 4 to 12. For some joints, other authors have described capsular patterns that differ from those of Cyriax.[33,42] Studies are needed to test the hypotheses regarding the cause of capsular patterns and to determine the capsular pattern for each joint.

Hertling and Kessler[42] have thoughtfully extended the concepts on causes of capsular patterns. They suggest that conditions resulting in a capsular pattern of limitation can be classified into two general categories: "(1) conditions in which there is considerable joint effusion or synovial in-

flammation, and (2) conditions in which there is relative capsular fibrosis."[42 (p. 36)]

Joint effusion and synovial inflammation accompany conditions such as traumatic arthritis, infectious arthritis, acute rheumatoid arthritis, and gout. In these conditions the joint capsule is distended by excessive intra-articular synovial fluid, causing the joint to maintain a position that allows the greatest intra-articular joint volume. Pain triggered by stretching the capsule, and muscle spasms that protect the capsule from further insult, inhibit movement, causing a capsular pattern of limitation.

Relative capsular fibrosis often occurs during chronic low-grade capsular inflammation, immobilization of a joint, and the resolution of acute capsular inflammation. These conditions increase the relative proportion of collagen as compared with mucopolysaccharide in the joint capsule or change the structure of the collagen. The resulting decrease in extensibility of the entire capsule causes a capsular pattern of limitation.

NONCAPSULAR PATTERNS OF RANGE-OF-MOTION LIMITATION

A limitation of passive motion that is not proportioned similarly to a capsular pattern is called a **noncapsular pattern** of limitation.[32,42] A noncapsular pattern is usually caused by a condition involving structures other than the entire joint capsule. Internal joint derangement, adhesion of a part of a joint capsule, ligament shortening, muscle strains, and muscle contractures are examples of conditions that typically result in noncapsular patterns of limitation. Noncapsular patterns usually involve only one or two motions of a joint, in contrast to capsular patterns, which involve all or most motions of a joint.

> **Example:** A strain of the biceps muscle may result in pain and limitation at the end of the range of passive elbow extension. The passive motion of elbow flexion would not be affected.

REFERENCES

1. MacConaill, MA and Basmajian, JV: Muscles and Movement: A Basis For Human Kinesiology, ed 2. Robert E. Krieger, New York, 1977.
2. Silver, D: Measurement of the range of motion in joints. J Bone Joint Surg 21:569, 1923.
3. Cave, EF and Roberts, SM: A method for measuring and recording joint function. J Bone Joint Surg 18:455, 1936.
4. Moore, ML: The measurement of joint motion. Part II: The technic of goniometry. Physical Therapy Review 29:256, 1949.
5. Moore, ML: Clinical assessment of joint motion. In Basmajian, JV (ed): Therapeutic Exercise, ed 4. Williams & Wilkins, Baltimore, 1984.

6. American Academy of Orthopaedic Surgeons: Joint Motion: Method of Measuring and Recording. AAOS, Chicago, 1965.
7. American Medical Association: Guides to the Evaluation of Permanent Impairment, ed 3. AMA, Milwaukee, 1990.
8. Clark, WA: A system of joint measurement. Journal of Orthopedic Surgery 2:687, 1920.
9. West, CC: Measurement of joint motion. Arch Phys Med Rehabil 26:414, 1945.
10. Waugh, KG, et al: Measurement of selected hip, knee and ankle joint motions in newborns. Phys Ther 63:1616, 1983.
11. Drews, JE, Vraciu, JK, and Pellino, G: Range of motion of the joints of the lower extremities of newborns. Physical and Occupational Therapy in Pediatrics 4:49, 1984.
12. Phelps, E, Smith, LJ, and Hallum, A: Normal range of hip motion of infants between nine and 24 months of age. Dev Med Child Neurol 27:785, 1985.
13. Wanatabe, H, et al: In Walker, JM: Musculoskeletal development: A review. Phys Ther 71:878, 1991.
14. Boone, DC and Azen, SP: Normal range of motion of joints in male subjects. J Bone Joint Surg Am 61:756, 1979.
15. Allander, E, et al: Normal range of joint movements in shoulder, hip, wrist and thumb with special reference to side: A comparison between two populations. Int J Epidemiol 3:253, 1974.
16. Roach, KE and Miles, TP: Normal hip and knee active range of motion: The relationship to age. Phys Ther 71:656, 1991.
17. Boone, DC, Walker, JM, and Perry, J: Age and sex differences in lower extremity joint motion. Presented at Annual Conference, American Physical Therapy Association, 1981.
18. Moll, JMH and Wright, V: Normal range of spinal mobility. Ann Rheum Dis 30:381, 1971.
19. Loebl, WY: Measurement of spinal posture and range of spinal movement. Annals of Physical Medicine 9:103, 1967.
20. Fitzgerald, GK, et al: Objective assessment with establishment of normal values for lumbar spinal range of motion. Phys Ther 63:1776, 1983.
21. Youdas, JW, et al: Normal range of motion of the cervical spine: An initial goniometric study. Phys Ther 72:770, 1992.
22. Beighton, P, Solomon, L, and Soskolne, CL: Articular mobility in an African population. Ann Rheum Dis 32:23, 1973.
23. O'Driscoll, SL and Thomenson, J: The cervical spine. Clinic in Rheumatic Diseases 8:617, 1982.
24. Kendall, FP and McCreary, EK: Muscles: Testing and Function, ed 3. Williams & Wilkins, Baltimore, 1983.
25. Hoppenfeld, S: Physical Examination of the Spine and Extremities. Appleton-Century-Crofts, New York, 1976.
26. Kapandji, IA: Physiology of the Joints, Vol 1, ed 2. Churchill Livingstone, London, 1970.
27. Kapandji, IA: Physiology of the Joints, Vol 2, ed 2. Williams & Wilkins, Baltimore, 1970.
28. Kapandji, IA: Physiology of the Joints, Vol 3, ed 2. Churchill Livingstone, London, 1970.
29. Esch, D and Lepley, M: Evaluation of Joint Motion: Methods of Measurement and Recording. University of Minnesota Press, Minneapolis, 1974.
30. Clarkson, HM and Gilewich, GB: Musculoskelatal Assessment: Joint Range of Motion and Manual Muscle Strength. Williams & Wilkins, Baltimore, 1989.
31. Palmer, ML and Epley, M: Clinical Assessment Procedures in Physical Therapy. JB Lippincott, Philadelphia, 1990.
32. Cyriax, J: Textbook of Orthopaedic Medicine: Diagnosis of Soft Tissue Lesions, ed 8. Bailliere Tindall, London, 1982.
33. Kaltenborn, FM: Mobilization of the Extremity Joints, ed 3. Olaf Norlis, Oslo, 1980.
34. Paris, SV: Extremity Dysfunction and Mobilization. Institute Press, Atlanta, 1980.
35. Cookson, JC and Kent, BE: Orthopedic manual therapy: An overview. Part I. Phys Ther 59:136, 1979.
36. Williams, P, et al: Gray's Anatomy of the Human Body, ed 37. Churchill Livingstone, Edinburgh, 1989.
37. Moore, KL: Clinically Oriented Anatomy. Williams & Wilkins, Baltimore, 1980.
38. Steindler, A: Kinesiology of the Human Body. Charles C. Thomas, Springfield, IL, 1955.
39. Gowitze, BA and Milner, M: Understanding the Scientific Basis for Human Movement, ed 3. Williams & Wilkins, Baltimore, 1988.
40. Norkin, CC and Levangie, PK: Joint Structure and Function, ed 2. FA Davis, Philadelphia, 1992.
41. Soderberg, GL: Kinesiology: Application to Pathological Motion. Williams & Wilkins, Baltimore, 1986.
42. Hertling, DH and Kessler, RM: Management of Common Musculoskeletal Disorders, ed 2. JB Lippincott, Philadelphia, 1990.

2

Procedures

Competency in goniometry requires that the examiner acquire the following knowledge and develop the following skills.

The examiner must have knowledge of the following for each joint and motion:

1. Recommended testing positions
2. Alternative positioning
3. Stabilization required
4. Joint structure and function
5. Normal end-feels
6. Anatomical bony landmarks
7. Instrument alignment

The examiner must have the skill to perform the following for each joint and motion:

1. Position and stabilize correctly
2. Move a body part through the appropriate range of motion
3. Determine the end of the range of motion (end-feel)
4. Palpate the appropriate bony landmarks
5. Align the measuring instrument with landmarks
6. Read the measuring instrument
7. Record measurements correctly

POSITIONING

Positioning is an important part of goniometry because it is used to place the joints in a zero starting position and to help stabilize the proximal joint segment. Positioning affects the amount of tension present in soft tissue structures

surrounding a joint (capsule, ligaments, and muscles). A testing position in which one or more of these soft tissue structures are or will became taut results in a more limited ROM than a position in which the same structures are or will become lax. As can be seen in the following example, the use of different testing positions alters the ROM obtained for hip flexion.

> **Example:** A testing position in which the knee is flexed yields a greater hip flexion ROM than a testing position in which the knee is extended. When the knee is extended, hip flexion is prematurely limited by tension in the hamstring muscles.

If examiners use the same position during successive measurements of a joint ROM, the relative amounts of tension in the soft tissue structures should be the same as in previous measurements. Therefore, a comparison of ROM measurements taken in the same position should yield similar results.[1] When different testing positions are used for successive measurements of a joint ROM, no basis for comparison exists.

Recommended testing positions refer to the positions of the body that we recommend for obtaining goniometric measurements. Standardized goniometric testing positions have not been established, and testing positions vary considerably among authors. The series of recommended testing positions that are presented in this text are designed to:

1. Place the joint in a starting position of 0 degrees
2. Permit a complete ROM
3. Provide stabilization for the proximal joint segment

If a recommended testing position cannot be attained because of restrictions imposed by the environment or limitations of the subject, the examiner must use creativity to decide how to obtain a particular joint measurement. The alternative testing position that is created must serve the same three functions as the recommended testing position. The examiner must describe the position precisely in the subject's records so that the same position can be used for all subsequent measurements.

Recommended testing positions involve a variety of positions. When an examiner intends to test several joints and motions during one testing session, the goniometric examination should be planned to avoid moving the subject unnecessarily. For example, if the subject is prone, all possible measurements in this position should be taken before the subject is moved into another position. The chart in Appendix B that lists joint measurements by body position has been designed to help the examiner plan a goniometric examination.

STABILIZATION

The recommended testing position helps to stabilize the subject's body and proximal joint segment so that a motion can be isolated to the joint being examined. Isolating the motion to one joint helps to ensure that a true measurement of the motion is obtained, rather than a measurement of combined motions that occur at a series of joints. Positional stabilization may be supplemented by manual stabilization provided by the examiner.

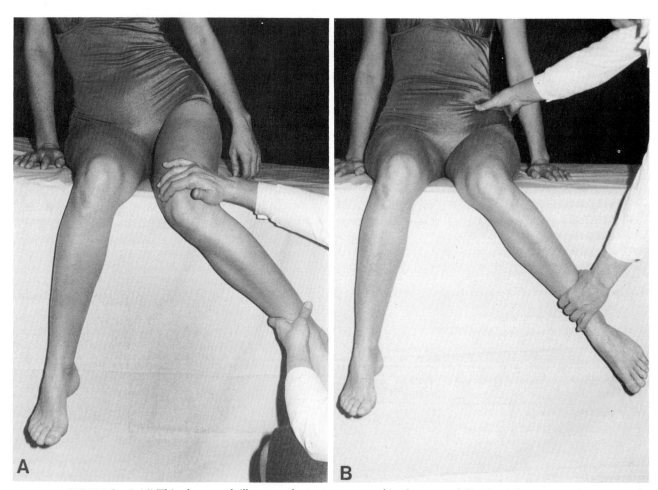

FIGURE 2–1. (A) This photograph illustrates the consequences of inadequate stabilization. The examiner has failed to stabilize the subject's pelvis and trunk; therefore, a lateral tilt of the pelvis and lateral flexion of the trunk accompany the motion of hip internal rotation. The range of internal rotation appears greater than it actually is because of the added motion from the pelvis and trunk. (B) This photograph illustrates the use of proper stabilization. The examiner is using her right hand to stabilize the pelvis (keep the pelvis from raising off the table) during the passive range of motion. The subject is instructed to assist in stabilizing the pelvis by placing her weight on the left side. The subject is asked to keep her trunk straight by placing both hands on the table.

Example: Measurement of medial (internal) rotation of the hip joint is performed with the subject in a recommended sitting position (Fig. 2–1A). The pelvis (proximal segment) is partially stabilized by the body weight, but the subject is moving her trunk and pelvis during hip rotation.

Additional stabilization should be provided by the examiner and the subject (Fig. 2–1B). The examiner provides manual stabilization for the pelvis by exerting a downward pressure on the iliac crest on the side being tested. The subject is instructed to shift her body weight over the hip being tested to help keep the pelvis stabilized.

For most measurements, the amount of manual stabilization applied by an examiner must be sufficient to keep the proximal joint segment fixed during movement of the distal joint component. If both the distal and proximal joint components are allowed to move during joint testing, the end of the ROM is difficult to determine. Learning how to stabilize requires practice because the examiner must stabilize with one hand while simultaneously moving the distal joint segment with the other hand. The techniques of stabilizing the proximal joint segment and of determining the end of a ROM (end-feel) are basic to goniometry and must be mastered prior to learning how to use the goniometer. Exercise 1 is designed to help the examiner learn how to stabilize and determine the end of the ROM (end-feel).

EXERCISE 1 ■ DETERMINING THE END OF THE RANGE OF MOTION AND END-FEEL

This exercise is designed to help the examiner determine the end of the ROM and to differentiate among the three normal end-feels: soft, firm, and hard.

ELBOW FLEXION: SOFT END-FEEL

Activities: See Figure 5–1 in Chapter 5.

1. Select a subject.
2. Position the subject supine with the arm placed close to the side of the body. A towel roll is placed under the distal end of the humerus to allow full elbow extension. The forearm is placed in full supination with the palm of the hand facing the ceiling. Move the subject's forearm toward the humerus (flex elbow).
3. With one hand, stabilize the distal end of the humerus (proximal joint segment) to prevent flexion of the shoulder.
4. With the other hand, slowly move the forearm through the full passive range of elbow flexion until you feel resistance limiting the motion.
5. Gently push against the resistance until no further flexion can be achieved. Carefully note the quality of the resistance. This soft end-feel is caused by compression of the muscle bulk of the anterior forearm with that of the anterior upper arm.
6. Compare this soft end-feel with the soft end-feel found in knee flexion (see the section on knee flexion in Chapter 8).

ANKLE DORSIFLEXION: FIRM END-FEEL

Activities: See Figure 9–1 in Chapter 9.

1. Select a subject.
2. Place the subject sitting so that the lower leg is over the edge of the supporting surface and the knee is flexed at least 30 degrees.
3. With one hand, stabilize the distal end of the tibia and fibula to prevent knee extension and hip motions.
4. With the other hand on the plantar surface of the metatarsals, slowly move the foot through the full passive range of ankle dorsiflexion until you feel resistance limiting the motion.
5. Push against the resistance until no further dorsiflexion can be achieved. Carefully note the quality of the resistance. This firm end-feel is caused by tension in the Achilles tendon, the posterior portion of the deltoid ligament, the posterior talofibular ligament, the calcaneofibular ligament, the

posterior joint capsule, and the wedging of the talus into the mortise formed by the tibia and fibula.

6. Compare this firm end-feel with the firm end-feel found in metacarpophalangeal extension of the fingers (see Chapter 6).

ELBOW EXTENSION: HARD END-FEEL

Activities

1. Select a subject.
2. Position the subject supine with the arm placed close to the side of the body. A small towel roll is placed under the distal end of the humerus to allow full elbow extension. The forearm is placed in full supination with the palm of the hand facing the ceiling. Move the subject's forearm toward the humerus (flex elbow).
3. With one hand resting on the towel roll and holding the posterior, distal end of the humerus, stabilize the humerus (proximal joint segment) to prevent extension of the shoulder.
4. With the other hand, slowly move the forearm through the full passive range of elbow extension until you feel resistance limiting the motion.
5. Gently push against the resistance until no further extension can be attained. Carefully note the quality of the resistance. When the end-feel is hard, it has no give to it. This hard end-feel is caused by contact between the olecranon process of the ulna and the olecranon fossa of the humerus.
6. Compare this hard end-feel with the hard end-feel usually found in radial deviation of the wrist (see radial deviation in Chapter 6).

MEASUREMENT INSTRUMENTS

A variety of instruments are used to measure joint motion. These instruments range from simple paper tracings and tape measures to elaborate electrogoniometers. An examiner may choose to use a particular instrument on the basis of the instrument's accuracy, cost, availability, and ease of use.

UNIVERSAL GONIOMETER

The most common instrument used to measure joint position and motion in the clinical setting is the **universal goniometer**. Moore[2,3] designated this type of goniometer as "universal" because of its versatility. It can be used to measure joint position and ROM at almost all joints of the body. The measurement techniques presented in this book demonstrate the use of the universal goniometer.

Universal goniometers may be constructed of metal or plastic. These instruments are produced in many sizes and shapes but adhere to the same basic design (Fig. 2–2). Typically the design includes a body and two thin extensions called arms—a stationary arm and a moving arm (Fig. 2–3).

The **body** of a universal goniometer resembles a protractor and may form a full or half-circle (Fig. 2–4). Measurement scales are located on one or both sides of the body.

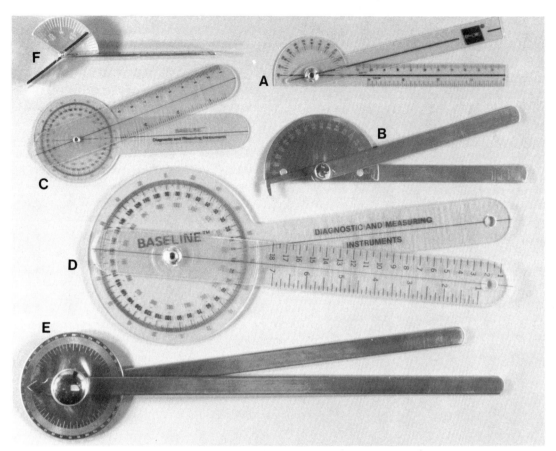

FIGURE 2-2. Metal and plastic universal goniometers are available in different sizes and shapes. Some goniometers have half-circle bodies and are made of plastic (*A*) or metal (*B*). Other goniometers have full-circle bodies and are made of plastic (*C* and *D*) or metal (*E*). Large goniometers (*D* and *E*) are used to measure large joints such as the hip and shoulder. The small metal goniometer (*F*) at the top left side of the photograph is specifically designed to measure the fingers and toes.

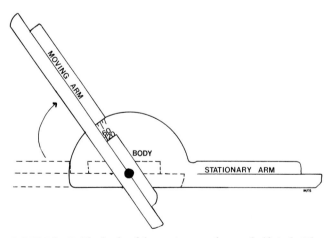

FIGURE 2-3. The body of the goniometer forms a half circle. The stationary arm is an integral part of the body of this particular type of goniometer and cannot be moved independently. The moving arm is attached to the body by either a screw or rivet, so that it can be moved with no accompanying movement of the body. In this example, the moving arm has a cut-out portion sometimes referred to as a "window." The window permits the examiner to read the scale on the body of the instrument.

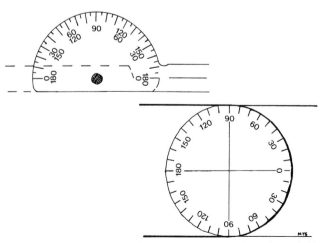

FIGURE 2-4. The body of the goniometer may be either a half circle (*top*) or a full circle (*bottom*).

Sometimes two scales are located on each body surface. The scales on a full-circle instrument extend either from 0 to 180 degrees and from 180 to 0 degrees, or from 0 to 360 degrees and from 360 to 0 degrees. The scales on a half-circle instrument extend from 0 to 180 degrees and from 180 to 0 degrees. The intervals on the scales may vary from 1 to 10 degrees.

Traditionally, the **arms** of a universal goniometer are designated as moving or stationary according to their method of attachment to the body of the goniometer. The **stationary arm** is a structural part of the body of the goniometer and cannot be moved independently of the body. The **moving arm** is attached to the fulcrum in the center of the body of the goniometer by a screwlike device that permits the arm to move freely on the body. In some instruments the screw may be tightened to hold the moving arm in a certain position or loosened to allow free movement. The moving arm may have one or more of the following features: a pointed proximal end, a black or white line extending the length of the arm, or a cut-out portion (window) (Fig. 2–5). These features help the examiner to read the scales.

The length of the arms varies among instruments from approximately 1 to 16 inches. These variations in length represent an attempt on the part of the manufacturers to adapt the size of the instrument to the size of the joints.

> **Example:** A universal goniometer with 16-inch arms is appropriate for measuring motion at the knee joint because the arms are long enough to permit alignment with the greater trochanter of the femur and the lateral malleolus of the tibia (Fig. 2–6A). A universal goniometer with short arms would be inappropriate because the arms do not extend a sufficient distance along either the femur or the tibia to permit accurate alignment with the bony landmarks (Fig. 2–6B). The same long arms would be inappropriate for measurement of the metacarpophalangeal joints of the hand because aligning the arms with the phalangeal and metacarpal bones would be awkward.

GRAVITY-DEPENDENT GONIOMETERS

Although not as common as the universal goniometer, several other types of manual goniometers may be found in the clinical setting. **Gravity-dependent goniometers** are

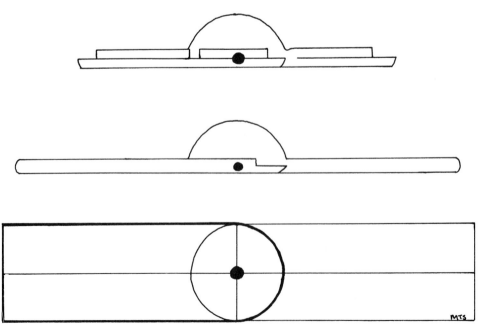

FIGURE 2–5. The top instrument is a half-circle goniometer with a number of features that make reading instruments easier. The moving arm has a black line that extends its length and cut-out areas at both ends and in the middle. The half-circle goniometer in the middle has a cut-out area only at the end of its moving arm. The full-circle plastic goniometer (*bottom*) has a black line extending along the middle of both the moving and stationary arms.

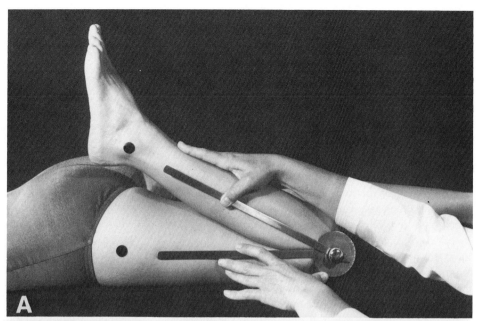

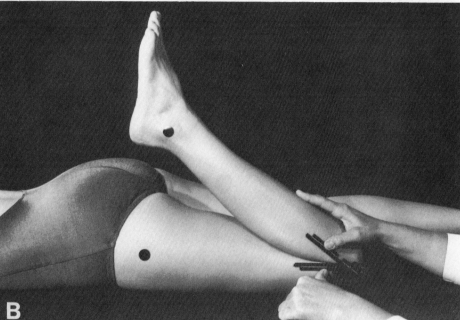

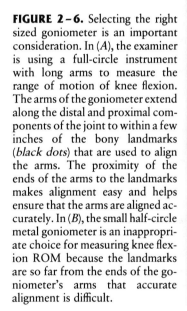

FIGURE 2 – 6. Selecting the right sized goniometer is an important consideration. In (*A*), the examiner is using a full-circle instrument with long arms to measure the range of motion of knee flexion. The arms of the goniometer extend along the distal and proximal components of the joint to within a few inches of the bony landmarks (*black dots*) that are used to align the arms. The proximity of the ends of the arms to the landmarks makes alignment easy and helps ensure that the arms are aligned accurately. In (*B*), the small half-circle metal goniometer is an inappropriate choice for measuring knee flexion ROM because the landmarks are so far from the ends of the goniometer's arms that accurate alignment is difficult.

sometimes called **inclinometers**. They use gravity's effect on pointers and fluid levels to measure joint position and motion (Fig. 2–7). The **pendulum goniometer** consists of a 360-degree protractor with a weighted pointer hanging from the center of the protractor. This device was first described by Fox and Van Breemen[4] in 1934. The **fluid (bubble) goniometer**, which was developed by Schenkar[5] in 1956, has a fluid-filled circular chamber containing an air bubble. It is similar to a carpenter's level, but being circular, has a 360-degree scale.

Both types of instrument are attached to or held on the distal segment of the joint being measured. The angle between the long axis of the distal segment and the line of gravity is noted. The pendulum and fluid goniometers may be easier to use in certain situations than the universal goniometer because they do not have to be aligned with bony landmarks. However, it is critical that the proximal segment of the joint being measured be positioned vertically or horizontally to obtain accurate measurements; otherwise, adjustments must be made in determining the measurement.[3,6] Pendulum and fluid goniometers are also difficult to use on small joints[7] and where there is soft tissue deformity or edema.[3,6]

Although universal, pendulum, and fluid goniometers may all be available within a clinical setting, they should not be used interchangeably.[8,9] For example, an examiner should not use a universal goniometer on Tuesday and a pendulum goniometer on Wednesday to measure a subject's knee ROM. The goniometers may provide slightly different results, making comparisons for judging changes in ROM inappropriate.

ELECTROGONIOMETERS

Electrogoniometers, introduced by Karpovich and Karpovich[10] in 1959, are used primarily in research to obtain dynamic joint measurements. Most devices have two arms, similar to those of the universal goniometer, which are attached to the proximal and distal segments of the joint being measured.[11-13] A potentiometer is connected to the two arms. Changes in joint position cause the resistance in the potentiometer to vary. The resulting change in voltage can be used to indicate the amount of joint motion.

Some electrogoniometers resemble pendulum goniometers.[14] Changes in joint position cause a change in contact between the pendulum and small resistors. Contact with the resistors produces a change in electric current, which is used to indicate the amount of joint motion. Electrogoniometers are expensive and take time to accurately calibrate and attach to the subject. Given these drawbacks, electrogoniometers are more often used in research than in

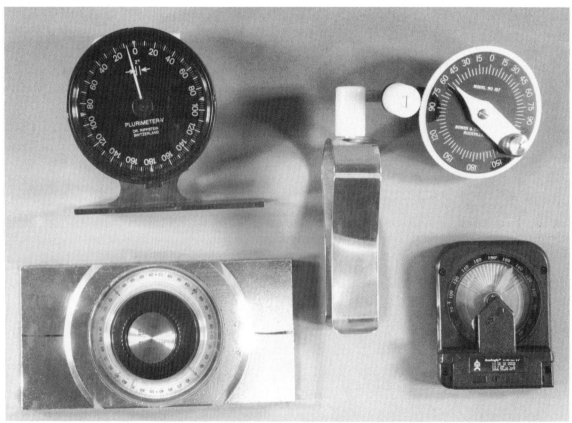

FIGURE 2–7. Each of these gravity-dependent, pendulum goniometers uses a weighted pointer to indicate the position of the goniometer relative to the vertical pull of gravity.

clinical settings. Radiographs, photographs, film, and videotapes are other joint measurement methods used more commonly in research settings.

VISUAL ESTIMATION

Although some examiners make **visual estimates** of joint position and motion rather than use a measuring instrument, we do not recommend this practice. Several authors suggest the use of visual estimates, especially in situations in which the subject has excessive soft tissue.[15,16] Most authorities report more accurate and reliable measurements using a goniometer in comparison to visual estimates.[17-22] Even when produced by a skilled examiner, visual estimates yield only subjective information, in contrast to goniometric measurements, which yield objective information. However, estimates are useful in the learning process. Such estimates made prior to goniometric measurements help to reduce errors attributable to reading the goniometer incorrectly. Goniometric measurements of a ROM can be compared with the approximate ROM obtained through observation. If the goniometric measurement is not in the same quadrant as the estimate, the examiner is alerted to the possibility that the wrong scale is being read.

After the examiner has read and studied this section on measurement instruments, Exercise 2 should be completed. Given the adaptability and widespread use of the universal goniometer in the clinical setting, this book focuses on teaching the measurement of joint motion using a universal goniometer.

EXERCISE 2 ■ THE UNIVERSAL GONIOMETER

The following activities are designed to help the examiner become familiar with the universal goniometer.

Equipment: Full-circle and half-circle universal goniometers made of plastic and metal.

Activities

1. Select a goniometer.
2. Identify the type of goniometer selected (full- or half-circle) by noting the shape of the body.
3. Differentiate between the moving and stationary arms of the goniometer. (Remember the stationary arm is an integral part of the body of the goniometer.)
4. Observe the moving arm to see if it has a cut-out portion.
5. Find the line in the middle of the moving arm and follow it to a number on the scale.
6. Study the face on the body of the goniometer and answer the following questions:
   Is the scale located on one or both sides?
   Is it possible to read the scale through the face of the goniometer?
   What intervals are used?
   Does the face contain one or two scales?
7. Hold the goniometer in both hands. Position the arms so that they form a continuous straight line. When the arms are in this position, the goniometer is at 0 degrees.
8. Keep the stationary arm fixed in place and shift the moving arm while watching the numbers on the scale, either at the tip of the moving arm or in the cut-out portion. Shift the moving arm from 0 to 45, 90, 150, and 180 degrees.
9. Keep the stationary arm fixed and shift the moving arm from 0 degrees through an estimated 45-degree arc of motion. Compare the estimate with the actual arc of motion by reading the scale on the goniometer. Try to estimate other arcs of motion and compare the estimates with the actual arc of motion.
10. Keep the moving arm fixed in place and move the stationary arm through different arcs of motion.
11. Repeat steps 2 to 10 using different goniometers.

ALIGNMENT

"Goniometer alignment" refers to the alignment of the arms of the goniometer with the proximal and distal segments of the joint being evaluated. Instead of depending on soft tissue contour, the examiner uses bony anatomical landmarks to more accurately visualize the joint segments. These landmarks, which have been identified for all joint measurements, should be exposed so that they may be identified easily (Fig. 2–8). Depending on the joint being evaluated, the subject may need to remove clothing to expose the anatomical landmarks. Use of these landmarks in conjunction with recommended testing positions should increase the accuracy and reliability of goniometric measurements. The landmarks and the test positions should be learned and adhered to whenever possible.

The stationary arm is often aligned parallel to the longitudinal axis of the proximal segment of the joint, and the moving arm is aligned parallel to the longitudinal axis of the distal segment of the joint (Fig. 2–9). In some situations,

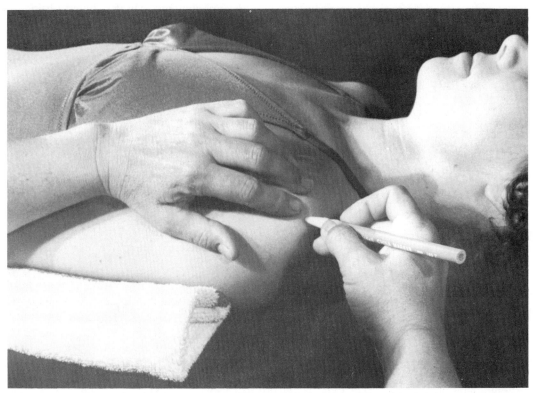

FIGURE 2–8. The examiner is using a grease pencil to mark the location of the subject's left acromion process. Note that the examiner is using the second and third digits of her left hand to palpate the bony landmark.

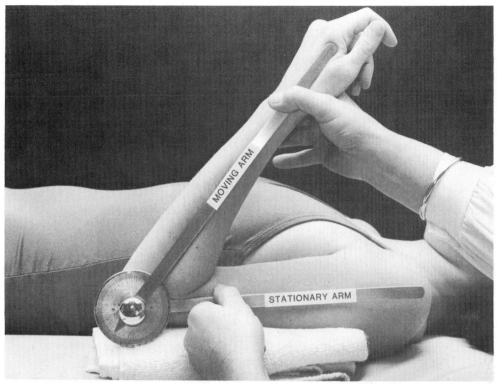

FIGURE 2 – 9. When using a full-circle goniometer to measure ROM of elbow flexion, align the stationary arm of the instrument parallel to the longitudinal axis of the proximal part (subject's left humerus) and align the moving arm parallel to the longitudinal axis of the distal part (subject's left forearm).

because of limitations imposed by either the goniometer or the subject (Fig. 2 – 10A), it may be necessary to reverse the alignment of the two arms so that the moving arm is aligned with the proximal part and the stationary arm is aligned with the distal portion (Fig. 2 – 10B). Therefore, we have decided to use the term **proximal arm** to refer to the arm of

the goniometer that is aligned with the proximal segment of the joint. The term **distal arm** refers to the arm aligned with the distal segment of the joint. The anatomical landmarks provide reference points that help to ensure that the alignment of the arms is correct.

The **fulcrum** of the goniometer may be placed over the

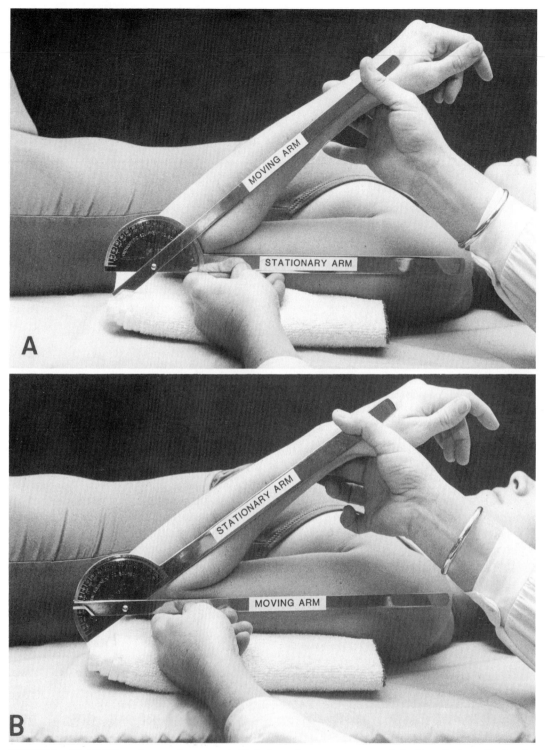

FIGURE 2–10. (*A*) When the examiner uses a half-circle goniometer to measure left elbow flexion, aligning the moving arm with the subject's forearm causes the pointer to move beyond the goniometer body, which makes it impossible to read the scale. (*B*) Reversing the arms of the instrument so that the stationary arm is aligned parallel to the moving (distal) part and the moving arm is aligned parallel to the proximal part means that the pointer remains on the body of the goniometer, enabling the examiner to read the scale along the pointer.

approximate location of the axis of motion of the joint being measured. However, because the axis of motion changes during movement, the location of the fulcrum must be adjusted accordingly. Moore[3] suggests that careful alignment of the proximal and distal arms ensures that the fulcrum of the goniometer is located at the approximate axis of motion. Therefore, alignment of the arms of the goniometer with the proximal and distal joint segments should be emphasized more than placement of the fulcrum over the approximate axis of motion.

Errors in measuring joint position and motion with a goniometer can occur if the examiner is not careful. When aligning the arms and reading the scale of the goniometer, the examiner must be at eye level with the goniometer to avoid parallax. If the examiner is higher or lower than the goniometer, the alignment and scales may be distorted. Often a goniometer will have several scales, one going from 0 to 180 degrees and another going from 180 to 0 degrees. Examiners must carefully determine which scale is correct for the measurement. If a visual estimate is made before the measurement is taken, gross errors caused by reading the wrong scale will be obvious. Another source of error is in misinterpreting the intervals on the scale. For example, the smallest interval of a particular goniometer may be 5 degrees, but an examiner may believe the interval represents 1 degree. In this case the examiner would incorrectly read 91 degrees instead of 95 degrees.

After the examiner has read this section on alignment, Exercise 3 should be completed.

EXERCISE 3 ■ GONIOMETER ALIGNMENT FOR ELBOW FLEXION

The following activities are designed to help the examiner learn how to align and read the goniometer.

Equipment: Full- and half-circle universal goniometers of plastic and metal in various sizes and a skin-marking pencil.

Activities: See Figures 5–1 to 5–3 in Chapter 5.

1. Select a goniometer and a subject.
2. Position the subject so that he or she is supine. The subject's right arm should be positioned so that it is close to the side of the body with the forearm in supination (palm of hand faces the ceiling). A towel roll placed under the distal humerus will help to ensure that the elbow is fully extended.
3. Locate and mark each of the following landmarks with the pencil: acromion process, lateral epicondyle of the humerus, radial head, and radial styloid process.
4. Align the proximal arm of the goniometer along the longitudinal axis of the humerus, using the acromion process and the lateral epicondyle as reference landmarks. Make sure that you are positioned so that the goniometer is at eye level during the alignment process.
5. Align the distal arm of the goniometer along the longitudinal axis of the radius, using the radial head and the radial styloid process as reference landmarks.
6. The fulcrum should be close to the lateral epicondyle. Check to make sure that the body of the goniometer is not being deflected by the supporting surface.
7. Recheck the alignment of the arms and readjust the alignment as necessary.
8. Read the scale on the goniometer.
9. Remove the goniometer from the subject's arm and place it nearby so it is handy for measuring the next joint position.
10. Move the subject's forearm into various positions in the flexion ROM, including the end of the flexion ROM. At each joint position, align and read the goniometer. Remember that you must support the subject's forearm while aligning the goniometer.
11. Repeat steps 3 to 10 on the subject's left upper extremity.
12. Repeat steps 4 to 10 using goniometers of different sizes and shapes.
13. Answer the following questions:
    Did the length of the goniometer arms affect the accuracy of the alignment? Explain.
    What length goniometer arms would you recommend as being the most appropriate for this measurement? Why?
    Did the type of goniometer used (full- or half-circle) affect either alignment or reading the scale? Explain.
    Did the side of the body that you were testing make a difference in your ability to align the goniometer? Why?

RECORDING

Goniometric measurements are recorded in numerical tables, in pictorial charts, or within the written text of an evaluation. Regardless of which method is used, recordings should provide enough information to permit an accurate interpretation of the measurement. The following items are recommended to be included in the recording:

1. Subject's name, age, and gender
2. Examiner's name
3. Date and time of measurement
4. Make and type of goniometer used
5. Side of the body, joint, and motion being measured, for example, left knee flexion
6. ROM, including the number of degrees at the beginning of the motion and the number of degrees at the end of the motion
7. Type of motion being measured, that is, passive or active motion
8. Any subjective information, such as discomfort or pain, that is reported by the subject during the testing
9. Any objective information obtained by the examiner during testing, such as a protective muscle spasm, crepitus, or capsular or noncapsular pattern of restriction
10. A complete description of any deviation from the recommended testing positions

If a subject has normal pain-free ROM during active or passive motion, the ROM may be recorded as normal (N) or within normal limits (WNL). To determine whether the ROM is normal, the examiner should compare the ROM of the joint being tested with ROM values from people of the same age and gender and from studies that used the same method of measurement. If this is not possible, the ROM of the joint being tested should be compared with the same joint of the subject's contralateral extremity. If the contralateral extremity is also impaired, the Average ROM Tables found in the beginnings of Chapters 4 to 12 or Appendix A may be consulted.

If passive ROM is decreased or increased as compared with the normal measurement, the ROM should be measured and recorded. Recordings should include both the starting and ending positions to define the ROM. A recording that includes only the total ROM, such as 50 degrees of flexion, gives no information as to where a motion begins and ends. Likewise, a recording that lists −20 degrees (minus 20 degrees) of flexion is open to misinterpretation because the lack of flexion could occur at either the end or the beginning of the ROM.

A motion, such as flexion, that begins at 0 degrees and ends at 50 degrees of flexion is recorded as 0 to 50 degrees of flexion (Fig. 2–11A). A motion that begins with the joint flexed at 20 degrees and ends at 70 degrees of flexion is recorded as 20 to 70 degrees of flexion (Fig. 2–11B). The total ROM is the same (50 degrees) in both instances. However, in the first instance the motion begins at 0 degrees of flexion, whereas in the second instance the motion begins at 20 degrees. Because both the starting and ending positions have been recorded, the measurement can be interpreted correctly. If we assume that the normal ROM for this movement is 0 to 150 degrees, the subject who has a 0- to 50-degree flexion ROM lacks motion at the end of the flexion ROM and is unable to complete the ROM. The subject with a 20- to 70-degree flexion ROM lacks the first portion of the flexion ROM (he or she is unable to begin in the zero starting position) and lacks motion at the end of the flexion ROM. The term **hypomobile** may be applied to both of these joints because both joints have a less-than-normal ROM.

Sometimes the opposite situation exists in which a joint has a greater-than-normal range of motion and is **hypermobile**. If an elbow joint is hypermobile, the starting position for measuring elbow flexion may be in hyperextension rather than at 0 degrees. If the elbow was hyperextended 20 degrees in the starting position, the beginning of the flexion ROM would be recorded as 20 degrees of hyperextension (Fig. 2–12). To clarify that the 20 degrees represents hyperextension rather than limited flexion, a zero representing the usual starting position, which is now within the ROM, is included. A range of motion that begins at 20 degrees of hyperextension and ends at 150 degrees of flexion is recorded as 20 to 0 to 150 degrees of flexion.

Some authorities have suggested using plus (+) and minus (−) signs to indicate hypomobility and hypermobility. However, the use of these signs varies depending on the authority consulted. To avoid confusion, we have omitted the use of plus and minus signs. A ROM that does not start with 0 degrees or ends prematurely indicates hypomobility. The addition of zero, representing the usual starting position, within the ROM indicates hypermobility.

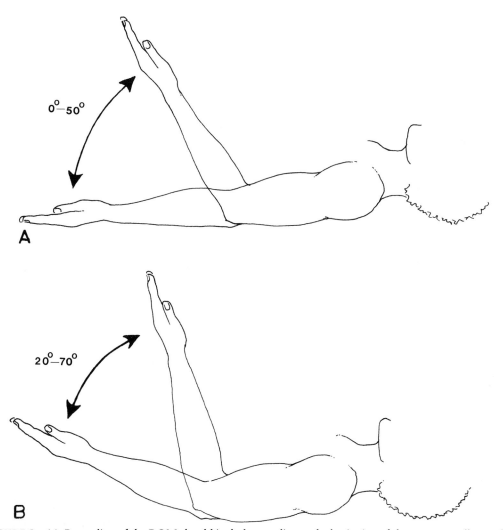

FIGURE 2–11. Recording of the ROM should include a reading at the beginning of the range as well as at the end. (*A*) In this illustration, the motion begins at 0 degrees and ends at 50 degrees so that the total ROM is 50 degrees. (*B*) In this subject, the motion begins at 20 degrees of flexion and ends at 70 degrees, so that the total ROM for this subject is 50 degrees. For both subjects, the total ROM is the same, 50 degrees, even though the arcs of motion are different.

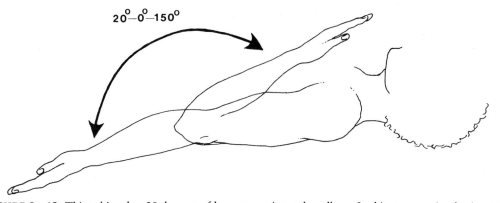

FIGURE 2–12. This subject has 20 degrees of hyperextension at her elbow. In this case, motion begins at 20 degrees of hyperextension and proceeds through the 0-degree position to 150 degrees of flexion.

Name *Paul Jones* Age *57* Gender *M*								
Left						Right		
		$\overline{Jw}$	$\overline{Jw}$	Examiner	$\overline{Jw}$			
		4/1/94	3/18/94	Date	3/18/94			
				Hip				
		0-98	0-75	Flexion	0-118			
		0-5	0-5	Extension	0-12			
		0-28	0-18	Abduction	0-32			
		0-12	0-6	Adduction	0-15			
		0-35	0-24	Medial Rotation	0-42			
		0-40	0-35	Lateral Rotation	0-44			
				Comments:				

FIGURE 2-13. This numerical table records the results of ROM measurements of a subject's left and right hips. The examiner has recorded her initials and the date of testing at the top of each column of ROM measurements. Note that the right hip was tested once on March 18, 1994, and the left hip was tested twice, once on March 18, 1994, and again on April 1, 1994.

NUMERICAL TABLES

Numerical tables typically list joint motions in a column down the center of the form (Fig. 2-13). Space to the left of the central column is reserved for measurements taken on the left side of the subject's body; space to the right is reserved for measurements taken on the right side of the body. The examiner's initials and the date of testing are noted at the top of the measurement columns. Subsequent measurements are recorded on the same form and identified by the examiner's initials and date at the top of the appropriate measurement column. This format makes it easy to compare a series of measurements to identify problem motions and then to track rehabilitative response over time. An example of a numerical recording table is included in Appendix C.

PICTORIAL CHARTS

Pictorial charts may be used in isolation or combined with numerical tables to record ROM measurements. Pictorial charts usually include a diagram of the normal starting and ending positions of the motion (Fig. 2-14). A scale is superimposed on the perimeter of the diagram. The examiner draws a line from the joint axis on the diagram to the scale to represent the beginning and the end of the subject's ROM. The examiner's initials and the testing date are noted beside the lines. The area on the diagram representing the ROM may be shaded in for emphasis. Subsequent measurements are recorded on the same chart using new

lines identified by the examiner's initials and the new testing date.

SAGITTAL-FRONTAL-TRANSVERSE-ROTATION METHOD

Another method of recording, which may be included in a written text or formatted into a table, is the **sagittal-frontal-transverse-rotation (SFTR) recording method,** developed by Gerhardt and Russe.[23,24] Although it is rarely used in the United States, its advantages have recently been described by Miller.[6] In the SFTR method three numbers are used to describe all motions in a given plane. The first and last numbers indicate the ends of the ROM in that plane. The middle number indicates the starting position, which would be 0 in normal motion.

In the sagittal plane, represented by S, the first number indicates the end of the extension ROM, the middle number the starting position, and the last number the end of the flexion ROM.

Example: If a subject has 50 degrees of shoulder extension and 170 degrees of shoulder flexion, these motions would be recorded: Shoulder S: 50-0-170 degrees.

In the frontal plane, represented by F, the first number indicates the end of the abduction ROM, the middle num-

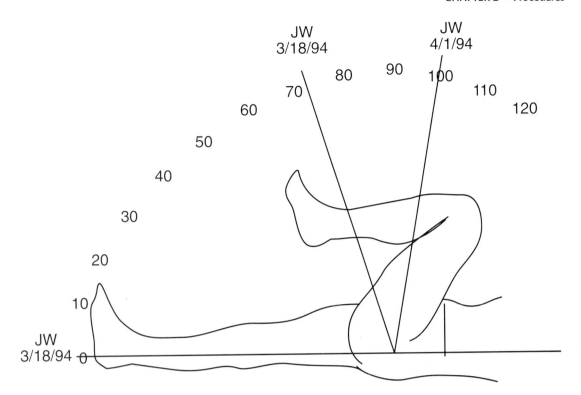

FIGURE 2 – 14. This pictorial chart records the results of flexion ROM measurements of a subject's left hip. For measurements taken on March 1, 1994, note the 0 to 73 degrees of left hip flexion; for measurements taken on April 1, 1994, note the 0 to 98 degrees of left hip flexion. (Adapted with permission from Range of Motion Test, New York University Medical Center, Rusk Institute of Rehabilitation Medicine.)

ber the starting position, and the last number the end of the adduction ROM. The ends of spinal ROMs in the frontal plane (lateral flexion) are listed to the left first and to the right last.

> **Example:** If a subject has 45 degrees of hip abduction and 15 degrees of hip adduction, these motions would be recorded: Hip F: 45 – 0 – 15 degrees.

In the transverse plane, represented by T, the first number indicates the end of the horizontal abduction ROM, the middle number the starting position, and the last number the end of the horizontal adduction ROM.

> **Example:** If a subject has 30 degrees of shoulder horizontal abduction and 135 degrees of shoulder horizontal adduction, these motions would be recorded: Shoulder T: 30 – 0 – 135 degrees.

Rotation is represented by R. Lateral rotation ROM, including supination and eversion, is listed first; medial rota-

tion ROM, including pronation and inversion, is listed last. Rotation ROM of the spine to the left is listed first; rotation ROM to the right is listed last. Limb position during measurement is noted if it varies from anatomical position. "F90" would indicate that a measurement was taken with the limb positioned in 90 degrees of flexion.

> **Example:** If a subject has 35 degrees of lateral rotation ROM of the hip and 45 degrees of medial rotation ROM of the hip, and these motions were measured with the hip in 90 degrees of flexion, these motions would be recorded: Hip R: (F90) 35 – 0 – 45 degrees.

Hypomobility is noted by the lack of zero as the middle number or by less-than-normal values for the first and last numbers, which indicate the ends of the ROM.

> **Example:** If elbow flexion ROM was limited and a subject could move only between 20 and 90 degrees of flexion, it would be recorded: Elbow S: 0 – 20 – 90 degrees. The starting position is 20 degrees of flexion, and the end of the ROM is 90 degrees of flexion.

A fixed-joint limitation, ankylosis is indicated by the use of only two numbers. The zero starting position is included to clarify in which motion the fixed position occurs.

> **Example:** An elbow fixed in 40 degrees of flexion would be recorded: Elbow S: 0–40 degrees.

AMERICAN MEDICAL ASSOCIATION GUIDE TO EVALUATION METHOD

Another system of recording restricted motion has been described by the American Medical Association in the *Guides to the Evaluation of Permanent Impairment*.[25] This book provides ratings of permanent impairment for all major body systems, including the respiratory, cardiovascular, digestive, and visual systems. The longest chapter focuses on impairment evaluation of the extremities, spine, and pelvis. Restricted active motion, ankylosis, amputation, sensory loss, vascular changes, loss of strength, pain, joint crepitation, joint swelling, joint instability, and deformity are measured and converted to percentage of impairment for the body part. The total percentage of impairment for the body part is converted to the percentage of impairment for the extremity, and finally to a percentage of impairment for the entire body. Often these permanent impairment ratings are used, along with other information, to determine disability and monetary compensation from employers or insurers. Physicians and therapists working with patients who have permanent impairments and are seeking compensation for their disabilities should refer to this book for more detail.

The system of recording restricted motion found in the *Guides to the Evaluation of Permanent Impairment* also uses the 0-to-180-degree notation method. The neutral starting position is recorded as 0 degrees; motions progress toward 180 degrees. However, the recording system proposed in the *Guides to the Evaluation of Permanent Impairment* does differ from other recording systems described in our text. In this system, when extension exceeds the neutral starting position, it is referred to as hyperextension and is expressed with the plus (+) symbol. For example, motion at the metacarpophalangeal joint of a finger from 15 degrees of hyperextension to 45 degrees of flexion would be recorded as +15 to 45 degrees. The plus symbol is used to emphasize the fact that the joint has hyperextension.

In this system, the minus (−) symbol is used to emphasize the fact that a joint has an extension lag. When the neutral (zero) starting position cannot be attained, an extension lag exists and is expressed with the minus symbol. For example, motion at the metacarpophalangeal joint of a finger from 15 degrees of flexion to 45 degrees of flexion would be recorded as −15 to 45 degrees.

PROCEDURES

Prior to beginning a goniometric evaluation, the examiner must:

- Determine which joints and motions need to be tested
- Organize the testing sequence by body position
- Gather the necessary equipment, such as goniometers, towel rolls, and recording forms
- Prepare an explanation of the procedure for the subject

EXPLANATION PROCEDURE

The steps listed below and the example that follows provide the examiner with a suggested format for explaining goniometry to a subject.

Steps

1. Introduction and explanation of purpose
2. Explanation and demonstration of goniometer
3. Explanation and demonstration of anatomical landmarks
4. Explanation and demonstration of recommended testing positions
5. Explanation and demonstration of examiner's and subject's roles
6. Confirmation of subject's understanding

Lay rather than technical terms are used in the example so that the subject can understand the procedure. During the explanation, the examiner should try to establish a good rapport with the subject and enlist the subject's participation in the evaluation process. After reading the example, the examiner should practice Exercise 4.

EXAMPLE: EXPLANATION OF GONIOMETRY

1. Introduction and Explanation of Purpose

Introduction: I am Jill Smith, a (occupational title).

Explanation: I am here to measure the amount of motion that you have at your joints, for example, how much motion you have at your elbow.

Demonstration: Jill flexes and extends her elbow so that the subject is able to observe a joint motion.

2. Explanation and Demonstration of Goniometer

Explanation: The instrument that I will be using to obtain the measurements is called a goniometer. It is similar to a protractor, but it has two extensions called arms.

Demonstration: Jill shows the goniometer to the subject. She lets the subject hold the goniometer and encourages the subject to ask questions. Jill shows the subject how the goniometer is used by holding it next to her own elbow.

3. Explanation and Demonstration of Anatomical Landmarks

Explanation: In order to obtain accurate measurements, I will need to identify some anatomical landmarks. These landmarks help me to align the arms of the goniometer. Because these landmarks are important, I may have to ask you to remove certain articles of clothing, such as your shirt or blouse. Also, I may have to use my fingers to press against your skin to locate some of the landmarks.

Demonstration: Jill shows the subject an easily identified anatomical landmark such as the ulnar styloid process, and a less easily identified landmark that requires palpation, such as the capitate.

4. Explanations and Demonstration of Recommended Testing Positions

Explanation: A series of recommended testing positions have been established to help make joint measurements easier and more accurate. Whenever possible, I would like you to assume these positions. I will be happy to help you get into a particular position. Please let my know if you need assistance.

Demonstration: Sitting and supine positions.

5. Explanation and Demonstration of Examiner's and Subject's Roles

Active Motion

Explanation: I will ask you to move your arm in exactly the same way that I move your arm.

Demonstration: Take the subject's arm through a passive ROM, then ask the subject to perform the same motion.

Passive Motion

Explanation: I will move your arm and take a measurement. You should relax and let me do all of the work. These measurements should not cause discomfort. Please let me know if you have any discomfort, and I will stop moving your arm.

Demonstration: Move the subject's arm gently and slowly through a range of elbow flexion.

6. Confirmation of Subject's Understanding

Explanation: Do you have any questions? Would you like me to show you any other measurements? Are you ready to begin?

EXERCISE 4 ■ EXPLANATION OF GONIOMETRY

Equipment: A universal goniometer.

Activities: Practice the following six steps with a subject.

1. Introduce yourself and explain the purpose of goniometric testing. Demonstrate a joint ROM on yourself.
2. Show the goniometer to your subject and demonstrate how it is used to measure a joint ROM.
3. Explain why bony landmarks must be located and palpated. Demonstrate how you would locate a bony landmark on yourself, and explain why clothing may have to be removed.
4. Explain and demonstrate why changes in position may be required.
5. Explain the subject's role in the procedure. Explain and demonstrate your role in the procedure.
6. Obtain confirmation of the subject's understanding of your explanation.

TESTING PROCEDURE

The testing process is initiated after the explanation of goniometry has been given and the examiner is assured that the subject understands the nature of the testing process.

The testing procedure consists of the following 12-step sequence of activities.

Steps

1. Place the subject in the recommended testing position.
2. Stabilize the proximal joint segment.
3. Move the distal joint segment through the available ROM. Make sure that the passive ROM is performed slowly and that the end of the range is attained and the end-feel determined.
4. Make a clinical estimate of the ROM.
5. Return the distal joint segment to the starting position.
6. Palpate bony anatomical landmarks.
7. Align the goniometer.
8. Read and record the starting position. Remove the goniometer.
9. Stabilize the proximal joint segment.
10. Move the distal segment through the full ROM.
11. Replace and realign the goniometer. Palpate the anatomical landmarks again if necessary.
12. Read and record ROM.

Exercise 5, which is based on the 12-step sequence, affords the examiner an opportunity to use the testing procedure for an evaluation of the elbow joint. This exercise should be practiced until the examiner is able to perform the activities sequentially without reference to the exercise.

EXERCISE 5 ■ TESTING PROCEDURE FOR GONIOMETRIC EVALUATION OF ELBOW FLEXION

Equipment: A universal goniometer, skin-marking pencil, recording form, and pencil.

Activities: See Figures 5–1 to 5–3 in Chapter 5.

1. Place the subject in a supine position, with the arm to be tested positioned close to the side of the body. Place a towel roll under the distal end of the humerus to allow full elbow extension. Position the forearm in full supination, with the palm of the hand facing the ceiling.
2. Stabilize the distal end of the humerus to prevent flexion of the shoulder.
3. Move the forearm through the full passive range of flexion. Evaluate the end-feel. Usually the end-feel is soft because of compression of the muscle bulk on the anterior forearm with that on the anterior humerus.
4. Make a clinical estimate of the beginning and end of the ROM.
5. Return the forearm to the starting position.
6. Palpate bony anatomical landmarks (acromion process, lateral epicondyle of the humerus, radial head, and radial styloid process) and mark with a skin pencil.
7. Align the arms and fulcrum of the goniometer. Align the proximal arm with the lateral midline of the humerus, using the acromion process and lateral epicondyle for reference. Align the distal arm along the lateral midline of the radius, using the radial head and radial styloid process for reference. The fulcrum should be close to the lateral epicondyle of the humerus.
8. Read the goniometer and record the starting position. Remove the goniometer.
9. Stabilize the proximal joint segment (humerus).
10. Perform the passive ROM, making sure that you complete the available range.
11. When the end of the ROM has been attained, replace and realign the goniometer. Palpate the anatomical landmarks again if necessary.
12. Read the goniometer and record your reading. Compare your reading with your clinical estimate to make sure that you are reading the correct scale on the goniometer.

REFERENCES

1. Rothstein, JM, Miller, PJ, and Roettger, F: Goniometric reliability in a clinical setting. Phys Ther 63:1611, 1983.
2. Moore, ML: The measurement of joint motion. Part II: The technic of goniometry. Physical Therapy Review 29:256, 1949.
3. Moore, ML: Clinical assessment of joint motion. In Basmajian, JV (ed): Therapeutic Exercise, ed 3. Williams & Wilkins, Baltimore, 1978.
4. Fox, RF and Van Breemen, J: Chronic Rheumatism, Causation and Treatment. Churchill, London, 1934, p 327.
5. Schenkar, WW: Improved method of joint motion measurement. New York Journal of Medicine 56:539, 1956.
6. Miller, PJ: Assessment of joint motion. In Rothstein, JM (ed): Measurement in Physical Therapy. Churchill Livingstone, New York, 1985.
7. Clarkson, HM and Gilewich, GB: Musculoskeletal Assessment: Joint Range of Motion and Manual Muscle Strength. Williams & Wilkins, Baltimore, 1989.
8. Petherick, M, et al: Concurrent validity and intertester reliability of universal and fluid-based goniometers for active elbow range of motion. Phys Ther 68:966, 1988.

9. Rheault, W, et al: Intertester reliability and concurrent validity of fluid-based and universal goniometers for active knee flexion. Phys Ther 68:1676, 1988.

10. Karpovich, PV and Karpovich, GP: Electrogoniometer: A new device for study of joints in action. Federation Proceedings 18:79, 1959.

11. Kettelkamp, DB, Johnson, RC, Smidt, GL, et al: An electrogoniometric study of knee motion in normal gait. J Bone Joint Surg Am 52:775, 1970.

12. Knutzen, KM, Bates, BT, and Hamill, J: Electrogoniometry of post-surgical knee bracing in running. Am J Phys Med Rehabil 62:172, 1983.

13. Carey, JR, Patterson, JR, and Hollenstein, PJ: Sensitivity and reliability of force tracking and joint-movement tracking scores in healthy subjects. Phys Ther 68:1087, 1988.

14. Clapper, MP and Wolf, SL: Comparison of the reliability of the orthoranger and the standard goniometer for assessing active lower extremity range of motion. Phys Ther 68:214, 1988.

15. American Academy of Orthopaedic Surgeons: Joint Motion: A Method of Measuring and Recording. AAOS, Chicago, 1965.

16. Rowe, CR: Joint measurement in disability evaluation. Clin Orthop 32:43, 1964.

17. Watkins, MA, et al: Reliability of goniometric measurements and visual estimates of knee range of motion obtained in a clinical setting. Phys Ther 71:90, 1991.

18. Youdas, JW, Carey, JR, and Garrett, TR: Reliability of measurements of cervical spine range of motion: Comparison of three methods. Phys Ther 71:98, 1991.

19. Low, JL: The reliability of joint measurement. Physiotherapy 62:227, 1976.

20. Moore, ML: The measurement of joint motion. Part I: Introductory review of the literature. Physical Therapy Review 29:195, 1949.

21. Salter, N: Methods of measurement of muscle and joint function. J Bone Joint Surg Br 34:474, 1955.

22. Minor, MA and Minor, SD: Patient Evaluation Methods for the Health Professional. Reston, VA, 1985.

23. Gerhardt, JJ and Russe, OA: International SFTR Method of Measuring and Recording Joint Motion. Hans Huber, Bern, 1975.

24. Gerhardt, JJ: Clinical measurement of joint motion and position in the neutral-zero method and SFTR: Basic principles. International Rehabilitation Medicine 5:161, 1983.

25. American Medical Association: Guides to the Evaluation of Permanent Impairment, ed 3. AMA, Milwaukee, 1990.

3

Validity and Reliability

VALIDITY

For goniometry to provide meaningful information, measurements must be valid and reliable. Currier[1] states that validity is "the degree to which an instrument measures what it is purported to measure; the extent to which it fulfills its purpose." Stated in another way, the validity of a measurement refers to how well the measurement represents the true value of the variable of interest. The purpose of goniometry is to measure the angle of joint position or range of joint motion. Therefore, a valid goniometric measurement is one that truly represents the actual joint angle or the total ROM.

Most support for the validity of goniometry is in the form of content validity. Content validity is determined by judging whether or not an instrument adequately measures and represents the content — the substance — of the variable of interest.[2-4] Much of the literature on goniometric measurement does not address the issue of validity. It is assumed that the angle created by aligning the arms of a universal goniometer with bony landmarks truly represents the angle created by the proximal and distal bones composing the joint. One infers that changes in goniometer alignment reflect changes in joint angle and represent a range of joint motion. Gajdosik and Bohannon[5] state, "Physical therapists judge the validity of most ROM measurements based on their anatomical knowledge and their applied skills of visual inspection, palpation of bony landmarks, and accurate alignment of the goniometer. Generally, the accurate application of knowledge and skills, combined with interpreting the results as measurement of ROM only, provide sufficient evidence to ensure content validity." [(p. 1871)]

Some studies have examined criterion-related validity for various types of goniometers used in the clinical setting. Criterion-related validity justifies the validity of the measuring instrument by comparing measurements made with the instrument to a well-established "gold standard" of measurement — the criterion.[2,3] On a very basic level, an examiner may question the construction of a particular goniometer and consider whether the degree units of the goniometer accurately represent the degree units of a circle. The angles of the goniometer can be compared with known angles of a protractor. Usually the construction of goniometers is adequate, and the issue of validity focuses on whether the goniometer accurately measures the angle of joint position and ROM in a subject.

The best gold standard used to establish criterion-related validity of goniometric measurements is radiography. Gogia et al.[6] measured the knee position of 30 subjects with radiography and with a large 360-degree plastic universal goniometer marked in 1-degree increments. Knee positions ranged from 0 to 120 degrees. High correlation and agreement were found between the two types of measurements. Therefore goniometric measurement of knee joint position was considered to be valid. Enwemeka[7] studied the validity of measuring knee ROM with a universal goniometer by comparing the goniometric measurements taken on 10 subjects with radiographs. No significant differences were found between the two types of measurements when ROM was within 30 to 90 degrees of flexion (mean difference between the two measurements ranged from 0.52 to 3.81 degrees). However, a significant difference was found when ROM was within 0 to 15 degrees of flexion (mean difference 4.59 degrees). Ahlbach and Lindahl[8] found that a joint-specific goniometer used to measure hip flexion and extension closely agreed with radiographic measurements.

35

Individual data on 14 of the subjects were presented, but summary statistics were not included. Herrmann,[9] in a study of 11 subjects, compared radiographs with pendulum goniometer measurements of head and neck flexion and extension. There was a high correlation and agreement between the two methods of measurement.

Some investigators have compared goniometric measurements with a photographic criterion. In a study by Fish and Wingate,[10] 46 physical therapy students using a universal goniometer measured a fixed elbow position with and without labeled landmarks and passive range of elbow flexion. Joint angles measured from still photographs were used as the criterion. Mean goniometric measurements differed 0.5 to 5 degrees from the means of measurements determined by still photography. Some of these differences were statistically significant. The authors call attention to errors in identifying landmarks, variations in external forces applied during passive ROM, visual obstruction of alignment when metal goniometers were used, parallax during photography, and a preferred alternative alignment of the proximal arm of the goniometer as possible causes of the discrepancies.

RELIABILITY

The reliability of a measurement refers to the amount of consistency between successive measurements of the same variable, on the same subject, under the same conditions. A goniometric measurement is highly reliable if successive measurements of a joint angle or ROM, on the same subject and under the same conditions, yield the same results. A highly reliable measurement contains little measurement error. Assuming that a measurement is valid, an examiner can confidently use the results of a highly reliable measurement to determine a true absence, presence, or change in dysfunction. For example, a highly reliable goniometric measurement could be used to determine the presence of joint ROM limitation, to evaluate patient progress toward rehabilitative goals, and to assess the effectiveness of therapeutic interventions.

A measurement with poor reliability contains a large amount of measurement error. An unreliable measurement is inconsistent and does not produce the same results when the same variable is measured on the same subject under the same conditions. A measurement that has poor reliability is not dependable and should not be used in the clinical decision-making process.

SUMMARY OF GONIOMETRIC RELIABILITY STUDIES

The reliability of goniometric measurement has been the focus of many research studies. Given the variety of study designs and measurement techniques, it is difficult to compare the results of many of these studies. However, some findings noted in several studies can be summarized. An overview of such findings is presented here. More information on reliability studies that pertain to the featured joint is reviewed in Chapters 4 to 12. Readers may also wish to refer to several review articles and book chapters on this topic.[5,11,12]

The measurement of joint position and ROM of the extremities with a universal goniometer has generally been found to have good-to-excellent reliability. Numerous reliability studies have been conducted on joints of the upper and lower extremities. Some studies have examined the reliability of measuring joints held in a fixed position, whereas others have examined the reliability of measuring passive or active ROM. Studies that measured a fixed joint position usually have reported higher reliability values than studies that measured ROM.[6,9,13,14] This is expected because more sources of variation or error are present in measuring ROM than in measuring a fixed joint position. Additional sources of error in measuring ROM include movement of the joint axis, variations in manual force applied by the examiner during passive ROM, and variations in a subject's effort during active ROM.

The reliability of goniometric ROM measurements varies somewhat depending on the joint and motion. ROM measurements of upper-extremity joints have been found to be more reliable than ROM measurements of lower-extremity joints.[15,16] Also, Hellebrandt et al.,[17] in a study of upper-extremity joints, noted that measurements of wrist flexion, medial rotation of the shoulder, and abduction of the shoulder were less reliable than measurements of other motions of the upper extremity. Low[18] found ROM measurements of wrist extension to be less reliable than measurements of elbow flexion. Reliability studies on ROM measurement of the cervical and thoracic spine using a universal goniometer generally report lower reliability values than studies of the extremity joints.[19-21] Many devices and techniques have been developed to try to improve the reliability of measuring spinal motions. Gajdosik and Bohannon[5] suggest that the reliability of measuring certain joints and motions may be adversely affected by the complexity of the joint. Measurement of motions that are influenced by movement of adjacent joints or multiple-joint muscles may be less reliable than measurement of motions of simple hinge joints. Difficulty palpating bony landmarks and passively moving heavy body parts may also play a role in reducing the reliability of measuring ROM of the lower extremity and spine.[5,15]

Many studies of joint measurement methods have found intratester reliability to be higher than intertester reliability.[13-29] Reliability was higher when successive measurements were taken by the same examiner than when successive measurements were taken by different examiners. This is true for studies that measured joint position and ROM of the extremities and spine with universal goniometers and other devices such as joint-specific goniometers, pendulum goniometers, tape measures, and flexible rulers. Only a few studies found intertester reliability to be higher than intratester reliability.[30-32] In all of these studies, the time interval between repeated measurements by the same examiner was considerably greater than the time interval between measurements by different examiners.

The reliability of goniometric measurements is affected by the measurement procedure. Several studies found that intertester reliability improved when all the examiners used consistent, well-defined testing positions and measurement methods.[23,25,26] Intertester reliability was lower if examiners used a variety of positions and measurement methods.

Several investigators have examined the reliability of using the mean (average) of several goniometric measurements as compared with using one measurement. Low[18] recommends using the mean of several measurements made with the goniometer to increase reliability over one measurement. Early studies by Cobe[33] and Hewitt[34] also used the mean of several measurements. However, Boone et al.[15] found no significant difference between repeated measurements made by the same examiner during one session and suggested that one measurement taken by an examiner is as reliable as the mean of repeated measurements. Rothstein et al.,[26] in a study on knee and elbow ROM, found that intertester reliability determined from the means of two measurements improved only slightly from the intertester reliability determined from single measurements.

The authors of some texts on goniometric methods suggest the use of universal goniometers with longer arms to measure joints with large body segments, such as the hip and shoulder.[11,35,36] Goniometers with shorter arms are recommended to measure joints with small body segments, such as the wrist and fingers. Robson,[37] using a mathematical model, determined that goniometers with longer arms are more accurate in measuring an angle than goniometers with shorter arms. Goniometers with longer arms reduce the effects of errors in the placement of the goniometer axis. However, Rothstein et al.[26] found no difference in reliability among large plastic, large metal, and small plastic universal goniometers when measuring knee and elbow ROM. Riddle et al.[24] also reported no difference in reliability between large and small plastic universal goniometers when measuring shoulder ROM.

Numerous studies have compared the measurement values and reliability of different types of devices used to measure joint ROM. Universal, pendulum, and fluid goniometers, joint-specific devices, and tape measures are some of the devices that have been compared. Studies comparing measurement devices have been conducted on the shoulder,[17] elbow,[13,17,38] wrist,[17] hand,[14] hip,[39,40] knee,[39,41] ankle,[39] cervical spine,[19,20,31,42] and thoracolumbar spine.[21,43-49] Many studies have found differences in values and reliability between measurement devices, while some studies have reported no differences.

In conclusion, on the basis of reliability studies and our clinical experience, we recommend the following procedures to improve the reliability of goniometric measurements. Examiners should use consistent, well-defined testing positions and anatomical landmarks to align the arms of the goniometer. During successive measurements of passive ROM, examiners should strive to apply the same amount of manual force to move the subject's body. During successive measurements of active ROM, the subject should be urged to exert the same effort to perform a motion. To reduce measurement variability, it is prudent to take repeated measurements on a subject with the same type of measurement device. For example, an examiner should take all repeated measurements of a ROM with a universal goniometer, rather than taking the first measurement with a universal goniometer and the second measurement with an inclinometer. We believe most examiners will find it easier and more accurate to use a large universal goniometer when measuring joints with large body segments, and a small goniometer when measuring joints with small body segments. Inexperienced examiners may wish to take several measurements and record the mean (average) of those measurements to improve reliability, but one measurement is usually sufficient for more experienced examiners using good technique. Finally, it is important to remember that successive measurements are more reliable if taken by the same examiner rather than different examiners.

MATHEMATICAL METHODS OF EVALUATING MEASUREMENT RELIABILITY

Clinical measurements are prone to three main sources of variation: (1) true biological variation, (2) temporal variation, and (3) measurement error.[50 (p. 39)] True **biological variation** refers to variation in measurements from one individual to another, caused by factors such as age, sex, race, genetics, medical history, and condition. **Temporal variation** refers to variation in measurements made on the same individual at different times, caused by changes in factors such as a subject's medical (physical) condition, activity level, emotional state, and circadian rhythms. **Measurement error** refers to variation in measurements made on the same individual under the same conditions at different times, caused by factors such as the examiners (testers), measuring instruments, and procedural methods. Reliability reflects the degree to which a measurement is free of measurement error; therefore, highly reliable measurements have little measurement error.

Taber's Cyclopedic Medical Dictionary[51] defines statistics as "the systematic collection, organization, analysis, and interpretation of numerical data." Statistics can be used to assess variation in numerical data and hence to assess measurement reliability.[50,52]

A digression into statistical methods of testing and expressing reliability is included to assist the examiner in correctly interpreting goniometric measurements and in understanding the literature on joint measurement. Several statistics—the **standard deviation, coefficient of variation, Pearson product moment correlation coefficient, intraclass correlation coefficient,** and **standard error of measurement**—are discussed. Examples that show the calculation of these statistical tests are presented. For additional information, including the assumptions underlying the use of these statistical tests, please refer to the cited references.

At the end of this chapter, two exercises are included for examiners to assess their reliability in obtaining goniometric measurements. Many authors recommend that clinicians conduct their own studies to determine reliability among their staff and patient population. Miller[12] has presented a step-by-step procedure for conducting such studies.

Standard Deviation

In the medical literature, the statistic most frequently used to indicate variation is the standard deviation.[50,52] The standard deviation is the square root of the mean of the squares of the deviations from the data mean. The standard deviation is symbolized as SD, s, or sd. If we denote each data observation as x, and the number of observations as n, and use the summation notation Σ, then the **mean**, which is denoted by $\bar{x}$, is

$$\text{mean} = \bar{x} = \frac{\Sigma x}{n}$$

Two formulas for the standard deviation are given below. The first is the definitional formula; the second is the computational formula. Both formulas give the same result. The definitional formula is easier to understand, but the computational formula is easier to calculate.

Standard deviation = SD

$$SD = \sqrt{\frac{\Sigma(x - \bar{x})^2}{n - 1}}$$

$$SD = \sqrt{\frac{\Sigma x^2 - (\Sigma x)^2/n}{n - 1}}$$

The standard deviation has the same units as the original data observations. If the data observations have a normal (bell-shaped) frequency distribution, one standard deviation above and below the mean includes about 68 percent of all the observations, and two standard deviations above and below the mean include about 95 percent of the observations.

It is important to note that several standard deviations may be determined from a single study and represent different sources of variation.[50] Two of these standard deviations are discussed here. One standard deviation that can be determined represents mainly *inter*subject variation around the mean of measurements taken of a group of subjects, indicating biological variation. This standard deviation may be of interest in deciding whether a subject has an abnormal ROM in comparison with other people of the same age and gender. Another standard deviation that can be determined represents *intra*subject variation around the mean of measurements taken of an individual, indicating measurement error. This is the standard deviation of interest to indicate measurement reliability.

An example of how to determine these two standard deviations is provided. Table 3–1 presents ROM measurements taken on five subjects. Three repeated measurements (observations) were taken on each subject by the same examiner.

The **standard deviation indicating biological variation** (intersubject variation) is determined by first calculating the mean ROM measurement for each subject. The mean ROM measurement for each of the five subjects is found in the last column of Table 3–1. The grand mean of the mean ROM measurement for each of the five subjects equals 56 degrees. The grand mean is symbolized by $\bar{X}$. The standard deviation is determined by finding the differences between each of the five subjects' means and the grand mean. The differences are squared and added together. The sum is used in the definitional formula for the standard deviation. Calculation of the standard deviation indicating biological variation is found in Table 3–2.

The standard deviation indicating biological variation equals 13.6 degrees. This standard deviation denotes primarily intersubject variation. Knowledge of intersubject variation may be helpful in deciding whether a subject has an abnormal ROM in comparison with other people of the

Table 3–1 **THREE REPEATED ROM MEASUREMENTS (IN DEGREES) TAKEN ON FIVE SUBJECTS**

Subject	First Measurement	Second Measurement	Third Measurement	Total	Mean of Three Measurements ($\bar{x}$)
1	57	55	65	177	59
2	66	65	70	201	67
3	66	70	74	210	70
4	35	40	42	117	39
5	45	48	42	135	45

Grand mean ($\bar{X}$) = (59 + 67 + 70 + 39 + 45)/5 = 56 degrees

Table 3-2 **CALCULATION OF THE STANDARD DEVIATION INDICATING BIOLOGICAL VARIATION IN DEGREES**

Subject	Mean of Three Measurements $(\bar{x})$	Grand Mean $(\bar{X})$	$(\bar{x} - \bar{X})$	$(\bar{x} - \bar{X})^2$
1	59	56	3	9
2	67	56	11	121
3	70	56	14	196
4	39	56	−17	289
5	45	56	−11	121

$$\Sigma(\bar{x} - \bar{X})^2 = 9 + 121 + 196 + 289 + 121 = 736 \text{ degrees}; \quad SD = \sqrt{\frac{(\bar{x} - \bar{X})^2}{(n-1)}} = \sqrt{\frac{736}{(5-1)}} = 13.6 \text{ degrees}$$

same age and gender. If a normal distribution of the measurements is assumed, one way of interpreting this standard deviation is to predict that about 68 percent of all the subjects' mean ROM measurements would fall between 42.4 degrees and 69.6 degrees (plus or minus one standard deviation around the grand mean). We would expect that about 95 percent of all the subjects' mean ROM measurements would fall between 28.8 degrees and 83.2 degrees (plus or minus two standard deviations around the grand mean).

The **standard deviation indicating measurement error** (intrasubject variation) also is determined by first calculating the mean ROM measurement for each subject. However, this standard deviation is determined by finding the differences between each of the three repeated measurements taken on a subject and the mean of that subject's measurements. The differences are squared and added together. The sum is used in the definitional formula for the standard deviation. Calculation of the standard deviation indicating measurement error for subject 1 is found in Table 3-3.

Referring to Table 3-1 and using the same procedure as in Table 3-3 for each subject:

Table 3-3 **CALCULATION OF THE STANDARD DEVIATION INDICATING MEASUREMENT ERROR IN DEGREES FOR SUBJECT 1**

Measurements (x)	Mean $(\bar{x})$	$(x - \bar{x})$	$(x - \bar{x})^2$
57	59	−2	4
55	59	−4	16
65	59	6	36

$\Sigma(x - \bar{x})^2 = 4 + 16 + 36 = 56$ degrees.

$$SD = \sqrt{\frac{(x - \bar{x})^2}{(n-1)}} = \sqrt{\frac{56}{2}} = 5.3 \text{ degrees.}$$

The standard deviation for subject 1 = 5.3 degrees.
The standard deviation for subject 2 = 2.6 degrees.
The standard deviation for subject 3 = 4.0 degrees.
The standard deviation for subject 4 = 3.6 degrees.
The standard deviation for subject 5 = 3.0 degrees.

The standard deviation for all of the subjects combined is determined by summing the five subjects' standard deviations and dividing by 5, which is the number of subjects:

$$SD = \frac{5.3 + 2.6 + 4.0 + 3.6 + 3.0}{5} = \frac{18.5}{5} = 3.7 \text{ degrees}$$

The standard deviation equals 3.7 degrees. This standard deviation denotes intrasubject variation and is appropriate for indicating measurement error, especially if the repeated measurements on each subject were taken within a short period of time. Note that in this example the standard deviation indicating measurement error (3.7 degrees) is much less than the standard deviation indicating biological variation (13.6 degrees). One way of interpreting the standard deviation for measurement error is to predict that about 68 percent of the repeated measurements on a subject would fall within 3.7 degrees (one standard deviation) above and below the mean of the repeated measurements of a subject because of measurement error. We would expect that about 95 percent of the repeated measurements on a subject would fall within 7.4 degrees (two standard deviations) above and below the mean of the repeated measurements of a subject, again because of measurement error. The smaller the standard deviation, the less the measurement error and the better the reliability.

Coefficient of Variation

Sometimes it is helpful to consider the percentage of variation rather than the standard deviation, which is expressed in the units of the data observation (measurement). The coefficient of variation is a measure of variation that is relative to the mean and standardized so that the variations of different variables can be compared. The coefficient of variation is the standard deviation divided by the mean and multiplied by 100 percent. It is a percentage and is not expressed in the units of the original observation. The coefficient of variation is symbolized by CV and the formula is:

$$\text{coefficient of variation} = CV = \frac{SD}{\bar{x}} (100\%)$$

For the example presented in Table 3-1, the coefficient of

variation indicating biological variation uses the standard deviation for biological variation (SD = 13.6 degrees).

$$CV = \frac{SD}{\bar{x}} (100\%) = \frac{13.6}{56} (100\%) = 24.3\%$$

The coefficient of variation indicating measurement error uses the standard deviation for measurement error (SD = 3.7 degrees).

$$CV = \frac{SD}{\bar{x}} (100\%) = \frac{3.7}{56} (100\%) = 6.6\%$$

In this example the coefficient of variation for measurement error (6.6 percent) is less than the coefficient of variation for biological variation (24.3 percent).

Another name for the coefficient of variation indicating measurement error is the **coefficient of variation of replication**.[53] The lower the coefficient of variation of replication, the lower the measurement error and the better the reliability. This statistic is especially useful in comparing the reliability of two or more variables that have different units of measurement, for example, comparing ROM measurement methods recorded in inches versus degrees.

Correlation Coefficients

Correlation coefficients are traditionally used to measure the relationship between two variables. They result in a number from −1 to +1, which indicates how well an equation can predict one variable from another variable.[2,4,50] A +1 describes a perfect positive linear (straight-line) relationship, whereas a −1 describes a perfect negative linear relationship. A correlation coefficient of 0 indicates that there is no linear relationship between the two variables. Correlation coefficients are used to indicate measurement reliability because it is assumed that two repeated measurements should be highly correlated and approach a +1. One interpretation of correlation coefficients used to indicate reliability is that 0.90 to 0.99 equals high reliability,

0.80 to 0.89 equals good reliability, 0.70 to 0.79 equals fair reliability, and 0.69 and below equals poor reliability.[54]

Because goniometric measurements produce ratio level data, the **Pearson product moment correlation coefficient** has been the correlation coefficient usually calculated to indicate the reliability of pairs of goniometric measurements. The Pearson product moment correlation coefficient is symbolized by r, and its formula is presented below. If this statistic is used to indicate reliability, x symbolizes the first measurement and y symbolizes the second measurement.

$$r = \frac{\Sigma(x - \bar{x})(y - \bar{y})}{\sqrt{\Sigma(x - \bar{x})^2}\ \sqrt{\Sigma(y - \bar{y})^2}}$$

Referring to the example in Table 3–1, the Pearson correlation coefficient can be used to determine the relationship between the first and second ROM measurements on the five subjects. Calculation of the Pearson product moment correlation coefficient for this example is found in Table 3–4. The resulting value of $r = 0.98$ indicates a highly positive linear relationship between the first and second measurements. In other words, the two measurements are highly correlated.

To decide whether the two measurements are identical, the equation of the straight line best representing the relationship should be determined. If the equation of the straight line representing the relationship includes a slope b equal to 1, and an intercept a equal to 0, then an r value which approaches +1 also indicates that the two measurements are identical. The equation of a straight line is $y = a + bx$, where x symbolizes the first measurement, y the second measurement, a the intercept, and b the slope. The equation for a slope is:

$$\text{slope} = b = \frac{\Sigma(x - \bar{x})(y - \bar{y})}{\Sigma(x - \bar{x})^2}$$

The equation for an intercept is:

$$\text{intercept} = a = \bar{y} - b\bar{x}$$

Table 3–4 CALCULATION OF THE PEARSON PRODUCT MOMENT CORRELATION COEFFICIENT FOR THE FIRST (x) AND SECOND (y) ROM MEASUREMENTS IN DEGREES

Subject	x	y	$x - \bar{x}$	$y - \bar{y}$	$(x - \bar{x})(y - \bar{y})$	$(x - \bar{x})^2$	$(y - \bar{y})^2$
1	57	55	3.2	−0.6	−1.92	10.24	0.36
2	66	65	12.2	9.4	114.68	148.84	88.36
3	66	70	12.2	14.4	175.68	148.84	207.36
4	35	40	−18.8	−15.6	293.28	353.44	243.36
5	45	48	−8.8	−7.6	68.88	77.44	57.76
					$\Sigma = 650.60;$	$\Sigma = 738.80;$	$\Sigma = 597.20.$

$\bar{x} = (57 + 66 + 66 + 35 + 45)/5 = 53.8$ degrees; $\bar{y} = (55 + 65 + 70 + 40 + 48)/5 = 55.6$ degrees.

$$r = \frac{\Sigma(x - \bar{x})(y - \bar{y})}{\sqrt{\Sigma(x - \bar{x})^2}\ \sqrt{\Sigma(y - \bar{y})^2}} = \frac{650.6}{\sqrt{738.8}\ \sqrt{597.2}} = \frac{650.6}{(27.2)\ (24.4)} = 0.98.$$

For our example, the slope and intercept are calculated as follows:

$$b = \frac{\Sigma(x - \bar{x})(y - \bar{y})}{\Sigma(x - \bar{x})^2} = \frac{650.6}{738.8} = 0.88$$

$$a = \bar{y} - b\bar{x} = 55.6 - 0.88(53.8) = 8.26$$

The equation of the straight line best representing the relationship between the first and second measurements in the example is $y = 8.26 + 0.88x$. Although the r value indicates high correlation, the two measurements are not identical given the linear equation.

One concern in interpreting correlation coefficients is that the value of the correlation coefficient is markedly influenced by the range of the measurements.[52] The greater the biological variation between individuals for the measurement, the more extreme the r value, so that r is closer to -1 or $+1$. Another limitation is the fact that the Pearson product moment correlation coefficient can evaluate the relationship between only two variables or measurements at a time.

To avoid the need for calculating and interpreting both the correlation coefficient and a linear equation, some investigators use the **intraclass correlation coefficient (ICC)** to evaluate reliability. The intraclass correlation coefficient is symbolized as ICC or ICCr. The intraclass correlation coefficient also allows the comparison of two or more measurements at a time. This statistic is determined from an analysis of variance model, which compares different sources of variation. The ICC is conceptually expressed as the ratio of the variance associated with the subjects over the sum of the variance associated with the subjects plus error variance.[56] Several different formulas for determining the values of the ICC have been described[55,56] and are not addressed here. Generally the ICC indicates the degree of agreement between the measurements. The theoretical limits of ICC between 0 and 1; 1 indicates perfect agreement (the repeated measurements are identical), whereas 0 indicates no agreement. Like the Pearson correlation coefficient, the ICC is also influenced by the range of the measurements between the subjects. As the group of subjects becomes more homogeneous, the ability of the ICC to detect agreement is reduced.[56,57]

Standard Error of Measurement

The standard error of measurement is the final statistic used to evaluate reliability that we review here. It has received support because of its practical interpretation in estimating measurement error.[2,58] According to DuBois,[58] "the standard error of measurement is the likely standard deviation of the error made in predicting true scores when we have knowledge only of the obtained scores."[(p. 401)] The true scores (measurements) are forever unknown, but a formula has been developed to estimate this statistic. The standard error of measurement is symbolized as s_{meas} or

SE_{meas}. If the standard deviation indicating biological variation is denoted SD_x, and the Pearson product moment correlation coefficient is denoted r, then the formula for the standard error of measurement (SE_{meas}) is:

$$SE_{meas} = SD_x \sqrt{1 - r}$$

Because the standard error of measurement is a special case of the standard deviation, one standard error of measurement above and below the observed measurement includes the true measurement 68 percent of the time. Expressed another way, about two thirds of the discrepancies between the observed measurement and the true measurement would be less than the standard error of measurement.

The standard error of measurement has occasionally been symbolized by some authors as SEM or SE_M, but it is not equivalent to, nor does it have the same interpretation as the standard error of the mean, which is symbolized as SEM, SE_M, or $SE(\bar{x})$.[2,50,52,59] The use of the same symbol to represent different statistics has added much confusion to the reliability literature. The standard error of the mean is the standard deviation of a distribution of means taken from samples of a population.[1,2,52] It describes how much variation can be expected in the means from future samples of the same size. Because we are interested in the variation of individual measurements when evaluating reliability rather than the variation of means, the standard deviation of the repeated measurements or the standard error of measurements are the appropriate statistical tests to use.[52,60]

Let us return to the example and calculate the standard error of the measurement. The value for r is the Pearson product moment correlation coefficient describing the relationship between the first and second measurements for the five subjects. The value for SD_x is the standard deviation indicating biological variation among the subjects.

$$SE_{meas} = SD_x \sqrt{1 - r} =$$
$$13.6 \sqrt{1 - 0.98} = 13.6 \sqrt{0.02} = 1.9 \text{ degrees.}$$

In this example, about two thirds of the time the true measurement would be within 1.9 degrees of the observed measurement.

EXERCISES TO EVALUATE RELIABILITY

The two exercises that follow (Exercises 6 and 7) have been included to help examiners assess their reliability in obtaining goniometric measurements. Calculations of the standard deviation and coefficient of variation are included in the belief that understanding is reinforced by practical application. Exercise 6 examines intratester reliability. **Intratester reliability** refers to the amount of agreement between repeated measurements of the same joint position or ROM by the same examiner (tester). An intratester reliability study answers the question: How accurately can an examiner reproduce his or her own measurements? Exercise 7 examines intertester reliability. **Intertester reliability** refers to the amount of agreement between repeated measurements of the same joint position or ROM by different examiners (testers). An intertester reliability study answers the question: How accurately can one examiner reproduce measurements taken by other examiners?

EXERCISE 6 ■ INTRATESTER RELIABILITY

1. Select a subject and a universal goniometer.
2. Measure elbow flexion ROM on your subject three times, following the steps outlined in Chapter 2, Exercise 5.
3. Record each measurement on the recording form (see opposite page) in the column labeled x. A measurement is denoted by x.
4. Compare the measurements. If a discrepancy of more than 5 degrees exist between measurements, recheck each step in the procedure to make sure that you are performing the steps correctly, and then repeat this exercise.
5. Continue practicing until you have obtained three successive measurements that are within 5 degrees of each other.
6. To gain an understanding of several of the statistics used to evaluate reliability, calculate the standard deviation and coefficient of variation by completing the following steps.
   a. Add the three measurements together to determine the sum of the measurements. Σ is the symbol for summation. Record the sum at the bottom of the column labeled x.
   b. To determine the **mean**, divide this sum by 3, which is the number of measurements. The number of measurements is denoted by n. The mean is denoted by $\bar{x}$. Space to calculate the mean is provided on the recording form.
   c. Subtract the mean from each of the three measurements and record the results in the column labeled $x - \bar{x}$.
   d. Square each of the numbers in the column labeled $x - \bar{x}$, and record the results in the column labeled $(x - \bar{x})^2$.
   e. Add the three numbers in column $(x - \bar{x})^2$ to determine the sum of the squares. Record the results at the bottom of the column labeled $(x - \bar{x})^2$.
   f. To determine the **standard deviation**, divide this sum by 2, which is the number of measurements minus 1 ($n - 1$). Then find the square root of this number. Space to calculate the standard deviation is provided on the recording form.
   g. To determine the **coefficient of variation**, divide the standard deviation by the mean. Multiply this number by 100 percent. Space to calculate the coefficient of variation is provided on the recording form.
7. Repeat this procedure with other joints and motions after you have learned the testing procedures.

RECORDING FORM FOR EXERCISE 6. INTRATESTER RELIABILITY

Subject's Name _____Date _____
Examiner's Name _____
Joint and Motion _____Right or Left Side _____
Passive or Active Motion _____Type of Goniometer _____

Measurement	x	$x - \bar{x}$	$(x - \bar{x})^2$	x^2
1				
2				
3				
$n = 3$	$\Sigma =$		$\Sigma =$	$\Sigma =$

Mean of the three measurements = $\bar{x} = \dfrac{\Sigma x}{n} =$

Standard deviation $= \sqrt{\dfrac{(x - \bar{x})^2}{n - 1}} =$

or use SD $= \sqrt{\dfrac{\Sigma x^2 - (\Sigma x)^2/n}{n - 1}} =$

Coefficient of variation $= \dfrac{SD}{\bar{x}} (100\%) =$

Recording form for Exercise 6: Intratester Reliability. Follow the steps outlined in Exercise 6 using this form to record your measurements and the results of your calculations.

EXERCISE 7 ■ INTERTESTER RELIABILITY

1. Select a subject and a universal goniometer.
2. Measure elbow flexion ROM on your subject once, following the steps outlined in Chapter 2, Exercise 5.
3. Ask two other examiners to measure the same elbow flexion ROM on your subject, using your goniometer and following the steps outlined in Chapter 2, Exercise 5.
4. Record each measurement on the recording form (see opposite page) in the column labeled x. A measurement is denoted by x.
5. Compare the measurements. If a discrepancy of more than 5 degrees exists between measurements, repeat this exercise. The examiners should observe one another's measurements to discover differences in technique that might account for variability, such as faulty alignment, lack of stabilization, or reading the wrong scale.
6. To gain an understanding of several of the statistics used to evaluate reliability, calculate the mean deviation, standard deviation, and coefficient of variation by completing the following steps.
   a. Add the three measurements together to determine the sum of the measurements. Σ is the symbol for summation. Record the sum at the bottom of the column labeled x.
   b. To determine the **mean**, divide this sum by 3, which is the number of measurements. The number of measurements is denoted by n. The mean is denoted by $\bar{x}$. Space to calculate the mean is provided on the recording form.
   c. Subtract the mean from each of the three measurements, and record the results in the column labeled $x - \bar{x}$.
   d. Square each of the numbers in the column labeled $x - \bar{x}$ and record the results in the column labeled $(x - \bar{x})^2$.
   e. Add the three numbers in column $(x - \bar{x})^2$ to determine the sum of the squares. Record the results at the bottom of column $(x - \bar{x})^2$.
   f. To determine the **standard deviation**, divide this sum by 2, which is the number of measurements minus 1 $(n - 1)$. Then find the square root of this number. Space to calculate the standard deviation is provided on the recording form.
   g. To determine the **coefficient of variation**, divide the standard deviation by the mean. Multiply this number by 100 percent. Space to calculate the coefficient of variation is provided on the recording form.
7. Repeat this exercise with other joints and motions after you have learned the testing procedures.

RECORDING FORM FOR EXERCISE 7. INTERTESTER RELIABILITY

Subject's Name _____ Date _____

Examiner 1. Name _____

Examiner 2. Name _____ Joint and Motion _____

Examiner 3. Name _____ Left or Right Side _____

Passive or Active Motion _____ Type of Goniometer_____

Examiner	x	$x - \bar{x}$	$(x - \bar{x})^2$	x^2
1				
2				
3				
$n = 3$	$\sum =$		$\sum =$	$\sum =$

Mean of the three measurements = $\quad \bar{x} = \dfrac{\sum x}{n}$

Standard deviation $\qquad = \sqrt{\dfrac{\sum(x - \bar{x})^2}{n - 1}} \ =$

or use SD $\qquad = \sqrt{\dfrac{\sum x^2 - (\sum x)^2/n}{n - 1}} \ =$

Coefficient of variation $\qquad = \dfrac{SD}{\bar{x}} (100\%) =$

Recording form for Exercise 7: Interester Reliability. Follow the steps outlined in Exercise 7 using this form to record your measurements and the results of your calculations.

REFERENCES

1. Currier, DP: Elements of Research in Physical Therapy, ed 3. Williams & Wilkins, Baltimore, 1990, p 171.
2. Kerlinger, FN: Foundations of Behavioral Research, ed 2. Holt, Rinehart, and Winston, New York, 1973.
3. American Psychological Association: Standards for Educational and Psychological Tests. Am Psych Assoc, Washington, DC, 1974.
4. Rothstein, JM: Measurement and clinical practice: Theory and application. In Rothstein, JM (ed): Measurement in Physical Therapy. Churchill Livingstone, New York, 1985.
5. Gajdosik, RL and Bohannon, RW: Clinical measurement of range of motion: Review of goniometry emphasizing reliability and validity. Phys Ther 67:1867, 1987.
6. Gogia, PP, et al: Reliability and validity of goniometric measurements at the knee. Phys Ther 67:192, 1987.
7. Enwemeka, CS: Radiographic verification of knee goniometry. Scand J Rehabil Med 18:47, 1986.
8. Ahlback, SO and Lindahl, O: Sagittal mobility of the hip-joint. Acta Orthop Scand 34:310, 1964.
9. Herrmann, DB: Validity study of head and neck flexion-extension motion comparing measurements of a pendulum goniometer and roentgenograms. J Orthop Sports Phys Ther 11:414, 1990.
10. Fish, DR and Wingate, L: Sources of goniometric error at the elbow. Phys Ther 65:1666, 1985.

11. Moore, ML: Clinical assessment of joint motion. In Basmajian, JV (ed): Therapeutic Exercise, ed 3. Williams & Wilkins, Baltimore, 1978.
12. Miller, PJ: Assessment of joint motion. In Rothstein, JM (ed): Measurement in Physical Therapy. Churchill Livingstone, New York, 1985.
13. Grohmann, JEL: Comparison of two methods of goniometry. Phys Ther 63:922, 1983.
14. Hamilton, GF and Lachenbruch, PA: Reliability of goniometers in assessing finger joint angle. Phys Ther 49:465, 1969.
15. Boone, DC, et al: Reliability of goniometric measurements. Phys Ther 58:1355, 1978.
16. Pandya, S, et al: Reliability of goniometric measurements in patients with Duchenne muscular dystrophy. Phys Ther 65:1339, 1985.
17. Hellebrandt, FA, Duvall, EN, and Moore, ML: The measurement of joint motion. Part III: Reliability of goniometry. Physical Therapy Review 29:302, 1949. 65:1339, 1985.
18. Low, JL: The reliability of joint measurement. Physiotherapy 62:227, 1976.
19. Tucci, SM, et al: Cervical motion assessment: A new, simple and accurate method. Arch Phys Med Rehabil 67:225, 1986.
20. Youdas, JW, Carey, JR, and Garrett, TR: Reliability of measurements of cervical spine range of motion: Comparison of three methods. Phys Ther 71:2, 1991.
21. Fitzgerald, GK, et al: Objective assessment with establishment of normal values for lumbar spine range of motion. Phys Ther 63:1776, 1983.
22. Mayerson, NH and Milano, RA: Goniometric measurement reliability in physical medicine. Arch Phys Med Rehabil 65:92, 1984.
23. Watkins, MA, et al: Reliability of goniometric measurements and visual estimates of knee range of motion obtained in a clinical setting. Phys Ther 71:90, 1991.
24. Riddle, DL, Rothstein, JM, and Lamb, RL: Goniometric reliability in a clinical setting: Shoulder measurements. Phys Ther 67:668, 1987.
25. Ekstrand, J, et al: Lower extremity goniometric measurements: A study to determine their reliability. Arch Phys Med Rehabil 63:171, 1982.
26. Rothstein, JM, Miller, PJ, and Roettger, RF: Goniometric reliability in a clinical setting: Elbow and knee measurements. Phys Ther 63:1611, 1983.
27. Solgaard, S, et al: Reproducibility of goniometry of the wrist. Scand J Rehabil Med 18:5, 1986.
28. Patel, RS: Intratester and intertester reliability of the inclinometer in measuring lumbar flexion [abstract]. Phys Ther 72:S44, 1992.
29. Lovell, FW, Rothstein, JM, and Personius, WJ: Reliability of clinical measurements of lumbar lordosis taken with a flexible rule. Phys Ther 69:96, 1989.
30. Defibaugh, JJ: Measurement of head motion. Part II: An experimental study of head motion in adult males. Phys Ther 44:163, 1964.
31. Balogun, JA, et al: Inter- and intratester reliability of measuring neck motions with tape measure and Myrin Gravity-Reference Goniometer. J Orthop Sports Phys Ther 10:248, 1989.
32. Capuano-Pucci, D, et al: Intratester and intertester reliability of the cervical range of motion. Arch Phys Med Rehabil 72:338, 1991.
33. Cobe, HM: The range of active motion at the wrist of white adults. J Bone Joint Surg Br 10:763, 1928.
34. Hewitt, D: The range of active motion at the wrist of women. J Bone Joint Surg Br 10:775, 1928.
35. Palmer, ML and Epler, M: Clinical Assessment Procedures in Physical Therapy. JB Lippincott, Philadelphia, 1990.
36. Clarkson, HM and Gilewich, GB: Musculoskeletal Assessment: Joint Range of Motion and Manual Muscle Strength. Williams & Wilkins, Baltimore, 1989.
37. Robson, P: A method to reduce the variable error in joint range measurement. Annals of Physical Medicine 8:262, 1966.
38. Petherick, M, et al: Concurrent validity and intertester reliability of universal and fluid-based goniometers for active elbow range of motion. Phys Ther 68:966, 1988.
39. Clapper, MP and Wolf, SL: Comparison of the reliability of the orthoranger and the standard goniometer for assessing active lower extremity range of motion. Phys Ther 68:214, 1988.
40. Ellison, JB, Rose, SJ, and Sahrman, SA: Patterns of hip rotation: A comparison between healthy subjects and patients with low back pain. Phys Ther 70:537, 1990.
41. Rheault, W, et al: Intertester reliability and concurrent validity of fluid-based and universal goniometers for active knee flexion. Phys Ther 68:1676, 1988.
42. White, DJ, et al: Reliability of three methods of measuring cervical motion [abstract]. Phys Ther 66:771, 1986.
43. Williams, R, et al: Reliability of the modified-modified Schober and double inclinometer methods for measuring lumbar flexion and extension. Phys Ther 73:26, 1993.
44. Reynolds, PMG: Measurement of spinal mobility: A comparison of three methods. Rheumatology and Rehabilitation 14:180, 1975.
45. Miller, MH, et al: Measurement of spinal mobility in the sagittal plane: New skin distraction technique compared with established methods. J Rheum 11:4, 1984.
46. Portek, I, et al: Correlation between radiographic and clinical measurement of lumbar spine movement. Br J Rheumatol 22:197, 1983.
47. Gill, K, et al: Repeatability of four clinical methods for assessment of lumbar spinal motion. Spine 13:50, 1988.
48. Lindahl, O: Determination of the sagittal mobility of the lumbar spine. Acta Orthop Scand 37:241, 1966.
49. White, DJ, et al: Reliability of three clinical methods of measuring lateral flexion in the thoracolumbar spine [abstract]. Phys Ther 67:759, 1987.
50. Colton, T: Statistics in Medicine. Little, Brown, Boston, 1974.
51. Thomas, CL (ed): Taber's Cyclopedic Medical Dictionary, ed 17. FA Davis, Philadelphia, 1993.
52. Dawson-Saunders, B and Trapp, RG: Basic and Clinical Biostatistics. Appleton & Lange, Norwalk, CT, 1990.
53. Francis, K: Computer communication: Reliability. Phys Ther 66: 1140, 1986.
54. Blesh, TE: Measurement in Physical Education, ed 2. Ronald Press, New York, 1974. Cited by Currier, DP: Elements of Research in Physical Therapy, ed 3. Williams & Wilkins, Baltimore, 1990.
55. Shout, PE and Fleiss, JL: Intraclass correlations: Uses in assessing rater reliability. Psychol Bull 86:420, 1979.
56. Lahey, MA, Downey, RG, and Saal, FE: Intraclass correlations: There's more there than meets the eye. Psychol Bull 93:586, 1983.
57. Mitchell, SK: Interobserver agreement, reliability, and generalizability of data collected in observational studies. Psychol Bull 86: 376, 1979.
58. DuBois, PH: An Introduction to Psychological Statistics. Harper & Row, New York, 1965, p 401.
59. Bartko, JJ and Carpenter, WJ: On the methods and theory of reliability. J Nerv Ment Dis 163:307, 1976.
60. Bartko, JJ: Rationale for reporting standard deviations rather than standard errors of the mean. Am J Psychiatry 142:1060, 1985.

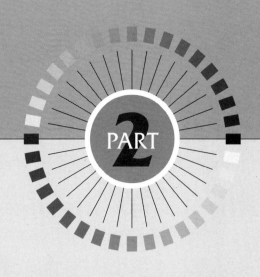

PART 2

Upper-Extremity Testing

OBJECTIVES

On completion of Part 2 the reader will be able to:

1. Identify:
   the appropriate planes and axes for each joint motion
   the structures that limit the end of the ROM at each joint and the expected normal end-feel

2. Describe:
   the recommended testing positions used for each joint motion
   goniometer alignment
   the capsular pattern of limitation
   the ROM necessary for functional activities

3. Explain:
   how age and gender can affect the ROM
   how sources of error in measurement can affect testing results

4. Perform a goniometric evaluation of any motion at the shoulder, elbow, wrist, or hand, including:

a clear explanation of the testing procedure
positioning of the subject in a recommended testing position
adequate stabilization of the proximal joint component
a correct determination of the end of the ROM
a correct identification of the end-feel
palpation of the correct bony landmarks
accurate alignment of the goniometer
correct reading and recording

5. Plan goniometric evaluations of the shoulder, elbow, wrist, and hand that are organized by body position

6. Assess intratester and intertester reliability of goniometric testing of the shoulder, elbow, wrist, and hand

The recommended testing positions, stabilization techniques, physiological end-feel, and goniometer alignment for the joints of the upper extremities are presented in Chapters 4 to 6. The goniometric evaluation should follow the 12-step sequence presented in Exercise 5 in Chapter 2.

4

The Shoulder

GLENOHUMERAL JOINT

STRUCTURE

The glenohumeral joint is a synovial ball-and-socket joint. The ball is the convex head of the humerus, which faces medially, superiorly, and posteriorly with respect to the shaft of the humerus. The socket is formed by the concave glenoid fossa of the scapula. The socket is shallow and smaller than the humeral head but is deepened and enlarged by the fibrocartilaginous glenoid labrum. The joint capsule is thin and lax, blends with the glenoid labrum, and is reinforced by the tendons of the rotator cuff muscles and by the glenohumeral (superior, middle, and inferior) and coracohumeral ligaments.

OSTEOKINEMATICS

The glenohumeral joint has 3 degrees of freedom. The motions permitted at the joint are flexion-extension, abduction-adduction, and medial-lateral rotation. Full ROM of the shoulder requires humeral, scapular, and clavicular motion at the glenohumeral, sternoclavicular, acromioclavicular, and scapulothoracic joints.

ARTHROKINEMATICS

Motion in flexion-extension and abduction-adduction occurs as a rolling and sliding of the head of the humerus on the glenoid fossa. The direction of the sliding is opposite to the movement of the shaft of the humerus. The humeral head slides posteriorly and inferiorly in flexion, anteriorly and superiorly in extension, inferiorly in abduction, and superiorly in adduction. In lateral rotation, the humeral head slides anteriorly on the glenoid fossa. In medial rotation, the humeral head slides posteriorly.

CAPSULAR PATTERN

The greatest limitation of passive motion is in lateral rotation, followed by abduction, with less limitation in medial rotation.[1]

STERNOCLAVICULAR JOINT

STRUCTURE

The sternoclavicular (SC) joint is a plane, synovial joint linking the medial end of the clavicle with the sternum and the cartilage of the first rib. The joint surfaces on each side of the joint are saddle shaped. The clavicular joint surface is convex cephalocaudally and concave anteroposteriorly. The opposing joint surface located at the notch formed by the manubrium of the sternum and the first costal cartilage is concave cephalocaudally and convex anteroposteriorly. An articular disc divides the joint into two separate compartments.

The associated joint capsule is strong and reinforced by anterior and posterior sternoclavicular ligaments. These ligaments limit anterior-posterior movement of the medial end of the clavicle. The costoclavicular ligament, which extends from the inferior surface of the medial end of the clavicle to the first rib, limits clavicular elevation and protraction. The interclavicular ligament extends from one clavicle to another and limits excessive inferior movement of the clavicle.

OSTEOKINEMATICS

The SC joint has 3 degrees of freedom, and motion consists of movement of the clavicle on the sternum. Clavicular motion at this joint includes elevation-depression, protraction-retraction, and rotation.[2]

ARTHROKINEMATICS

During clavicular elevation and depression, the convex surface of the clavicle slides on the concave manubrium in a direction opposite the movement of the lateral end of the clavicle. In protraction and retraction, the concave portion of the clavicular joint surface slides on the convex surface of the costal cartilage in the same direction as the lateral end of the clavicle. In rotation, the clavicular joint surface spins on the opposing joint surface. Therefore, the clavicle slides inferiorly in elevation, superiorly in depression, anteriorly in protraction, and posteriorly in retraction.

ACROMIOCLAVICULAR JOINT

STRUCTURE

The acromioclavicular (AC) joint is a plane synovial joint linking the scapula and the clavicle. The scapular joint surface is a concave facet located on the acromion of the scapula. The clavicular joint surface is a convex facet located on the lateral end of the clavicle. The joint contains a fibrocartilaginous disc and is surrounded by a weak joint capsule. The superior and inferior acromioclavicular ligaments reinforce the capsule. The coracoclavicular ligament, which extends between the clavicle and the scapular coracoid process, provides additional stability.

OSTEOKINEMATICS

The AC joint has 3 degrees of freedom and permits movement of the scapula on the clavicle in three planes. The primary motions are upward and downward rotation of the scapula in the frontal plane.[3] The other two motions are tipping and winging of the scapula. Tipping (tilting) is movement of the glenoid fossa and inferior angle of the scapula in the sagittal plane. Winging (abduction) is a posterior lateral movement of the vertebral border of the scapula in the transverse plane.[3]

ARTHROKINEMATICS

Motion of the joint surfaces consists of a sliding of the concave acromial facet on the convex clavicular facet. Acromial sliding on the clavicle occurs in the same direction as movement of the scapula.

SCAPULOTHORACIC JOINT

STRUCTURE

The scapulothoracic joint is considered to be a functional rather than an anatomical joint. The joint surfaces are the anterior surface of the scapula and the posterior surface of the thorax.

OSTEOKINEMATICS

The motions that occur at this joint are scapular abduction-adduction, elevation-depression, upward and downward rotation, tipping, and winging.

ARTHROKINEMATICS

Motion consists of a gliding of the scapula on the thorax.

RANGE OF MOTION

Table 4–1 shows the mean values of ROM measurements obtained from various sources. The age, gender, and number of subjects that were measured to obtain the values reported for the American Academy of Orthopedic Surgeons (AAOS) and the American Medical Association (AMA) are unknown. Boone and Azen[6] measured active ROM in males using a universal goniometer.

FUNCTIONAL RANGE OF MOTION

Table 4–2 summarizes the shoulder ROM required for various self-feeding activities.

EFFECTS OF AGE AND GENDER

Table 4–3 shows the relationship between age and shoulder ROM for newborns through adolescents. Values from the study by Wanatabe et al.[8] were derived from measurements of passive ROM of males and females. The mean values listed from Boone[9] were derived from measurements of active ROM taken with a universal goniometer on healthy males.

A review of mean values presented in Table 4–3 for the

Table 4–1 **SHOULDER MOTION: MEAN VALUES (IN DEGREES) FROM SELECTED SOURCES**

Motion	AMERICAN ACADEMY OF ORTHOPAEDIC SURGEONS[4]	AMERICAN MEDICAL ASSOCIATION[5]	BOONE AND AZEN[6] $N = 109$* Mean	Standard Deviation
Flexion	180.0	150.0	166.7	4.7
Extension	60.0	50.0	62.3	9.5
Abduction	180.0	180.0	184.0	7.0
Medial rotation	70.0	90.0	68.8	4.6
Lateral rotation	90.0	90.0	103.7	8.5

*Values are for male subjects 18 mo–54 yr of age.

Table 4–2 **SHOULDER RANGE OF MOTION NECESSARY FOR FUNCTIONAL ACTIVITIES**

Activity	Motion	Range (Degrees)
Eating with a spoon[7]	Flexion	7.8–36.1
	Abduction	6.6–21.8
	Medial rotation	4.8–16.8
Eating with a fork	Flexion	10.7–35.2
	Abduction	7.1–18.6
	Medial rotation	5.1–18.1
Drinking from a cup	Flexion	15.8–43.2
	Abduction	12.7–31.2
	Medial rotation	5.2–23.4

different age groups shows very slight differences among age groups. The largest values are found in the youngest age group. Wanatabe et al.[8] found that the ROM in shoulder extension and lateral rotation was greater in Japanese infants than the average values obtained for adults. Boone and Azen[6] found a significantly greater active ROM in shoulder extension and lateral rotation in male children 12 years and under than in male subjects in the other age groups. However, Boone and Azen found no significant differences in shoulder abduction among the same male

subjects in the following six age groups tested: 1 to 5 years, 6 to 12 years, 13 to 19 years, 20 to 29 years, 30 to 39 years, and 40 to 54 years.

Table 4–4 summarizes the effects of age on shoulder ROM in adults. Values cited from Boone[9] were obtained from measurements of active ROM in male subjects using a universal goniometer. The values from the study by Walker et al.[10] also were obtained from measurements of male subjects using a universal goniometer. The values from Downey et al.[11] were obtained from measurements of active ROM using a universal goniometer on 70 female and 30 male subjects.

The mean values in Table 4–4 show a trend for the older groups (60 years of age and older) to have lower mean values than younger groups (20 to 39 years of age) for the motion of extension. Although changes in the mean values are slight among the other motions, the standard deviations for the oldest groups are much larger than the values reported for the younger groups (20 to 45 years of age). The larger standard deviations appear to indicate that the ROM is more variable in the older group than in the younger groups. However, the fact that the measurements of the two oldest groups were obtained by different investigators should be considered when drawing conclusions from this information.

Table 4–3 **EFFECTS OF AGE ON SHOULDER MOTION: MEAN VALUES (IN DEGREES) FOR NEWBORNS THROUGH ADOLESCENTS**

Motion	WANATABE ET AL.[8] 0–2 YR ($N = 45$) Range of Means*	BOONE[9] 1–5 YR ($N = 19$) Mean	Standard Deviation	6–12 YR ($N = 17$) Mean	Standard Deviation	13–19 YR ($N = 17$) Mean	Standard Deviation
Flexion	172–180	168.8	3.7	169.0	3.5	167.4	3.9
Extension	79–89	68.9	6.6	69.6	7.0	64.0	9.3
Medial rotation	72–90	71.2	3.6	70.0	4.7	70.3	5.3
Lateral rotation	118–134	110.0	10.0	107.4	3.6	106.3	6.1
Abduction	177–187	186.3	2.6	184.7	3.8	185.1	4.3

*Ranges of mean values for passive range of motion.

Table 4 – 4 **EFFECTS OF AGE ON SHOULDER MOTION: MEAN VALUES IN DEGREES FOR YOUNG AND OLD ADULTS 20 – 93 YR OF AGE**

| | BOONE[9] | | | | | | WALKER ET AL.[10] | | DOWNEY ET AL.[11] | |
| | 20 – 29 YR (N = 19) | | 30 – 39 YR (N = 18) | | 40 – 54 YR (N = 19) | | 60 – 85 YR (N = 30) | | 61 – 93 YR (N = 106) | |
Motion	Mean	Standard Deviation	Mean	Standard Deviation	Mean	Standard Deviation	Mean	Standard Deviation	Mean	Standard Deviation
Flexion	164.5	5.9	165.4	3.8	165.1	5.2	160.0	11.0	165.0	10.7
Extension	58.3	8.3	57.5	8.5	56.1	7.9	38.0	11.0		
Medial rotation	65.9	4.0	67.1	4.2	68.3	3.8	59.0	16.0	65.0	11.7
Lateral rotation	100.0	7.2	101.5	6.9	97.5	8.5	76.0	13.0	80.6	11.0
Abduction	182.6	9.8	182.8	7.7	182.6	9.8	155.0	22.0	157.9	17.4

In addition to the evidence for age-related changes presented in Tables 4 – 3 and 4 – 4, West,[12] Clarke et al.,[13] Allander et al.,[14] and Walker et al.[10] have identified either age- or gender-related trends, or both. West[12] found that older subjects had slightly less ROM in flexion and extension than younger subjects. Clarke et al.[13] found age and gender differences in a study in which they used a hydrogoniometric technique to measure passive ROM in the following three groups: normal individuals, current patients with stiff and painful shoulders, and discharged shoulder patients. These authors found that in the normal group consisting of 60 males and females aged 21 to 80 years, the older subgroups had less passive ROM than the younger groups. Males in the normal group had on an average 92 percent of the ROM of their female counterparts, the difference being most marked in abduction. In the group consisting of current shoulder patients (15 males and 15 females) aged 31 to 71 years, males had a greater reduction in ROM than their female counterparts.

Allander et al.,[14] in a study of passive ROM of the shoulder in 517 females and 203 males aged 33 to 70 years, found that joint mobility was affected by age, gender, and side (left or right). According to these authors, the ROM in shoulder rotation decreased with increasing age, but the decrease was small, averaging only 2.2 degrees for each 5-year interval between 45 and 60 years of age. Males had a smaller ROM in shoulder rotation than females. Independently of gender, the right side showed a smaller range of motion than the left for some age groups.

Walker et al.[10] found that women aged 60 to 84 years had greater ROM in shoulder abduction and shoulder extension than their male counterparts. The mean differences for women were 20 degrees greater than males for shoulder abduction, and 11 degrees greater than males for shoulder extension.

RELIABILITY AND VALIDITY

The intratester and intertester reliability of measurements of shoulder motion have been studied by Helle-brandt et al.,[15] Boone et al.,[16] Pandya et al.[17] and Riddle et al.[18] All of these studies, with the exception of the study by Boone et al.,[16] were conducted on patient populations, and all studies presented evidence that intratester reliability was better than intertester reliability. In most studies, reliability varied according to the motion being measured. In other words, reliability of measurements of some motions was better than the reliability of measurements of other motions.

Hellebrandt et al.[15] in a study of 77 patients, found the intratester reliability of measurements of active ROM of shoulder abduction and medial rotation to be less than the intratester reliability of other shoulder motions, irrespective of the goniometer used. The authors concluded that the difficulties lay in the structural and functional peculiarities of the joint rather than in a lack of reliability of the testers. Intratester reliability for other shoulder motions was high.

Boone et al.,[16] in a study in which four physical therapists used universal goniometers to measure the passive ROM in shoulder lateral rotation in 12 normal male subjects once a week for 4 weeks, found that intratester reliability was higher than intertester reliability. Variations in measurements of shoulder lateral rotation were small in comparison with variations in measurements of flexion-extension at the knee, which were large.

Pandya et al.,[17] in a study in which five testers measured the range of shoulder abduction of 150 children and young adults (1 to 20 years of age) with Duchenne muscular dystrophy, found that the intratester ICC for measurements of shoulder abduction was 0.84. The intertester measurement of shoulder abduction was considerably lower (ICC = 0.67). In comparison with measurements of elbow and wrist extension, the measurement of shoulder abduction was less reliable. This finding is similar to that of Hellebrandt et al.,[15] who found the intratester reliability of shoulder abduction to be less than intratester reliability for other shoulder motions.

Riddle et al.[18] conducted a two-part study to determine intratester and intertester reliability for passive ROM measurements of the following shoulder motions: flexion-extension, abduction, horizontal abduction-adduction, and lateral-medial rotation. The testers used two different-sized universal goniometers (large and small) for their measurements. Fifty patients (24 men and 26 women), ranging in age from 21 to 77 years, participated in the first part of the study, which measured the motions of flexion, extension, and abduction. Intratester reliability was greater than intertester reliability, but ICC values varied according to the motion being measured. ICC values for intratester reliability of measurements of flexion, extension, and abduction, obtained with either a large or a small goniometer, ranged from 0.94 to 0.98. This finding differs from those of Hellebrandt et al.[15] and Pandya et al.,[17] who found lower intratester reliability for abduction. The ICC values for intertester reliability for flexion and abduction ranged from 0.84 to 0.89. ICC values for intertester reliability of measurements of extension were poor, ranging from 0.26 with the small goniometer to 0.27 with the large goniometer. Fifty patients (30 men and 20 women), ranging in age from 19 to 77 years, participated in the second part of the study. ICC values for intratester reliability of measurements of horizontal abduction-adduction and lateral-medial rotation ranged from 0.87 to 0.99. Intertester reliability was considerably lower for measurements of horizontal abduction, horizontal adduction, and medial rotation, with ICC values ranging from 0.28 to 0.55. ICC values for intertester reliability for measurement of lateral rotation were high: 0.88 for the large goniometer and 0.90 for the small goniometer. The authors recommended that because repeated measurements of horizontal abduction, horizontal adduc-

tion, medial rotation, and extension were unreliable when taken by more than one tester, these measurements should be taken by the same therapist.[18] Neither the size of the goniometer nor the patient's diagnosis appeared to affect reliability.

TESTING PROCEDURES

Full ROM of the shoulder requires movement at the glenohumeral, scapulothoracic, acromioclavicular, and sternoclavicular joints. In an attempt to make measurements more informative and to help identify glenohumeral joint problems within the shoulder complex, we suggest using two methods of measuring the ROM of the shoulder. One method measures passive motion primarily at the glenohumeral joint. The other method measures passive ROM at all the joints.

We have found the method that measures primarily glenohumeral motion to be helpful in teaching students how to identify components of motion at the shoulder complex. We are not aware of any studies that have been done to assess either the reliability or the validity of this method of measuring the average ROM.

The second method measures full motion of the shoulder and is useful in evaluating the functional ROM of the shoulder complex. ROM values for shoulder complex motion are presented in Tables 4–1 to 4–4. Both methods of measuring the ROM of the shoulder are presented in the discussions of stabilization techniques and end-feels that follow.

FLEXION

Motion occurs in the sagittal plane around a medial-lateral axis.

Recommended Testing Position

Position the subject supine, with the knees flexed to flatten the lumbar spine. The shoulder is positioned in 0 degrees of abduction, adduction, and rotation. The forearm is positioned in 0 degrees of supination and pronation so that the palm of the hand faces the body.

Stabilization

Glenohumeral Motion

Stabilize the scapula to prevent elevation, posterior tilting (inferior angle presses against rib cage), and upward rotation of the scapula (Fig. 4–1).

Shoulder Complex Motion

Stabilize the thorax to prevent extension of the spine.

Normal End-Feel

Glenohumeral Motion

The end-feel is firm because of tension in the posterior band of the coracohumeral ligament, the posterior joint capsule, and the teres minor, teres major, and infraspinatus muscles.

Shoulder Complex Motion

The end-feel is firm because of tension in the latissimus dorsi muscle and the costosternal fibers of the pectoralis major muscle.

Goniometer Alignment

See Figures 4–2 and 4–3.

1. Center the fulcrum of the goniometer close to the acromial process.
2. Align the proximal arm with the midaxillary line of the thorax.
3. Align the distal arm with the lateral midline of the humerus, using the lateral epicondyle of the humerus for reference.

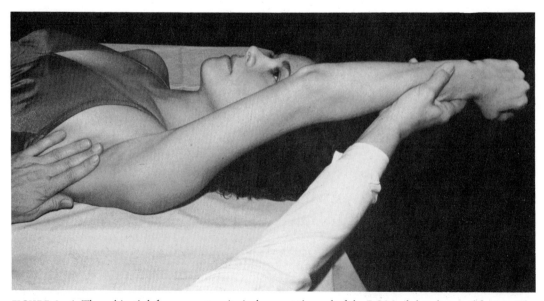

FIGURE 4–1. The subject's left upper extremity is shown at the end of the ROM of glenohumeral flexion. The examiner's left hand, which is placed over the lateral border of the subject's scapula, is the stabilizing hand. The examiner is able to determine that the end of the ROM has been reached, because any attempt to move the extremity into additional flexion causes the lateral border of the scapula to move anteriorly and laterally. The stabilizing hand detects and prevents scapular motion.

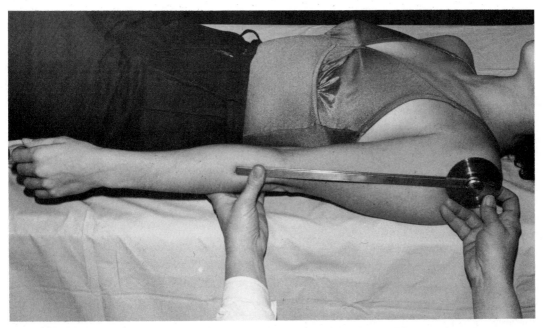

FIGURE 4 – 2. The subject is shown at the beginning of the ROM of glenohumeral flexion. The body of the full-circle metal goniometer is aligned with the subject's acromion process. The two arms of the goniometer are aligned along the lateral midline of the thorax and the lateral midline of the humerus and extend over the lateral epicondyle of the humerus.

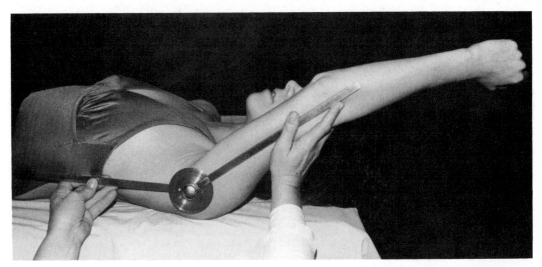

FIGURE 4 – 3. The alignment of the goniometer at the end of the ROM of glenohumeral flexion. The examiner's right hand supports the subject's extremity and maintains the goniometer's distal arm in correct alignment over the lateral epicondyle. The examiner's left hand aligns the goniometer's proximal arm with the lateral midline of the thorax.

EXTENSION

Motion occurs in the sagittal plane around a medial-lateral axis.

Recommended Testing Position

Position the subject prone, with the head facing away from the shoulder being tested. No pillow is used under the head. The shoulder is positioned in 0 degrees of abduction and rotation. The elbow is positioned in slight flexion so that tension in the long head of the biceps brachii muscle will not restrict the motion. The forearm is positioned in 0 degrees of supination and pronation so that the palm of the hand faces the body.

Stabilization

Glenohumeral Motion

Stabilize the scapula to prevent elevation and anterior tilting (inferior angle protrudes posteriorly) of the scapula (Fig. 4–4).

Shoulder Complex Motion

Stabilize the thorax to prevent forward flexion of the spine.

Normal End-Feel

Glenohumeral Motion

The end-feel is firm because of tension in the anterior band of the coracohumeral ligament and the anterior joint capsule.

Shoulder Complex Motion

The end-feel is firm because of tension in the clavicular fibers of the pectoralis major muscle and the serratus anterior muscle.

Goniometer Alignment

See Figures 4–5 and 4–6.

1. Center the fulcrum of the goniometer close to the acromial process.
2. Align the proximal arm with the midaxillary line of the thorax.
3. Align the distal arm with the lateral midline of the humerus, using the lateral epicondyle of the humerus for reference.

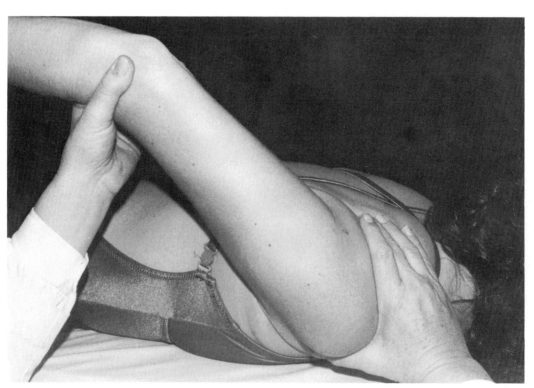

FIGURE 4–4. The subject's right upper extremity at the end of the ROM of extension. The examiner's right is holding the scapula. The examiner is able to determine that the end of the ROM in extension has been attained because additional extension causes the scapula to elevate and tilt anteriorly. The examiner's stabilizing hand detects and prevents scapular motion.

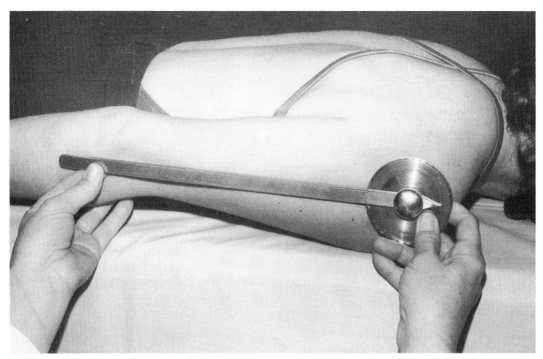

FIGURE 4 – 5. The subject is at the beginning of the ROM of extension with her head turned away from the joint being tested. The body of the goniometer is aligned with the acromion process, and the arms are aligned along the lateral midline of the thorax and the lateral midline of the humerus and extend over the lateral epicondyle.

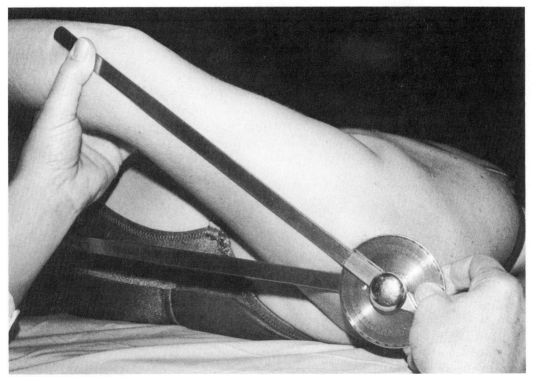

FIGURE 4 – 6. This photograph shows the goniometer alignment at the end of the ROM in extension. The examiner's left hand supports the subject's extremity and holds the distal arm of the goniometer in correct alignment over the lateral epicondyle of the humerus. The goniometer body is held over the subject's acromion process, while the proximal arm is aligned along the lateral midline of the thorax.

ABDUCTION

Motion occurs in the frontal plane around an anterior-posterior axis.

Recommended Testing Position

Position the subject supine. As an alternative, measurements may be taken with the subject sitting or prone. The shoulder is positioned in 0 degrees of flexion and extension and full lateral rotation so that the palm of the hand faces anteriorly. If the humerus is not laterally rotated, contact between the greater tubercle of the humerus and the upper portion of the glenoid fossa or acromial process will restrict the motion. The elbow should be extended so that tension in the long head of the triceps will not restrict the motion.

Stabilization

Glenohumeral Motion

Stabilize the scapula to prevent upward rotation and elevation of the scapula (Figs. 4–7 and 4–8). Figure 4–8 shows an alternative testing position.

Shoulder Complex Motion

Stabilize the thorax to prevent lateral flexion of the trunk.

Normal End-Feel

Glenohumeral Motion

The end-feel is usually firm because of tension in the middle and inferior bands of the glenohumeral ligament, the inferior joint capsule, and the latissimus dorsi and pectoralis major muscles.

Shoulder Complex Motion

The end-feel is firm because of tension in the major and minor rhomboid muscles and the middle and inferior portions of the trapezius muscle.

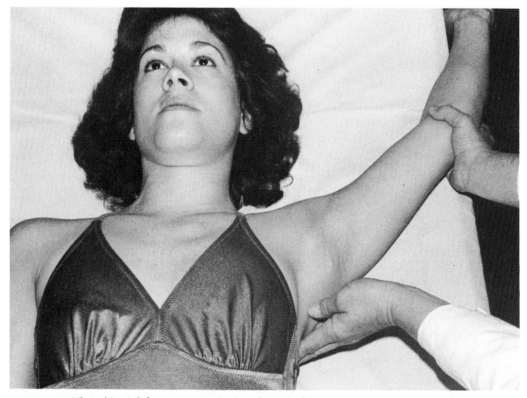

FIGURE 4–7. The subject's left upper extremity is at the end of the ROM of glenohumeral abduction. The examiner's left hand stabilizes the scapula. The end of the ROM in abduction occurs at the point where attempts to move the extremity into further abduction result in lateral scapular motion. This scapular motion can be detected by the stabilizing hand. The supine testing position is somewhat easier to use than the alternative sitting position, because in the former position extremity and trunk are supported by the table.

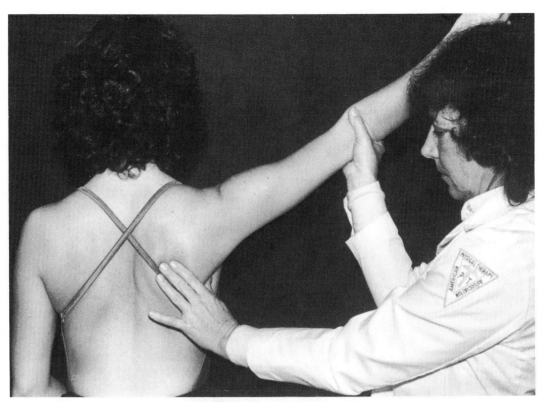

FIGURE 4–8. The right upper extremity at the end of the ROM in abduction. The examiner's left hand stabilizes the scapula. The end of the ROM in abduction occurs at the point where attempts to move the extremity into further abduction cause the inferior angle of the scapula to move laterally away from the rib cage. The examiner's left hand is able to detect the lateral scapular motion. In the sitting position, the trunk is not as well stabilized as it is in the supine position; therefore, the examiner must be alert to lateral bending of the thorax. In addition, the examiner can ask the subject to try to keep the back straight.

Goniometer Alignment (Supine Position)

See Figures 4–9 and 4–10.

1. Center the fulcrum of the goniometer close to the anterior aspect of the acromial process.

2. Align the proximal arm so that it is parallel to the midline of the anterior aspect of the sternum.
3. At the end of the ROM, align the distal arm with the medial midline of the humerus.

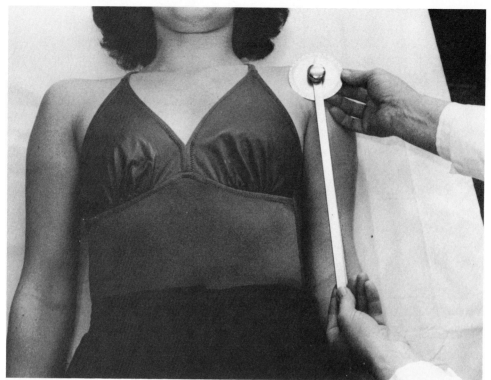

FIGURE 4–9. The supine starting position for measuring ROM of shoulder abduction; the body of the goniometer is aligned over the anterior aspect of the acromion process. The arms of the goniometer are aligned along the anterior midline of the humerus and parallel to the sternum.

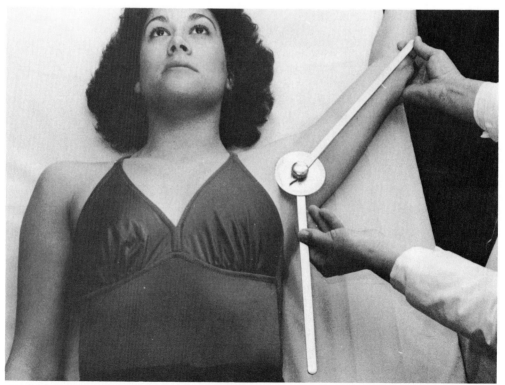

FIGURE 4–10. At the end of the ROM in shoulder abduction, the proximal arm of the goniometer is aligned parallel to the sternum. The distal arm of the goniometer is held in position along the medial midline of the humerus by the examiner. Note that the humerus is laterally rotated.

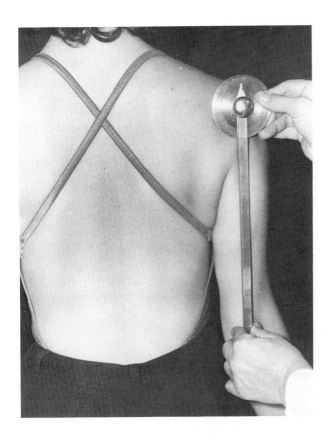

Alternative Goniometer Alignment

Sitting Position

See Figures 4–11 and 4–12.

1. Center the fulcrum of the goniometer close to the posterior aspect of the acromial process.
2. Align the proximal arm parallel to the spinous processes of the vertebral column.
3. At the end of the ROM, align the distal arm with the lateral midline of the humerus, using the lateral epicondyle for reference.

ADDUCTION

Motion occurs in the frontal plane around an anterior-posterior axis.

Recommended Testing Position, Stabilization, and Goniometer Alignment

The testing position, stabilization, and alignment are the same as for shoulder abduction.

FIGURE 4–11. The examiner positions the body of the goniometer over the posterior aspect of the acromion process when measuring shoulder abduction in the sitting position. The two arms of the goniometer are aligned along the posterior midline of the humerus and parallel to the spinous processes of the vertebral column.

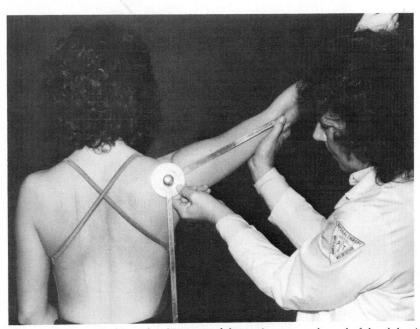

FIGURE 4–12. This photograph shows the alignment of the goniometer at the end of the abduction ROM in the sitting position. The examiner's right hand supports the subject's right upper extremity and holds the distal arm of the goniometer aligned along the lateral midline of the humerus. The proximal arm should be free to hang perpendicular to the floor and parallel to the subject's vertebral column. Sometimes the sitting position is more awkward than the supine position, because the examiner must support the weight of the subject's arm during passive ROM and watch the subject's thorax constantly to ensure that no lateral flexion occurs.

MEDIAL (INTERNAL) ROTATION

Motion occurs in the transverse plane around a vertical axis when the subject is in the anatomical position.

Recommended Testing Position

Position the subject supine, with the arm being tested in 90 degrees of shoulder abduction. The forearm is perpendicular to the supporting surface and is in 0 degrees of supination and pronation so that the palm of the hand faces the feet. The full length of the humerus rests on the supporting surface. The elbow is not supported. A pad is placed under the humerus so that the humerus is positioned level with the acromial process.

Stabilization

Glenohumeral Motion

In the beginning of the ROM, stabilization is often needed at the distal end of the humerus to keep the shoulder in 90 degrees of abduction. Toward the end of the ROM, the scapula is stabilized to prevent elevation and anterior tilting (inferior angle protrudes posteriorly) of the scapula (Fig. 4–13).

Shoulder Complex Motion

In the beginning of the ROM, stabilization is often needed at the distal end of the humerus to keep the shoulder in 90 degrees of abduction. Toward the end of the ROM, the thorax is stabilized to prevent flexion of the spine.

Normal End-Feel

Glenohumeral Motion

The end-feel is firm because of tension in the posterior joint capsule and the infraspinatus and teres minor muscles.

Shoulder Complex Motion

The end-feel is firm because of tension in the major and minor rhomboid muscles and the middle and inferior portions of the trapezius muscle.

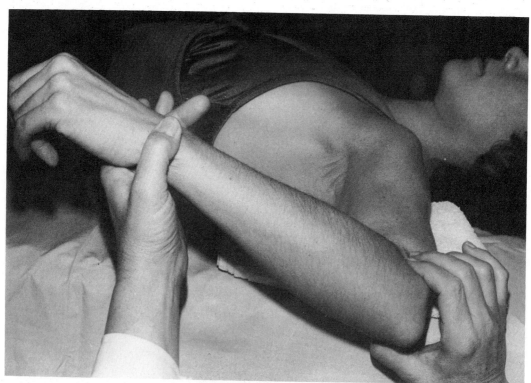

FIGURE 4–13. This photograph shows the left upper extremity at the end of the ROM of medial (internal) rotation of the shoulder. The glenohumeral joint is positioned at 90 degrees of abduction, and the elbow is maintained in 90 degrees of flexion. The examiner's right hand stabilizes the distal end of the humerus to maintain the abducted shoulder position. The end of the ROM in medial rotation occurs when continuation of the motion causes the scapula to tilt anteriorly. The scapular motion may be observed at the anterior and superior aspects of the shoulder.

Goniometer Alignment

See Figures 4–14 and 4–15.

1. Center the fulcrum of the goniometer over the olecranon process.
2. Align the proximal arm so that it is either parallel to or perpendicular to the floor.
3. Align the distal arm with the ulna, using the olecranon process and ulnar styloid for reference.

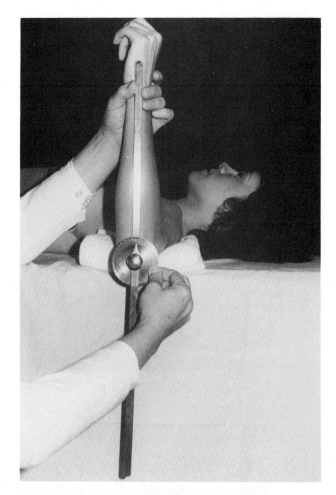

FIGURE 4–14. The examiner places the body of the goniometer over the olecranon process and aligns the distal arm with the ulnar styloid process in the testing positions for both medial and lateral rotation at the glenohumeral joint. The proximal arm of the goniometer should be freely movable so that gravity causes it to hang perpendicular to the floor.

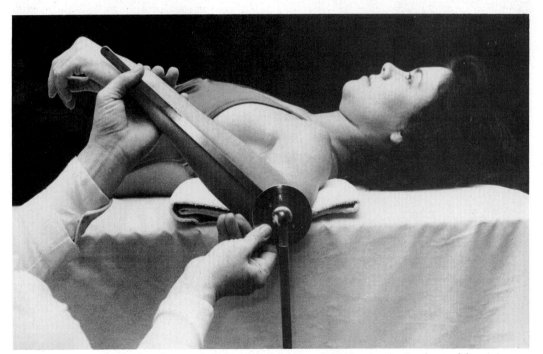

FIGURE 4–15. The examiner supports the subject's left forearm and maintains the distal arm of the goniometer over the ulnar styloid process at the end of the ROM of medial rotation. The examiner's right hand holds the body of the goniometer over the olecranon process. The freely moving proximal arm of the goniometer hangs perpendicular to the floor.

LATERAL (EXTERNAL) ROTATION

Motion occurs in the transverse plane around a vertical axis when the subject is in the anatomical position.

Recommended Testing Position

The testing position is the same as for medial rotation of the shoulder.

Stabilization

Glenohumeral Motion

In the beginning of the ROM, stabilization is often needed at the distal end of the humerus to keep the shoulder in 90 degrees of abduction. Toward the end of the ROM, the scapula is stabilized to prevent its tilting posteriorly (the inferior angle presses against the rib cage) (Fig. 4–16).

Shoulder Complex Motion

In the beginning of the ROM, stabilization is often needed at the distal end of the humerus to keep the shoulder in 90 degrees of abduction. Toward the end of the ROM, the thorax is stabilized to prevent extension of the spine.

Normal End-Feel

Glenohumeral Motion

The end-feel is firm because of tension in the three bands of the glenohumeral ligament, the coracohumeral ligament, the anterior joint capsule, and the subscapularis, pectoralis major, latissimus dorsi, and teres major muscles.

Shoulder Complex Motion

The end-feel is firm because of tension in the serratus anterior and pectoralis minor muscles.

Goniometer Alignment

See Figures 4–17 and 4–18.
The alignment is the same as for medial rotation of the shoulder.

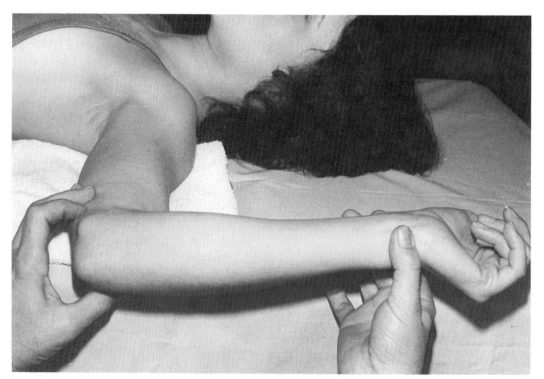

FIGURE 4–16. The subject's left upper extremity is at the end of the ROM of glenohumeral lateral rotation. The examiner stabilizes the distal humerus to prevent abduction beyond 90 degrees. The examiner uses her right hand to move the subject's forearm while preventing either supination or elbow extension. The end of the ROM in lateral rotation is reached when additional motion causes the scapula to press against the posterior rib cage.

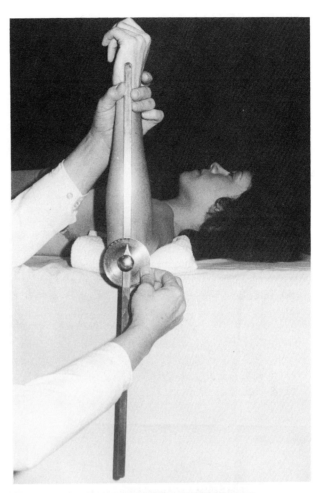

FIGURE 4–17. The goniometer alignment for ROM in lateral rotation is the same as the alignment for medial rotation. The examiner, however, has to change hand positions so that the left hand rather than the right hand holds the body of the goniometer (as shown in Fig. 4–18).

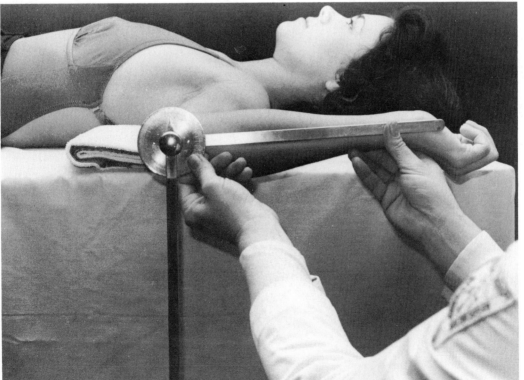

FIGURE 4–18. The alignment of the goniometer at the end of the ROM in lateral rotation may require the examiner to sit on a chair or stool to read the goniometer at eye level.

REFERENCES

1. Cyriax, JH and Cyriax, PJ: Illustrated Manual of Orthopaedic Medicine. Butterworths, London, 1983.
2. Culham, E and Peat, M: Functional anatomy of the shoulder complex. J Orthop Sports Phys Ther 18:342, 1993.
3. Norkin, C and Levangie, P: Joint Structure and Function: A Comprehensive Analysis, ed 2. FA Davis, Philadelphia, 1992.
4. American Academy of Orthopaedic Surgeons: Joint Motion: Method of Measuring and Recording. AAOS, Chicago, 1965.
5. American Medical Association: Guides to the Evaluation of Permanent Impairment, ed 3. AMA, Chicago, 1988.
6. Boone, DC and Azen, SP: Normal range of motion in male subjects. J Bone Joint Surg Am 61:756, 1979.
7. Safee-Rad, R, et al: Normal functional range of motion of upper limb joints during performance of three feeding activities. Arch Phys Med Rehabil 71:505, 1990.
8. Wanatabe, H, et al: The range of joint motions of the extremities in healthy Japanese people: The difference according to age. Phys Ther 71:878, 1991.
9. Boone, DC: Techniques of measurement of joint motion. (Unpublished supplement to Boone, DC and Azen, SP: Normal range of motion in male subjects. J Bone Joint Surg Am 61:756, 1979.)
10. Walker, JM, et al: Active mobility of the extremities in older subjects. Phys Ther 64:919, 1984.
11. Downey, PA, Fiebert, I, and Stackpole-Brown, JB: Shoulder range of motion in persons aged sixty and older [abstract]. Phys Ther 71:S75, 1991.
12. West, CC: Measurement of joint motion. Arch Phys Med Rehabil 26:414, 1945.
13. Clarke, GR, et al: Preliminary studies in measuring range of motion in normal and painful stiff shoulders. Rheumatology and Rehabilitation 14:39, 1975.
14. Allander, E, et al: Normal range of joint movement in shoulder, hip, wrist and thumb with special reference to side: A comparison between two populations. Int J Epidemiol 3:253, 1974.
15. Hellebrandt, FA, Duvall, EN, and Moore, ML: The measurement of joint motion. Part III: Reliability of goniometry. Physical Therapy Review 29:302, 1949.
16. Boone, DC, et al: Reliability of goniometric measurements. Phys Ther 58:1355, 1978.
17. Pandya, S, et al: Reliability of goniometric measurements in patients with Duchenne muscular dystrophy. Phys Ther 65:1339, 1985.
18. Riddle, DL, Rothstein, JM, and Lamb, RL: Goniometric reliability in a clinical setting: Shoulder measurements. Phys Ther 67:668, 1987.

5

The Elbow and Forearm

HUMEROULNAR AND HUMERORADIAL JOINTS

STRUCTURE

The humeroulnar and humeroradial joints between the upper arm and the forearm are considered to be a hinged compound synovial joint. The proximal joint surface of the humeroulnar joint consists of the convex trochlea located on the anterior medial surface of the distal humerus. The distal joint surface is the concave trochlear notch on the proximal ulna.

The proximal joint surface of the humeroradial joint is the convex capitulum located on the anterior lateral surface of the distal humerus. The concave radial head on the proximal end of the radius is the opposing joint surface.

The joints are enclosed in a fairly large, loose, weak joint capsule that also encloses the superior radioulnar joint. Medial and lateral collateral ligaments reinforce the sides of the capsule and help to provide medial-lateral stability.[1]

When the arm is in the anatomical position, the long axes of the humerus and the forearm form an acute angle at the elbow. The angle is called the "carrying angle." This angle is about 5 degrees in men and approximately 10 to 15 degrees in women. An angle that is larger (more acute) than average is called "cubitus valgus."

OSTEOKINEMATICS

The humeroulnar and humeroradial joints have 1 degree of freedom; flexion-extension in the sagittal plane around a coronal axis. In elbow flexion and extension, the axis of rotation lies approximately at the center of the trochlea.[2]

ARTHROKINEMATICS

At the humeroulnar joint, sliding of the ulna on the trochlea continues during extension until the ulnar olecranoid process enters the humeral olecranon fossa. In flexion, the trochlear ridge of the ulna slides along the trochlear groove until the ulnar coronoid process reaches the floor of the coronoid fossa of the humerus.

At the humeroradial joint, the concave radial head slides posteriorly on the convex surface of the capitulum during extension. In flexion, the rim of the radial head slides anteriorly in the capitulotrochlear groove to enter the radial fossa.

CAPSULAR PATTERN

The capsular pattern is rather variable, but usually the ROM in flexion is more limited than in extension. For example, 30 degrees of limitation in flexion would correspond to 10 degrees of limitation in extension.[3]

SUPERIOR AND INFERIOR RADIOULNAR JOINTS

STRUCTURE

Superior Radioulnar Joint

The ulnar portion of the superior radioulnar joint includes both the radial notch located on the lateral aspect of the proximal ulna and the annular ligament. The radial notch and the annular ligament form a concave joint surface. The radial aspect of the joint is the convex head of the radius.

Inferior Radioulnar Joint

The ulnar component of the inferior radioulnar joint is the convex ulnar head. The opposing articular surfaces are the ulnar notch of the radius and an articular disc.

The interosseous membrane, a broad sheet of collagenous tissue linking the radius and ulna, provides stability for both joints. The following three structures provide stability for the superior radioulnar joint: the annular and quadrate ligaments and the oblique cord. Stability of the inferior radioulnar joint is provided by the joint disc and the anterior and posterior radioulnar ligaments.[1]

OSTEOKINEMATICS

The superior and inferior radioulnar joints are mechanically linked. Therefore, motion at one joint is always accompanied by motion at the other joint. The axis for motion is a longitudinal axis extending from the radial head to the ulnar head. The mechanically linked joint is a synovial pivot joint with 1 degree of freedom. The motions permitted are pronation and supination. In pronation the radius crosses over the ulna, whereas in supination the radius and ulna lie parallel to one another.

ARTHROKINEMATICS

At the superior radioulnar joint, the convex rim of the head of the radius spins within the annular ligament and the concave radial notch during pronation and supination. The convex articular surface on the head of the radius spins posteriorly during pronation and anteriorly during supination.

At the inferior radioulnar joint, the concave surface of the ulnar notch on the radius slides over the ulnar head and articulates with the disc. The concave articular surface of the radius slides anteriorly (in the same direction as the hand) during pronation and slides posteriorly (in the same direction as the hand) during supination.

CAPSULAR PATTERN

According to Cyriax and Cyriax[3] and Magee,[4] the capsular pattern is equal limitation of pronation and supination.[3,4] However, according to Hertling and Kessler,[5] a greater limitation of supination than pronation occurs at the superior radioulnar joint, whereas involvement of the inferior radioulnar joint produces little loss of movement.

RANGE OF MOTION

Table 5–1 shows the mean values of ROM for various motions at the elbow. The age, gender, and number of subjects that were measured to obtain the values reported by the AAOS and AMA in Table 5–1 are unknown. Boone and Azen[8] measured active ROM in males using a universal goniometer.

Table 5 – 1 **MOTION AT THE ELBOW AND FOREARM: MEAN VALUES IN DEGREES FROM SELECTED SOURCES**

Motion	AMERICAN ACADEMY OF ORTHOPAEDIC SURGEONS[6]	AMERICAN MEDICAL ASSOCIATION[7]	BOONE AND AZEN[8] 18 MO–54 YR (N = 109)	
			Mean	Standard Deviation
Flexion	150.0	140.0	142.9	5.6
Extension	0.0	0.0	0.6	3.1
Pronation	80.0	80.0	75.8	5.1
Supination	80.0	80.0	82.1	3.8

FUNCTIONAL RANGE OF MOTION

Table 5–2, which shows the ROM required of the elbow and forearm for various functional activities, has been adapted from the works of Safaee-Rad et al.[9] and Morrey et al.[10] Safaee-Rad et al.[9] used a three-dimensional measurement system to quantify the ROM required at four upper-limb joints during the following three feeding activities: eating with a spoon, eating with a fork, and drinking from a handled cup. Ten healthy male subjects 20 and 29 years of age participated in the study. Subjects were seated at a table at the start of each activity, with elbows flexed to 90 degrees and the forearm and wrist in neutral position. The drinking task required the greatest arc of elbow flexion (57.7 degrees) among the three activities, and eating with a spoon required the least (22 degrees).

Morrey et al.[10] used a triaxial electrogoniometer to measure elbow motion in 33 normal individuals (15 males and 18 females) ranging in age from 21 to 75 years. According to Morrey et al., most of the activities of daily living that were measured required a total arc of about 100 degrees (30 to 130 degrees) of elbow flexion and about 100 degrees of rotation (50 degrees of supination and 50 degrees of pronation). Approximately 140 degrees of flexion were required to reach the back of the head and about 15 degrees of flexion to reach the shoes. Using a telephone required the greatest ROM among the activities studied by Morrey et al.[10]

Table 5–2 **ELBOW AND FOREARM MOTION DURING FUNCTIONAL ACTIVITIES: MEAN VALUES IN DEGREES FOR STARTING AND ENDING POSITIONS AND ARC OF MOTION[9,10]**

| | FLEXION | | | PRONATION | SUPINATION | |
| | START | END | ARC | START | END | ARC |
Activity	Mean	Mean	Mean	Mean	Mean	Mean
Put on a shirt	15.0	140.0	125.0[10]			
Use the telephone	42.8	135.6	92.8	40.9	22.6	63.5[10]
Rise from a chair	94.5	20.3	74.2	33.8	− 9.5*	24.3[10]
Drink from a cup	71.5	129.2	57.7[9]			
Open a door	24.0	57.4	33.4	35.4	23.4	58.8[10]
Eat with a fork	93.8	122.3	28.5[9]			
Read a newspaper	77.9	104.3	26.4	48.8	− 7.3*	41.5[10]
Pour from a pitcher	35.6	58.3	22.7	42.9	21.9	64.8[10]
Eat with a spoon	101.2	123.2	22.0[9]			
Cut with a knife	89.2	106.7	17.5	41.9	− 26.9*	15.0[10]

*The minus sign indicates pronation.

EFFECTS OF AGE AND GENDER

Tables 5–3 and 5–4 summarize the effects of age and gender on ROM of various movements of the elbow and forearm. A comparison of the values in Table 5–3 with the values in Table 5–4 shows that male and female infants have more ROM in flexion and pronation-supination than older individuals. Boone and Azen[8] found that male children in the youngest group studied (1 to 5 years of age) had a significantly greater amount of pronation and supination than other age groups. However, the differences appear to be very slight because they are less than one standard deviation.

Walker et al.[13] found that the older males in their study were unable to extend their elbows to attain a neutral starting position of 0 degrees. The mean value for the starting position was 6 degrees instead of 0 degrees. Bergstrom et al.,[14] in a study of 52 women and 37 men aged 79 years, found that 11% had flexion contractures of greater than 5 degrees of the right elbow, and 7% had bilateral flexion contractures.

RELIABILITY AND VALIDITY

Reliability studies involving the elbow have been conducted by many authors, including Hellebrandt et al.,[15] Boone et al.,[16] Rothstein et al.,[17] Fish and Wingate,[18] Grohmann,[19] and Petherick, et al.[20] Hellebrandt et al.[15] found statistically significant intratester differences between the means of duplicate measurements of active elbow flexion on 77 patients using the universal goniometer. Boone et al.[16] found that intratester reliability was higher than intertester reliability for the measurement of active ROM of elbow flexion.

In contrast to Boone et al.,[16] Rothstein et al.[17] found high ICCs (above 0.90) for both intratester and intertester reliability for passive ROM of elbow flexion and extension. Their study involved 12 testers who measured 24 subjects using three different commonly used universal goniometers (large and small plastic and large metal).

Fish and Wingate[18] found that the standard deviation of passive ROM goniometric measurements (2.4 to 3.4 degrees) was larger than the standard deviation from photographic measurements (0.7 to 1.1 degrees). These authors postulated that measurement error was due to improper identification of bony landmarks, inaccurate alignment of

Table 5–3 **EFFECTS OF AGE ON ELBOW AND FOREARM MOTION: MEAN VALUES IN DEGREES FOR NEWBORNS, CHILDREN, AND ADOLESCENTS 2 WK–19 YR OF AGE**

| | WANATABE ET AL.[11] | | | BOONE[12] | | | | |
| | 2 WK–2 YR (N = 45) | 18 MO–5 YR (N = 19) | | 6–12 YR (N = 17) | | 13–19 YR (N = 17) | |
Motion	Range of Means	Mean	Standard Deviation	Mean	Standard Deviation	Mean	Standard Deviation
Flexion	148–158	144.9	5.7	146.5	4.0	144.9	6.0
Extension		0.4	3.4	2.1	3.2	0.1	3.8
Pronation	90–96	78.9	4.4	76.9	3.6	74.1	5.3
Supination	81–93	84.5	3.8	82.9	2.7	81.8	3.2

Table 5–4 **EFFECTS OF AGE ON ELBOW AND FOREARM MOTION: MEAN VALUES IN DEGREES FOR ADULTS 20–85 YR OF AGE**

| | BOONE[12] | | | | | | WALKER ET AL.[13] | |
| | 20–29 YR (N = 19) | | 30–39 YR (N = 18) | | 40–54 YR (N = 19) | | 60–85 YR (N = 30) | |
Motion	Mean	Standard Deviation	Mean	Standard Deviation	Mean	Standard Deviation	Mean	Standard Deviation
Flexion	140.1	5.2	141.7	3.2	139.7	5.8	139.0	14.0
Extension	0.7	3.2	0.7	1.7	− 0.4*	3.0	− 6.0*	5.0
Pronation	76.2	3.9	73.6	4.3	75.0	7.0	68.0	9.0
Supination	80.1	3.7	81.7	4.2	81.4	4.0	83.0	11.0

*Values indicate mean number of degrees from neutral or zero starting position.

the goniometer, and variations in the amount of torque applied by the tester.

Grohmann,[19] in a study involving 40 testers and one subject, found that no significant differences existed between measurements obtained using an over-the-joint method for goniometer alignment and the traditional lateral method. Differences between the means of the measurements were less than 2 degrees.

Petherick et al.,[20] in a study involving 10 male and 20 female subjects, found that intertester reliability using a fluid-based goniometer was higher than with a universal goniometer. The authors determined that no concurrent validity existed between the fluid-based and universal goniometers, and that therefore these instruments could not be used interchangeably.

TESTING PROCEDURES
FLEXION

Motion occurs in the sagittal plane around a medial-lateral axis.

Recommended Testing Position

Position the subject supine, with the shoulder in 0 degrees of flexion, extension, and abduction so that the arm is close to the side of the body. A pad is placed under the distal end of the humerus to allow full elbow extension. The forearm is positioned in full supination with the palm of the hand facing the ceiling.

Stabilization

Stabilize the distal end of the humerus to prevent flexion of the shoulder (Fig. 5–1).

Normal End-Feel

Usually the end-feel is soft because of compression of the muscle bulk of the anterior forearm with that of the anterior upper arm. If the muscle bulk is atrophied, the end-feel may be hard because of contact between the coronoid process of the ulna and coronoid fossa of the humerus and contact between the head of the radius and the radial fossa of the humerus. The end-feel may be firm because of tension in the posterior joint capsule and the triceps brachii muscle.

Goniometer Alignment

See Figures 5–2 and 5–3.

1. Center the fulcrum of the goniometer over the lateral epicondyle of the humerus.
2. Align the proximal arm with the lateral midline of the humerus, using the center of the acromial process for reference.
3. Align the distal arm with the lateral midline of the radius, using the radial head and radial styloid process for reference.

EXTENSION

Motion occurs in the sagittal plane around a medial-lateral axis.

Recommended Testing Position, Stabilization, and Goniometer Alignment

The testing position, stabilization, and alignment are the same as for elbow flexion.

Normal End-Feel

Usually the end-feel is hard because of contact between the olecranon process of the ulna and the olecranon fossa of the humerus. Sometimes the end-feel is firm because of tension in the anterior joint capsule, the collateral ligaments, and the biceps brachii and brachialis muscles.

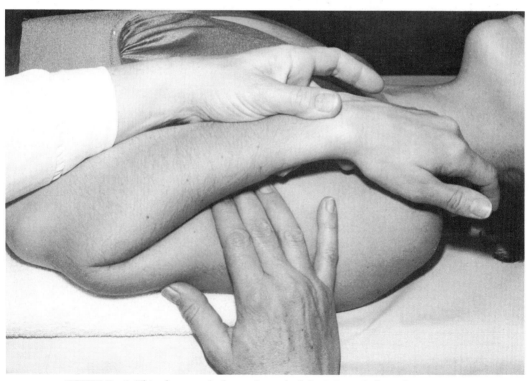

FIGURE 5–1. This photograph shows the end of the ROM of elbow flexion.

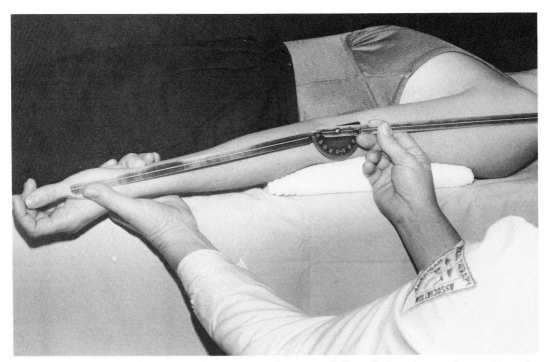

FIGURE 5–2. In the starting position for measuring the ROM of elbow flexion, the examiner positions the proximal arm of the half-circle metal goniometer along the lateral midline of the subject's left humerus. The distal arm of the goniometer is positioned along the lateral midline of the forearm and aligned with the radial styloid process. A towel placed under the distal humerus and elbow ensures that the supporting surface does not prevent the full ROM of elbow extension. As can be seen in this photograph, the subject's elbow is in about 10 degrees of hyperextension.

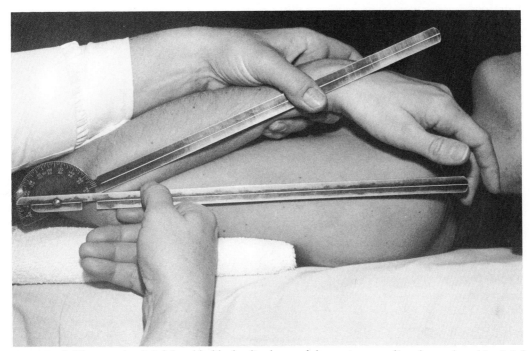

FIGURE 5–3. The examiner's left hand holds the distal arm of the goniometer aligned over the subject's left radial styloid process at the end of elbow flexion. With her right hand, the examiner holds the proximal arm in alignment along the lateral midline of the subject's humerus.

PRONATION

Motion occurs in the transverse plane around a vertical axis when the subject is in the anatomical position.

Recommended Testing Position

Position the subject sitting, with the shoulder in 0 degrees of flexion, extension, abduction, adduction, and rotation so that the upper arm is close to the side of the body. The elbow is flexed to 90 degrees and the forearm is supported by the examiner. The forearm is initially positioned midway between supination and pronation so that the thumb points toward the ceiling.

Stabilization

Stabilize the distal end of the humerus to prevent medial rotation and abduction of the shoulder (Fig. 5–4).

Normal End-Feel

The end-feel may be hard because of contact between the ulna and the radius, or it may be firm because of tension in the dorsal radioulnar ligament of the inferior radioulnar joint, the interosseous membrane, and the supinator and biceps brachii muscles.

Goniometer Alignment

See Figures 5–5 and 5–6.

1. Center the fulcrum of the goniometer lateral to the ulnar styloid process.
2. Align the proximal arm parallel to the anterior midline of the humerus.
3. Place the distal arm across the dorsal aspect of the forearm, just proximal to the styloid processes of the radius and ulna, where the forearm is most level and free of muscle bulk.

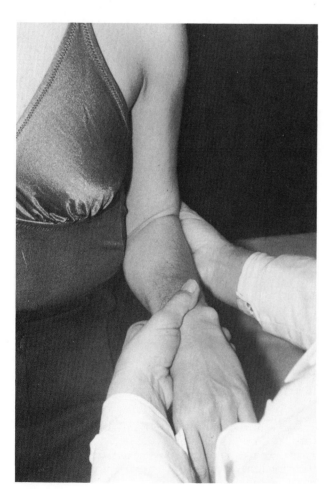

FIGURE 5–4. The end of the ROM of pronation of the left forearm. The subject is sitting on the edge of a table, and the examiner is standing facing the subject. The examiner's right hand, which is cupped around the subject's elbow, helps to prevent both medial rotation and abduction of the shoulder. The examiner's left hand grasps the radius rather than the subject's wrist or hand. If the examiner grasps either the subject's wrist or hand, movement of the wrist may be mistaken for movement at the radioulnar joints. The end of the ROM in pronation occurs when resistance prevents further motion from occurring at the forearm.

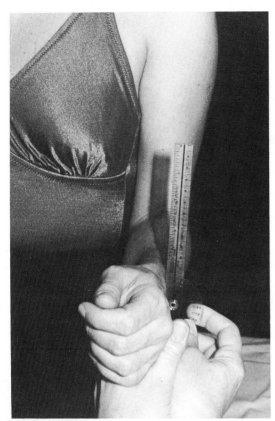

FIGURE 5–5. In the starting position for pronation, the goniometer is placed lateral to the distal radioulnar joint. The arms of the goniometer are aligned parallel to the anterior midline of the humerus.

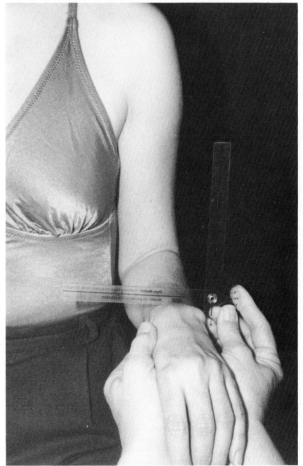

FIGURE 5–6. At the end of pronation, the proximal arm of the goniometer is aligned parallel to the anterior midline of the humerus, while the distal arm lies across the dorsum of the forearm just proximal to the radial and ulnar styloid process. The fulcrum of the goniometer is aligned so that it is proximal and lateral to the ulnar styloid process.

SUPINATION

Motion occurs in the transverse plane around a longitudinal axis when the subject is in the anatomical position.

Recommended Testing Position

The testing position is the same as for pronation of the forearm.

Stabilization

Stabilize the distal end of the humerus to prevent lateral rotation and adduction of the shoulder (Fig. 5–7).

Normal End-Feel

The end-feel is firm because of tension in the palmar radioulnar ligament of the inferior radioulnar joint, oblique cord, interosseous membrane, and pronator teres and pronator quadratus muscles.

Goniometer Alignment

See Figures 5–8 and 5–9.

1. Center the goniometer medial to the ulnar styloid process.
2. Align the proximal arm parallel to the anterior midline of the humerus.
3. Place the distal arm across the ventral aspect of the forearm, just proximal to the styloid processes, where the forearm is most level and free of muscle bulk.

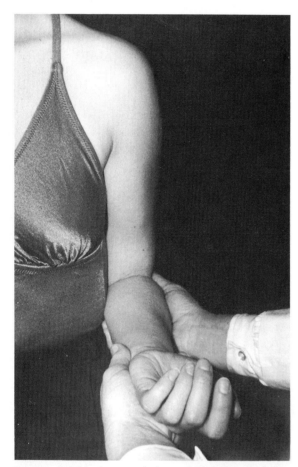

FIGURE 5–7. This photograph shows the left forearm at the end of the ROM in supination. The examiner's right hand holds the elbow close to the subject's body and in 90 degrees of elbow flexion. The examiner's left hand pushes on the distal radius while supporting the forearm. The end of the ROM of supination is reached when attempts to move the subject's forearm into further supination meet with resistance and cause either adduction or lateral rotation at the shoulder.

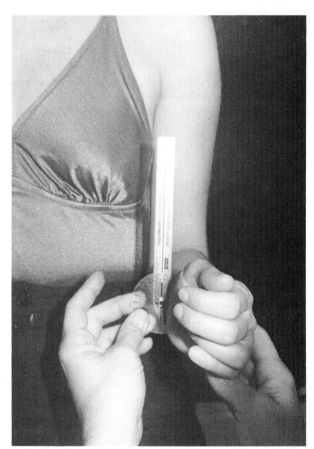

FIGURE 5–8. In the starting position for measuring the ROM in supination, the examiner places the goniometer body on the medial aspect of the forearm at the level of the distal radioulnar joint and aligns the arms of the instrument parallel to the anterior midline of the humerus. Above, the examiner's right hand supports the subject's forearm and helps to keep the elbow at 90 degrees of flexion.

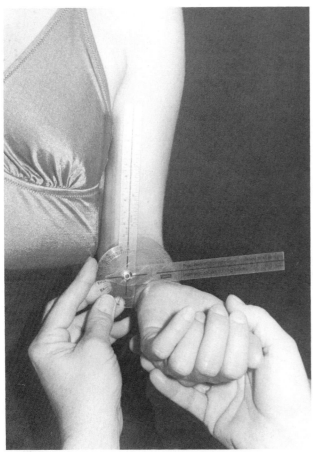

FIGURE 5–9. At the end of the ROM of supination, the distal arm of the goniometer rests on the medial aspect of the forearm at the level of the distal radioulnar joint. The position of the examiner's right hand is incorrect because it was altered for this photograph. The examiner's right hand should be grasping the subject's radius rather than the subject's hand.

REFERENCES

1. Norkin, CC and Levangie, PK: Joint Structure and Function: A Comprehensive Analysis, ed 2. FA Davis, Philadelphia, 1993.
2. Morrey, BF and Chao, EYS: Passive motion of the elbow joint. J Bone Joint Surg Am 58:50, 1976.
3. Cyriax, JH and Cyriax, PJ: Illustrated Manual of Orthopaedic Medicine. Butterworths, London, 1983.
4. Magee, DJ: Orthopedic Physical Assessment. WB Saunders, Philadelphia, 1987.
5. Hertling, D and Kessler, RM: Management of Common Musculoskeletal Disorders, ed 2. JB Lippincott, Philadelphia, 1993.
6. American Academy of Orthopaedic Surgeons: Joint Motion: Methods of Measuring and Recording. AAOS, Chicago, 1965.
7. American Medical Association: Guides to the Evaluation of Permanent Impairment, ed 3. AMA, Chicago, 1988.
8. Boone, DC and Azen, SP: Normal range of motion in male subjects. J Bone Joint Surg Am 61:756, 1979.
9. Safaee-Rad, R, et al: Normal functional range of motion of upper limb joints during performance of three feeding activities. Arch Phys Med Rehabil 71:505, 1990.
10. Morrey, BF, Askew, KN, and Chao, EYS: A biomechanical study of normal functional elbow motion. J Bone Joint Surg Am 63:872, 1981.
11. Wanatabe, H, et al: The range of joint motions of the extremities in healthy Japanese people: The difference according to age. Cited in Walker, JM: Musculoskeletal development: A review. Phys Ther 71:878, 1991.
12. Boone, DC: Techniques of measurement of joint motion. (Unpublished supplement to Boone, DC and Azen, SP: Normal range of motion in male subjects. J Bone Joint Surg Am 61:756, 1979.)
13. Walker, JM, et al: Active mobility of the extremities in older subjects. Phys Ther 64:919, 1984.
14. Bergstrom, G, et al: Prevalence of symptoms and signs of joint impairment. Scand J Rehabil Med 17:173, 1985.
15. Hellebrandt, FA, Duvall, EN, and Moore, ML: The measurement of joint motion. Part III: Reliability of Goniometry. Physical Therapy Review 29:302, 1949.
16. Boone, DC, et al: Reliability of goniometric measurements. Phys Ther 58:1355, 1978.
17. Rothstein, JM, Miller, PJ, and Roettger, RF: Goniometric reliability in a clinical setting: Elbow and knee measurements. Phys Ther 63:1611, 1983.
18. Fish, DR and Wingate, L: Sources of goniometric error at the elbow. Phys Ther 65:1666, 1985.
19. Grohmann, JEL: Comparison of two methods of goniometry. Phys Ther 63:922, 1983.
20. Petherick, M, et al: Concurrent validity and intertester reliability of universal and fluid-based goniometers for active elbow range of motion. Phys Ther 68:966, 1988.

6

The Wrist and Hand

RADIOCARPAL AND MIDCARPAL JOINTS

STRUCTURE

The condyloid radiocarpal joint attaches the hand to the forearm. The proximal articulating surfaces consist of lateral and medial facets on the distal radius and the radioulnar disc. The proximal surface of the disc forms a portion of the distal radioulnar joint. The distal surface of the disc forms a portion of the articular surface of the radiocarpal joint.[1] The radial facets and the disc form a continuous concave surface.[2] The distal joint surfaces are the three carpal bones: the scaphoid, lunate, and triquetrum. The carpal bones, which are connected by interosseous ligaments, form a convex surface. The joint is enclosed by a strong capsule and reinforced by capsular ligaments.

The midcarpal joint is considered to be a functional rather than an anatomical joint. It has a joint capsule that is continuous with each intercarpal joint. The joint surfaces are reciprocally convex and concave and consist of the scaphoid, lunate, and triquetrum proximally and the trapezium, trapezoid, capitate, and hamate bones distally. The radiocarpal and midcarpal joints are of the condyloid type, with 2 degrees of freedom.[2]

OSTEOKINEMATICS

The wrist complex (radiocarpal and midcarpal joints) permits flexion-extension in the sagittal plane around a medial-lateral axis, and radial-ulnar deviation (abduction-adduction or radial-ulnar flexion) in the frontal plane around an anterior-posterior axis. Both joints contribute to these motions in varying amounts.

ARTHROKINEMATICS

Motion at the radiocarpal joint occurs because the convex surfaces of the proximal row of carpals slide on the concave surfaces of the radius and radioulnar disc. The proximal row of carpals slides in a direction opposite to the movement of the hand. The carpals move dorsally on the radius and disc during wrist flexion and ventrally toward the palm during wrist extension. During ulnar deviation, the carpals slide in a radial direction. During radial deviation, they slide in an ulnar direction.

Motion at the midcarpal joint occurs because the distal row of carpals slides on the proximal row. During flexion, the convex surfaces of the capitate and hamate slide dorsally on the concave surfaces of portions of the scaphoid, lunate, and triquetrum. The surfaces of the trapezium and trapezoid are concave and slide volarly on the convex surface of the scaphoid. During extension, the capitate and hamate slide volarly on the scaphoid, lunate, and triquetrum; the trapezium and the trapezoid slide dorsally on the scaphoid. During radial deviation, the capitate and hamate slide ulnarly, and the trapezium and trapezoid slide dorsally. In ulnar deviation, the capitate and hamate slide radially; the trapezium and trapezoid slide volarly.[3]

CAPSULAR PATTERN

The capsular pattern at the wrist is an equal limitation of flexion and extension. A slight limitation in both radial and ulnar deviation also is present.[4]

Table 6–1 **WRIST MOTION: MEAN VALUES IN DEGREES FROM SELECTED SOURCES**

Motion	AMERICAN ACADEMY OF ORTHOPAEDIC SURGEONS[5]	AMERICAN MEDICAL ASSOCIATION[6]	BOONE AND AZEN[7] 18 MO–54 YR (N = 109)	
			Mean	Standard Deviation
Flexion	80.0	60.0	76.4	6.3
Extension	70.0	60.0	74.9	6.4
Radial deviation	20.0	20.0	21.5	4.0
Ulnar deviation	30.0	30.0	36.0	3.8

WRIST RANGE OF MOTION

Table 6–1 provides ROM information for all wrist motions. The age, gender, and number of subjects from which the values for the AAOS[5] and AMA[6] were obtained are unknown. The values presented in Table 6–1 for Boone and Azen[7] were obtained from measurements of active ROM using a universal goniometer on healthy male subjects.

FUNCTIONAL RANGE OF MOTION

Table 6–2 provides wrist ROM values for various functional activities. The mean values in Table 6–2 were derived from measurements of wrist ROM of 12 men and seven women ranging from 25 to 60 years of age. Each person performed three repetitions of each activity. A review of the table shows that the majority of activities require wrist extension. Only cutting with a knife and using a telephone require flexion. Bringing a glass to the mouth requires the least amount of extension (arc = 12.8 degrees),

whereas rising from a chair requires the largest amount of extension (arc = 62.8 degrees). An extension arc greater than 60 degrees is higher than the average AMA value for the total ROM in extension (see Table 6–1). Therefore, if getting out of a chair was a necessary activity for a patient, the full ROM in wrist extension would be needed. However, according to the table, most of the other activities can be completed with a flexion range of 0 to 5 degrees and an extension range of 0 to 37 degrees.

Table 6–3 provides wrist ROM values required for various personal care activities. The mean values in Table 6–3 show that the majority of positions assumed during personal care activities require wrist flexion. Also, the positions appear to require less overall wrist motion than the activities of daily living presented in Table 6–2. The maximum amount of flexion for hand to chest is only 27.8 degrees (mean plus standard deviation), slightly less than one half of the average values presented in Table 6–1. The mean extension values are less than the values required for daily living activities. According to Table 6–3, all of the positions could be assumed with 0 to 28 degrees of flexion

Table 6–2 **AMOUNTS OF WRIST MOTION REQUIRED TO PERFORM SELECTED ACTIVITIES OF DAILY LIVING: MEAN EXTENSION VALUES IN DEGREES OBTAINED USING A UNIAXIAL ELECTROGONIOMETER**

Activity	BRUMFIELD AND CHAMPOUX[8] 25–60 YR (N = 19)		
	Start	End	Arc of Motion
Lift glass to mouth	11.2	24.0	12.8
Pour from a pitcher	8.7	29.7	21.0
Cut with a knife	− 3.5*	20.2	23.7
Lift fork to mouth	9.3	36.5	27.2
Read a newspaper	1.7	34.9	33.2
Use a telephone	− 0.1*	42.6	42.7
Rise from a chair	0.6	63.4	62.8

*The minus sign indicates flexion.
Adapted from Brumfield and Champoux,[8] with permission.

Table 6–3 **POSITION OF THE WRIST ASSUMED DURING PERSONAL CARE ACTIVITIES: MEAN VALUES IN DEGREES OBTAINED WITH A UNIAXIAL ELECTROGONIOMETER**

	BRUMFIELD AND CHAMPOUX[8]			
	25–60 YR (N = 19)			
	FLEXION		EXTENSION	
Activity Position	Mean	Standard Deviation	Mean	Standard Deviation
Hand to waist	15.6	8.3		
Hand to neck	4.6	8.5		
Hand to chest	18.9	8.9		
Hand to sacrum	0.6	9.8		
Hand to occiput			12.7	9.9
Hand to shoe			14.2	10.6
Hand to vertex (head)	2.3	12.5		

Adapted from Brumfield and Champoux,[8] with permission.

(mean plus standard deviation) and 25 degrees of extension (mean plus standard deviation).

EFFECTS OF AGE AND GENDER

Table 6–4 provides wrist ROM values for newborns and children. Although caution must be used in drawing conclusions from comparisons of the findings of Wanatabe et al.[9] with the findings of Boone,[10] the mean values from Wanatabe et al.[10] are larger in flexion and extension than values reported for the males in both the 1- to 5-year-old group and in the 6- to 12-year-old group studied by Boone.[10] The ROM values for both ulnar and radial deviation for the two youngest groups studied by Boone[10] are larger than the values reported for the other age groups presented in Table 6–5. Values for ulnar deviation are larger than values for radial deviation.

Table 6–4 **EFFECTS OF AGE ON WRIST MOTION: MEAN VALUES IN DEGREES FOR NEWBORNS AND CHILDREN 2 WK–12 YR OF AGE**

| | WANATABE ET AL.[9] | BOONE[10] | | | |
| | 2 WK–2 YR (N = 45) | 18 MO–5 YR (N = 19) | | 6–12 YR (N = 17) | |
Motion	Range of Means	Mean	Standard Deviation	Mean	Standard Deviation
Flexion	88–96	82.2	3.8	76.3	5.6
Extension	82–89	76.1	4.9	78.4	5.9
Radial deviation		24.2	3.7	21.3	4.1
Ulnar deviation		38.7	3.6	35.4	2.4

Table 6–5 **EFFECTS OF AGE ON WRIST MOTION: MEAN VALUES IN DEGREES FOR ADOLESCENTS AND ADULTS 13–85 YR OF AGE**

| | BOONE[10] | | | | | | | | WALKER ET AL.[11] | |
| | 13–19 YR (N = 17) | | 20–29 YR (N = 19) | | 30–39 YR (N = 18) | | 40–54 YR (N = 19) | | 60–85 YR (N = 30) | |
Motion	Mean	Standard Deviation	Mean	Standard Deviation	Mean	Standard Deviation	Mean	Standard Deviation	Mean	Standard Deviation
Flexion	75.4	4.5	76.8	5.5	74.9	4.0	72.8	8.9	62.0	12.0
Extension	72.9	6.4	77.5	5.1	72.8	6.9	71.6	6.3	61.0	6.0
Radial deviation	19.7	3.0	21.4	3.6	20.3	3.1	21.6	5.1	20.0	6.0
Ulnar deviation	35.7	4.2	35.1	3.8	36.1	2.9	34.7	4.5	28.0	7.0

Table 6–5 provides wrist ROM values for adolescents and adults. The values from Boone[10] and from Walker et al.[11] presented in Table 6–5 were obtained from male subjects using a universal goniometer. The effects of age on wrist motion from 13 to 54 years of age appear to be very slight. Although the values for flexion, extension, and ulnar deviation in the oldest group (60 to 85 years of age) are less than values for other age groups, little change appears for radial deviation. However, caution must be used in making comparisons between values obtained by different researchers, because their measurement methods may have differed.

Two other studies offer additional information on the effects of age on wrist motion. Hewitt,[12] in a study of 112 individuals between 11 and 45 years of age, found slight differences in the average amount of active motion in different age groups. A group of 17 individuals ranging in age from 11 to 15 years had slightly less flexion and radial deviation but more ulnar deviation and extension than the general average. Allander et al.,[13] in a study of 309 Icelandic females, 208 Swedish females, and 203 Swedish males ranging in age from 33 to 70 years, found a decrease in flexion and extension ROM at both wrists with increasing age. Males lost an average of 2.2 degrees of motion every 5 years.

The following two studies offer evidence of gender- and side-related effects on the wrist joint. Cobe,[14] in a study of 100 college males and 15 women ranging in age from 20 to 30 years, found women to have a greater active ROM in all motions at the wrist. Another difference was found between the genders. Men had greater ROM in their left wrist than they did in their right wrist in all motions except ulnar deviation. In contrast, the total average ROM for women was found to be greater on the right side than on the left side except for radial deviation. Cobe suggests that the heavy work that men performed using their right extremities might account for the decrease in right-side motion in comparison with left-side motion.

Allander et al.[13] also found differences between right and left sides, but these authors found that both men and women had less ROM on the right than on the left. However, men had less motion on the right than women and generally had less motion than women.

RELIABILITY AND VALIDITY

In early studies of wrist motion conducted by Hewitt[12] and Cobe,[14] both authors observed considerable differences in repeated measurements of active wrist motion. The greatest fluctuations occurred in radial and ulnar deviation, which Hewitt[12] attributed to a lack of motor control on the part of the subjects.

Cobe[14] found "amazing differences" in successive measurements of active ROM in the same individual, although the person was cooperating fully in attempting to perform the motion. Cobe attributed these variations in wrist motion to the fact that motions at the wrist are not limited by bony contact and that people are not skilled in expending maximum effort to overcome the soft tissue resistance that is present. Cobe suggested that only average values have much validity and that changes in ROM should exceed 5 degrees to be considered significant.

Later studies of intratester and intertester reliability have been conducted by Hellebrandt et al.,[15] Low,[16] Allander et al.,[13] Boone et al.,[17] Bird and Stowe,[18] Solgaard et al.,[19] Horger,[20] and La Stayo and Wheeler.[21] The majority of these investigators found that intratester reliability was greater than intertester reliability and that reliability varied according to the motion being tested.

Hellebrandt et al.[15] concluded that wrist flexion was one of the less reliable measurements, although the mean difference between successive measurements was only 1.07 degrees for the universal goniometer and 2.13 degrees for a joint-specific measurement device.

Low[16] found that intratester reliability for wrist extension was greater than intertester reliability. In Low's study, in which 50 testers measured the author's active wrist extension using a universal goniometer, motion varied more on a day-to-day basis than elbow flexion. Intertester variation for measurements of wrist extension was 10.5 degrees. Low suggested that one tester should make all the measurements because intratester error was considerably less than intertester error.

Boone et al.[17] conducted a study in which four testers measured ulnar deviation using a universal goniometer on 12 male volunteers (26 to 54 years of age). Measurements were repeated over a period of 4 weeks. Intratester reliability was found to be greater than intertester reliability. The authors concluded that when more than one tester measures the same motion, increases in motion should exceed 5 degrees to determine actual changes.

Bird and Stowe[18] concluded that the error for passive ROM measurements was greater than the error for measurements of active ROM.

Solgaard et al.[19] found intratester standard deviations of 5.2 to 8 degrees and intertester standard deviations of 6 to 10.1 degrees, in a study of wrist and forearm motions involving 31 healthy subjects (eight men and 23 women) with a median age of 37 years. Measurements were taken with a universal goniometer. The coefficients of variation (percent variation) between testers were greater for ulnar and radial deviation than for flexion, extension, pronation, and supination. Differences in ROM between right and left wrists were negligible. The authors concluded that the opposite wrist could be used for reference when evaluating restrictions in ROM.

Horger[20] conducted a study that included 33 men and 15 women referred to either occupational therapy or hand management clinics for evaluation or treatment. The patients ranged in age from 18 to 71 years, with a mean age of 38.8 years. Measurements of both active and passive range of wrist motions were taken with a universal goniometer by 11 occupational therapists and two physical therapists. Six of the therapists were specialized in hand therapy and performed measurements of wrist motion five times per day. The remaining therapists performed wrist measurements about three times per month. Therapists were free to select their own method of measurement. The specialized therapists used an ulnar alignment for flexion and extension, whereas the nonspecialized therapists used a radial goniometer alignment.

Horger[20] found ICCs for intratester reliability of both active and passive wrist motion to be highly reliable (above 0.90) for all motions. Agreements between measurements in the sagittal plane (flexion-extension) were higher than for measurements in the frontal plane (radial and ulnar deviation). The author determined that the presence of pain reduced the intratester reliability of both active and passive measurements, but active measurements were affected more than passive measurements. Overall, intratester reliability was greater than intertester reliability. However, intertester reliability was excellent among specialized therapists for all motions except passive radial deviation. In contrast, intertester reliability among nonspecialized therapists was only fair for active extension, flexion, and adduction, and for passive extension and flexion. Intertester reliability coefficients for measurements of active motion were higher than coefficients for passive motion except for ra-

dial deviation. Reliability was relatively unaffected by such factors as variations in external force and anatomical changes due to trauma or deformity.

La Stoya and Wheeler[21] studied the intratester and intertester reliability of passive ROM measurements of wrist flexion and extension using three different goniometric alignments (ulnar, radial, and dorsal-volar). The testers included 32 therapists from eight hand–upper extremity clinical sites in the United States. Therapists used 6-inch plastic universal goniometers to measure 140 wrists using all three techniques. Six of the eight clinics showed significant differences among techniques. Intratester mean ICCs for passive ROM for wrist flexion were 0.86 for radial, 0.87 for ulnar, and 0.90 for dorsal alignment. Intratester mean ICCs for passive ROM for extension were 0.80 for radial, 0.89 for ulnar, and 0.93 for volar alignment. The factors identified that affected reliability were listed in order of importance: patient, unexplained error, diagnostic category, prior treatment, technique, and therapist. The authors recommended that, because of differences among the goniometer alignments, these techniques should not be used interchangeably. Also, because the dorsal-volar technique was found to be more reliable in this study, the authors suggested that it should be the technique of choice for measuring passive ROM of wrist flexion and extension. This particular technique is recommended by the AMA for measurements of wrist motion used for permanent disability ratings.

TESTING PROCEDURES: THE WRIST

FLEXION

Motion occurs in the sagittal plane around a medial-lateral axis.

Recommended Testing Position

Position the subject so that he or she is sitting next to a supporting surface. The shoulder is abducted to 90 degrees and the elbow is flexed to 90 degrees. The forearm is positioned midway between supination and pronation so that the palm of the hand faces the ground. The forearm rests on the supporting surface, but the hand is free to move. Avoid radial or ulnar deviation of the wrist and flexion of the fingers. (If the fingers are flexed, tension in the extensor digitorum communis, extensor indicis, and extensor digiti minimi muscles will restrict the motion.)

Stabilization

Stabilize the radius and ulna to prevent supination or pronation of the forearm (Fig. 6–1).

Normal End-Feel

The end-feel is firm because of tension in the dorsal radiocarpal ligament and the dorsal joint capsule.

Goniometer Alignment

See Figures 6–2 and 6–3.

1. Center the fulcrum of the goniometer over the lateral aspect of the wrist over the triquetrum.
2. Align the proximal arm with the lateral midline of the ulna, using the olecranon and ulnar styloid processes for reference.
3. Align the distal arm with the lateral midline of the fifth metacarpal.

Alternative Goniometer Alignment

This alternative goniometer alignment is recommended by the AMA *Guides to the Evaluation of Permanent Impairment.*[6]

1. Center the fulcrum of the goniometer over the capitate on the dorsal aspect of the wrist joint.
2. Align the proximal arm along the dorsal midline of the forearm.
3. Align the distal arm with the dorsal aspect of the third metacarpal.

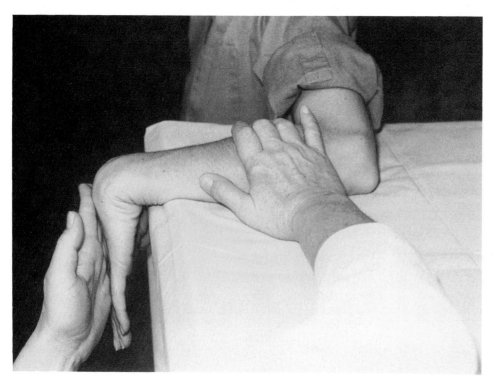

FIGURE 6–1. This photograph shows the end of wrist flexion (palmar flexion) ROM. The subject sits on a low stool so that her humerus rests on the supporting surface when the glenohumeral joint is at 90 degrees of abduction. The subject's elbow is flexed at 90 degrees of flexion, and about three quarters of her forearm is supported by the table. There must be sufficient space for the hand to move freely. The examiner's hand exerts pressure over the dorsum of the hand to complete the ROM.

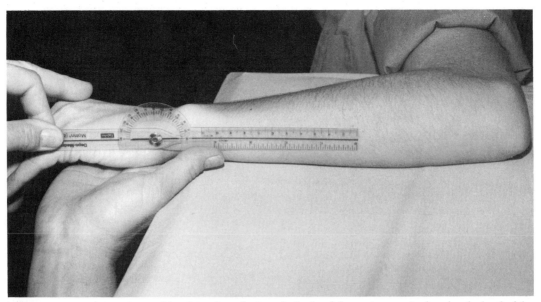

FIGURE 6–2. In the starting position for palmar flexion, the body of the goniometer is placed at the level of the triquetrum. The proximal goniometer arm is aligned along the ulna in line with the olecranon process and the ulnar styloid process. The distal arm is aligned along the fifth metacarpal.

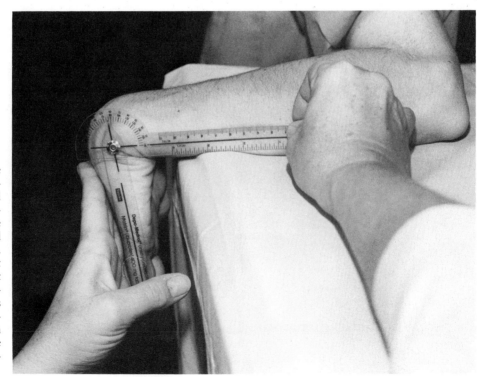

FIGURE 6–3. At the end of the ROM in palmar flexion, the goniometer body lies over the lateral aspect of the carpal bones just distal to the ulnar styloid process. The distal goniometer arm is aligned with the subject's fifth metacarpal. The examiner maintains the wrist in palmar flexion by using her left hand to exert pressure on the middle of the dorsum of the subject's hand. The examiner avoids exerting pressure directly on the fifth metacarpal because such pressure will distort the goniometer alignment.

EXTENSION (DORSAL FLEXION)

Recommended Testing Position and Stabilization

The testing position and stabilization are similar to those used for measuring wrist flexion. Avoid extension of the fingers so that tension in the flexor digitorum superficialis and profundus muscles will not restrict the motion (Fig. 6-4).

Normal End-Feel

Usually the end-feel is firm because of tension in the palmar radiocarpal ligament and the palmar joint capsule, but it may be hard because of contact between the radius and the carpal bones.

Goniometer Alignment

The alignment is the same as for wrist flexion (Figs. 6-5 and 6-6).

Alternative Positioning and Goniometer Alignment

This alternative positioning is recommended by the AMA *Guides to the Evaluation of Permanent Impairment.*[6] Position the forearm in supination.

1. Center the fulcrum over the wrist joint at the level of the capitate.
2. Align the proximal arm with the volar midline of the forearm.
3. Align the distal arm with the volar midline of the third metacarpal.

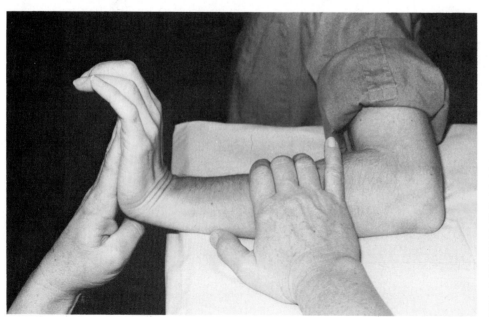

FIGURE 6-4. At the end of the wrist extension (dorsal flexion) ROM, the examiner's right hand stabilizes the subject's elbow at 90 degrees of flexion and helps to prevent lateral rotation at the glenohumeral joint. The examiner's left hand holds the subject's left wrist in extension. The examiner is careful to distribute pressure equally across the subject's four metacarpals.

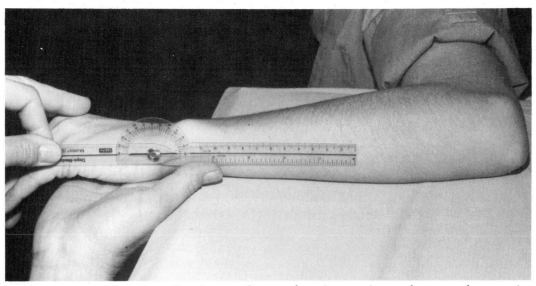

FIGURE 6–5. Starting position and goniometer alignment for wrist extension are the same as for measuring wrist flexion.

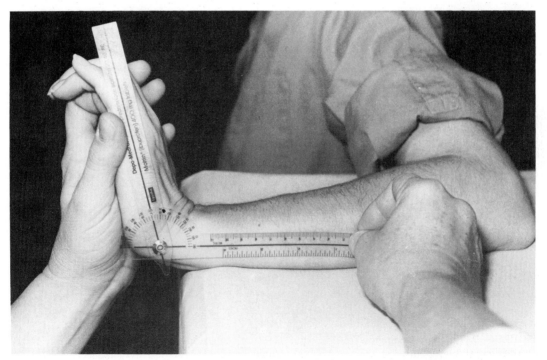

FIGURE 6–6. At the end of the ROM of wrist extension, the examiner's left hand maintains the alignment of the distal goniometer arm with the fifth metacarpal while holding the wrist in extension. The examiner avoids exerting pressure on the fifth metacarpal.

RADIAL DEVIATION (RADIAL FLEXION)

Motion occurs in the frontal plane around an anterior-posterior axis.

Recommended Testing Position

The testing position is the same as for wrist flexion.

Stabilization

Stabilize the distal ends of the radius and ulna to prevent pronation or supination of the forearm and elbow flexion beyond 90 degrees (Fig. 6–7).

Normal End-Feel

Usually the end-feel is hard because of contact between the radial styloid process and the scaphoid, but it may be firm because of tension in the ulnar collateral ligament, ulnocarpal ligament, and ulnar portion of the joint capsule.

Goniometer Alignment

See Figures 6–8 and 6–9.

1. Center the fulcrum of the goniometer over the middle of the dorsal aspect of the wrist over the capitate.
2. Align the proximal arm with the dorsal midline of the forearm, using the lateral epicondyle of the humerus for reference.
3. Align the distal arm with the dorsal midline of the third metacarpal. Do not use the third phalanx for reference.

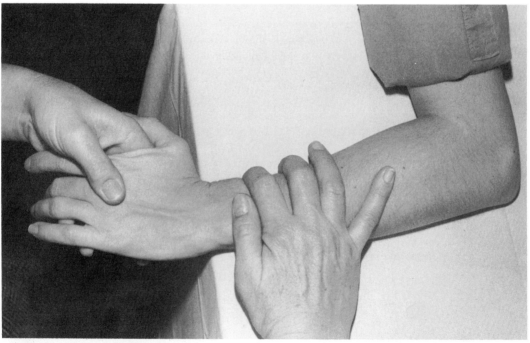

FIGURE 6–7. This photograph shows the end of the ROM in radial deviation. The subject sits on a low stool so that her humerus is supported on the table with the glenohumeral joint in 90 degrees of abduction. The examiner's right hand prevents flexion of the subject's elbow beyond 90 degrees when the wrist is moved into radial deviation. The examiner's left hand supports the weight of the subject's hand. The examiner avoids moving the wrist into either flexion or extension.

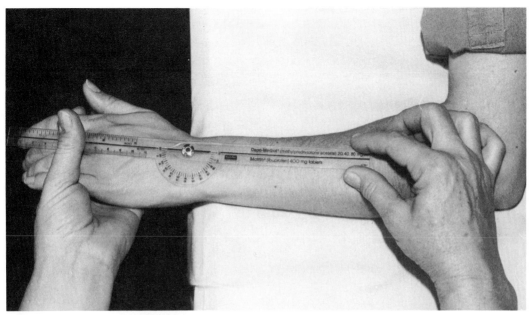

FIGURE 6–8. The starting positions for measuring radial and ulnar deviation are the same. The examiner centers the goniometer body on the dorsal aspect of the wrist, close to the capitate. The examiner aligns the proximal goniometer arm with the dorsal midline of the subject's forearm and the distal arm with the third metacarpal. The examiner's left hand supports the weight of the subject's hand under the metacarpals and holds the proximal goniometer arm in correct alignment. The examiner keeps the subject's hand in the same plane as the forearm and avoids wrist flexion and extension.

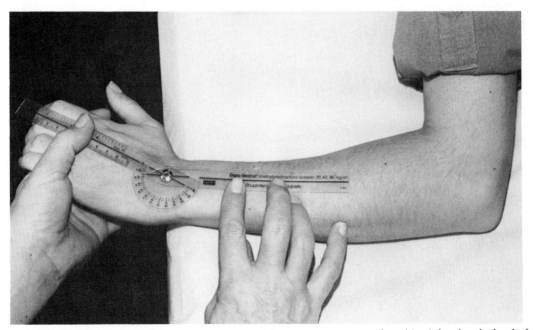

FIGURE 6–9. At the end of the radial deviation ROM, the examiner supports the subject's hand at the level of metacarpals so that the wrist is maintained in a neutral position relative to flexion and extension. The examiner's right hand maintains the goniometer's proximal arm in alignment with the dorsal midline of the subject's forearm using the left lateral epicondyle as a reference.

ULNAR DEVIATION (ULNAR FLEXION)

Recommended Testing Position and Stabilization

The testing position is the same as for radial deviation of the wrist (Fig. 6–10).

Normal End-Feel

The end-feel is firm because of tension in the radial collateral ligament and the radial portion of the joint capsule.

Goniometer Alignment

The alignment is the same as for radial deviation of the wrist (Figs. 6–11 and 6–12).

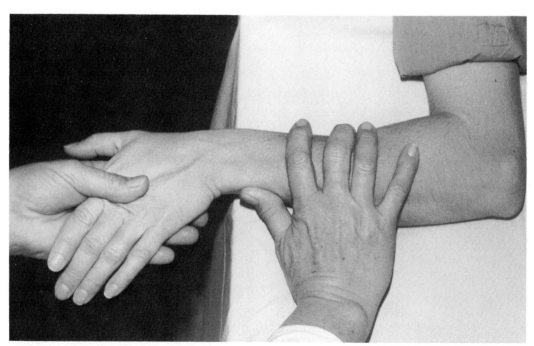

FIGURE 6–10. At the end of the ulnar deviation ROM, the examiner's right hand maintains the subject's elbow in 90 degrees of flexion by preventing elbow extension. The examiner's left hand supports the weight of the subject's hand and maintains the wrist in a neutral position relative to flexion and extension. By firmly grasping the subject's second and third metacarpals, the examiner is able to control motion at the wrist.

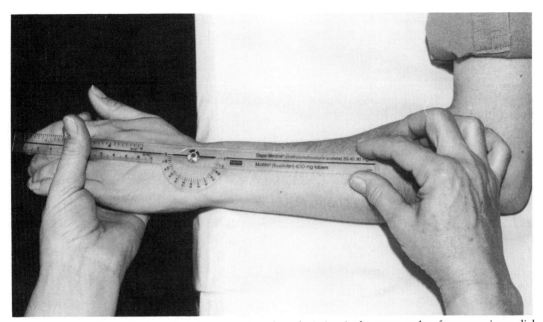

FIGURE 6–11. The starting position for measuring ulnar deviation is the same as that for measuring radial deviation.

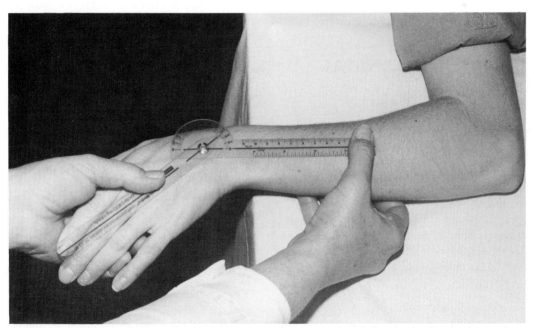

FIGURE 6–12. At the end of the ulnar deviation ROM, the examiner's right hand maintains the proximal goniometer arm in alignment with the dorsal midline of the forearm and the lateral epicondyle of the humerus. The examiner's left hand keeps the distal goniometer arm aligned with the subject's third metacarpal.

METACARPOPHALANGEAL JOINTS (FINGERS)

STRUCTURE

The metacarpophalangeal (MCP) joints are composed of the convex distal end of each metacarpal (second to fifth) and the concave end of each proximal phalanx. The joints are enclosed in fibrous capsules, and ligamentous support is provided by collateral, and the deep transverse metacarpal ligaments. Additional support is provided by the volar plates and interosseus and extensor tendons.

OSTEOKINEMATICS

The MCP joints are biaxial condyloid joints that have 2 degrees of freedom, allowing flexion-extension in the sagittal plane and abduction-adduction in the frontal plane.

ARTHROKINEMATICS

The concave base of the phalanx glides over the convex head of the metacarpal in the same direction as the shaft of the phalanx. In flexion the base of the phalanx glides toward the palm, whereas in extension the base glides dorsally on the metacarpal head. In abduction the base of the phalanx glides in the same direction as the movement of the finger.

CAPSULAR PATTERN

Motion is equally restricted in flexion and extension.[4]

PROXIMAL INTERPHALANGEAL AND DISTAL INTERPHALANGEAL JOINTS (FINGERS)

STRUCTURE

The structure of both the proximal interphalangeal (PIP) and distal interphalangeal (DIP) joints is very similar. Each phalanx has a concave base and a convex head. The joint surfaces comprise the head of the more proximal phalanx and the base of the adjacent more distal phalanx. Each joint is supported by two lateral collateral ligaments and a volar plate.

OSTEOKINEMATICS

The PIP and DIP joints of the digits are classified as synovial hinge joints with 1 degree of freedom: flexion-ex-

tension in the sagittal plane. In addition, some passive hyperextension is possible at the DIP joints.

ARTHROKINEMATICS

Motion of the joint surfaces includes a sliding of the concave base of the more distal phalanx on the convex head of the proximal phalanx. Sliding of the base of the moving phalanx occurs in the same direction as the movement of the shaft. For example, in PIP flexion, the base of the middle phalanx slides toward the palm. In PIP extension the base of the middle phalanx slides toward the dorsum of the hand.

CAPSULAR PATTERN

Motion is equally restricted in both flexion and extension.[3,4]

FINGER RANGE OF MOTION

The ROM at the MCP joints varies with each joint but generally increases from the second digit to the fifth digit. The index finger has approximately 90 degrees of flexion, and the fifth finger has approximately 110 degrees.[2] The amount of hyperextension is variable, and the opposite extremity should be used as a basis for comparison. Hyperextension of 20 to 45 degrees is common.[20] The ROM in abduction-adduction is greatest in extension and least in full flexion. The index and fifth fingers have a greater ROM in abduction-adduction than the second and third fingers.

The PIP joints of the fingers have the greatest ROM in flexion of any digital joints. The ROM increases from the second to fifth digits, ranging from 105 degrees for the second digit to 135 degrees for the fifth digit. DIP flexion ranges from 80 degrees at the second digit to 90 degrees at the fifth digit. The PIP joints have less hyperextension than the MCP and DIP joints. Table 6–6 provides a summary of mean ROM values for the fingers and thumb.

FUNCTIONAL RANGE OF MOTION

The wrist and hand work together to perform personal care tasks, activities of daily living, and a multitude of occupational and recreational activities. Mobility, muscular strength and control, and sufficient sensation are necessary for a hand that is capable of adequate performance. Classification systems for describing and defining hand function

Table 6–6 **MOTION AT THE FINGERS: MEAN VALUES IN DEGREES**

Joint	Motion	American Academy of Orthopaedic Surgeons[5]	American Medical Association[6]
MCP (2–5)	Flexion	0–90	0–90
	Extension	0–45	0–20
	Abduction		
PIP (2–5)	Flexion	0–100	0–100
DIP (2–5)	Flexion	0–90	0–70
	Extension	0–10	0–30
CMC (1)	Abduction	0–70	0–50
	Flexion	0–15	
	Extension		
MCP (1)	Flexion	0–50	0–60
DIP (1)	Flexion	0–80	0–80

are too numerous to be reviewed in this publication, but Stanley and Tribuzi[22] have reviewed many functional tests for the hand in their textbook.

EFFECTS OF AGE AND GENDER

Goniometric studies focusing on the effects of age and gender on ROM typically exclude the joints of the fingers, and therefore not much information is available on these joints. However, Beighton et al.[23] used passive hyperextension of the MCP joint of the fifth finger (beyond 90 degrees) and passive opposition of the thumb (to the flexor aspect of the forearm) as indicators of hypermobility in a study of 456 men and 625 women in an African village. They found that joint laxity decreased with age, but that females at any age had more joint laxity than males.

Allander et al.,[13] in a study of 517 women and 208 men (33 to 70 years of age) found that the MCP joint of the thumb showed greater biological variation than the shoulder, hip, and wrist joints. Measurements of the thumb MCP joint ROM demonstrated no consistent pattern of age-related effects. In some of the age groups, females showed more mobility in the MCP joint than their male counterparts, and right-side motion was less than left-side motion.[13]

Fairbank et al.,[24] in a study of the joint mobility of 446 normal adolescents, found that females tended to have more joint laxity than males. These authors suggest that the most convenient joint motions for measuring joint mobility were thumb abduction and finger extension.

RELIABILITY AND VALIDITY

As was the case with effects of age and gender, very few studies have been conducted to assess the reliability and validity of goniometric measurements in the hand. Hamilton and Lachenbruch[25] had seven testers measure MCP, PIP, and DIP flexion of the fingers with three types of goniometer. Measurements were taken daily for 4 days. These authors found that intertester reliability was less than intratester reliability. No significant differences existed between a dorsal (over-the-joint) goniometer, a pendulum goniometer, and the universal goniometer. According to Bear-Lehman and Abreu,[26] a 5-degree margin of error is acceptable for goniometric measurement of joints in the hand by an experienced examiner using standardized protocols.

TESTING PROCEDURES: METACARPOPHALANGEAL JOINTS (FINGERS)

Included in this and the following sections are the common clinical techniques for measuring motions of the fingers and thumb. These techniques are appropriate for evaluating most people. However, swelling and bony deformities sometimes require the examiner to create alternative evaluation techniques. Photocopies, photographs, and tracings of the hand at the beginning and end of the ROM may be especially helpful.

FLEXION

Motion occurs in the sagittal plane around a medial-lateral axis.

Recommended Testing Position

Position the subject sitting, with the forearm midway between pronation and supination. The wrist is positioned in 0 degrees of flexion, extension, and radial and ulnar deviation. The forearm and hand rest on a supporting surface. The MCP joint being examined should be in a neutral posi-

tion relative to abduction and adduction. Avoid extreme flexion of the PIP and DIP joints of the finger being examined.

Stabilization

Stabilize the metacarpal to prevent wrist motion. Do not hold the MCP joints of the other fingers in extension, because tension in the transverse metacarpal ligament will restrict the motion (Fig. 6–13).

Normal End-Feel

The end-feel may be hard because of contact between the palmar aspect of the proximal phalanx and metacarpal, or it may be firm because of tension in the dorsal joint capsule and the collateral ligaments.

Goniometer Alignment

See Figures 6–14 and 6–15.

1. Center the fulcrum of the goniometer over the dorsal aspect of the MCP joint.
2. Align the proximal arm over the dorsal midline of the metacarpal.
3. Align the distal arm over the dorsal midline of the proximal phalanx.

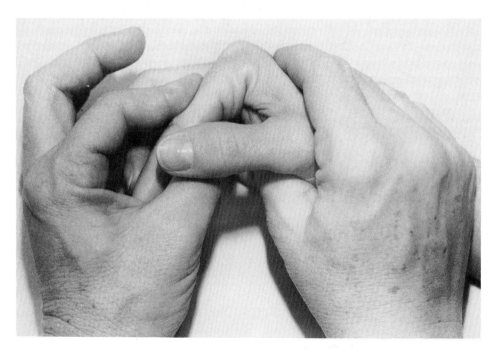

FIGURE 6–13. At the end of the flexion ROM of the second MCP joint, the examiner's right hand stabilizes the subject's second metacarpal and maintains the wrist in a neutral position relative to flexion and extension. The examiner's left index finger and thumb grasp the subject's proximal phalanx and maintain the second MCP joint in flexion.

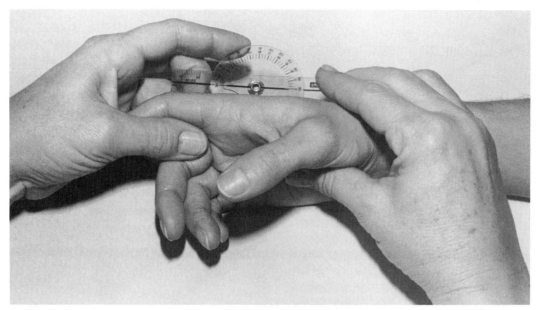

FIGURE 6-14. In the starting position for MCP flexion, the body of the plastic half-circle goniometer is positioned over the dorsal aspect of the subject's second MCP joint. The proximal arm of the goniometer is held on the dorsal midline of the subject's second metacarpal by the examiner's right hand. The distal goniometer arm is aligned on the dorsal midline of the subject's second proximal phalanx. The examiner's left thumb supports the subject's proximal phalanx and helps to maintain the second MCP joint in a neutral position relative to abduction and adduction.

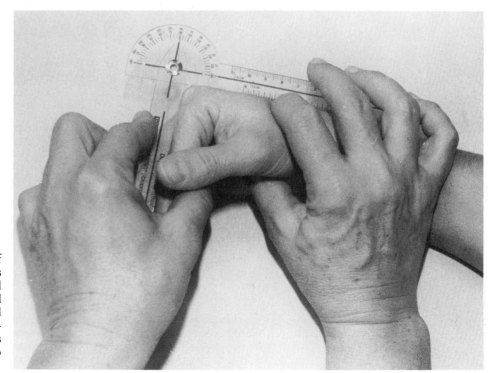

FIGURE 6-15. At the end of MCP flexion, the examiner's right hand holds the proximal goniometer arm in alignment and stabilizes the subject's second metacarpal. Note that the fulcrum of the goniometer lies somewhat distal and superior to the MCP joint.

EXTENSION

Motion occurs in the sagittal plane around a medial-lateral axis.

Recommended Testing Position

Position the subject sitting, with the forearm midway between pronation and supination. The wrist is positioned in 0 degrees of flexion, extension, and radial and ulnar deviation. The forearm and hand rest on a supporting surface. The MCP joint being examined should be in a neutral position relative to abduction and adduction. Avoid extension or extreme flexion of the PIP and DIP joints of the finger being tested. (If the PIP and DIP joints are positioned in extension, tension in the flexor digitorum superficialis and profundus muscles may restrict the motion. If the PIP and DIP joints are positioned in full flexion, tension in the lumbricalis and interosseus muscles will restrict the motion.)

Stabilization

Stabilize the metacarpal to prevent wrist motion. Do not hold the MCP joints of the other fingers in full flexion, because tension in the transverse metacarpal ligament will restrict the motion (Fig. 6–16).

Normal End-Feel

The end-feel is firm because of tension in palmar joint capsule and palmar fibrocartilaginous plate (palmar ligament).

Goniometer Alignment

The alignment is the same as for flexion of the MCP joint (Figs. 6–17 and 6–18).

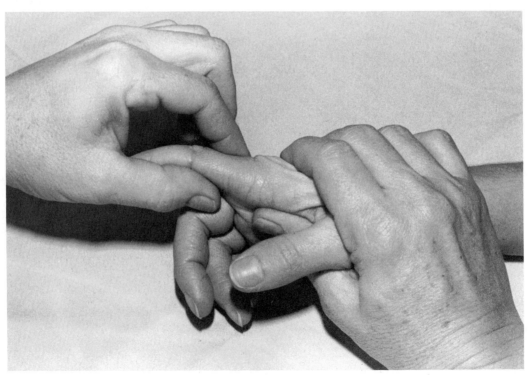

FIGURE 6–16. At the end of MCP extension, the examiner's left index finger and thumb grasp the subject's second proximal phalanx and maintain MCP extension. The examiner's right hand maintains the subject's wrist in neutral and stabilizes the second metacarpal.

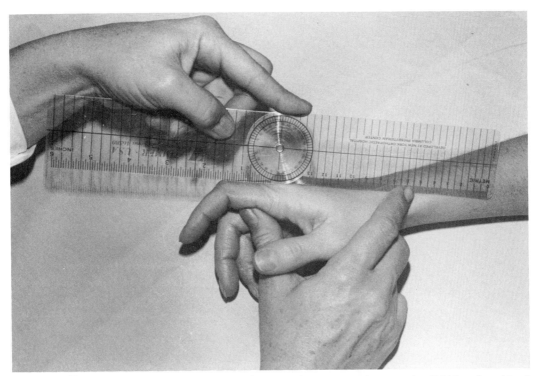

FIGURE 6 – 17. A full-circle plastic goniometer is being used to measure the extension ROM at the subject's second MCP joint. The proximal arm of the instrument is slightly longer than necessary for optimal alignment. If a goniometer of the right size is not available, the examiner can cut the arm of a plastic model to suitable length.

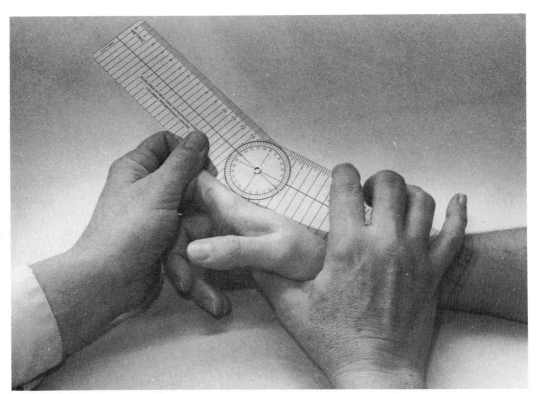

FIGURE 6 – 18. At the end of MCP extension, the body of the goniometer is aligned over the dorsal aspect of the subject's second MCP joint. The examiner's right hand maintains the subject's wrist in a neutral position and holds the proximal arm of the goniometer aligned over the subject's second metacarpal. It is easy to see that the subject's ROM in extension is smaller than her ROM in flexion.

ABDUCTION

Motion occurs in the frontal plane around an anterior-posterior axis.

Recommended Testing Position

Position the subject sitting, with the wrist in 0 degrees of flexion, extension, and radial and ulnar deviation. The forearm is fully pronated so that the palm of the hand faces the ground. The MCP joint is in 0 degrees of flexion and extension. The forearm and hand rest on a supporting surface.

Stabilization

Stabilize the metacarpal to prevent wrist motions (Fig. 6–19).

Normal End-Feel

The end-feel is firm because of tension in the collateral ligaments of the MCP joints, the fascia of the web space between the fingers, and the palmar interosseus muscles.

Goniometer Alignment

See Figures 6–20 and 6–21.

1. Center the fulcrum of the goniometer over the dorsal aspect of the MCP joint.
2. Align the proximal arm over the dorsal midline of the metacarpal.
3. Align the distal arm over the dorsal midline of the proximal phalanx.

ADDUCTION

Motion occurs in the frontal plane around an anterior-posterior axis.

Recommended Testing Position, Stabilization, and Goniometer Alignment

The testing position, stabilization, and alignment are the same as for measuring abduction of the MCP joints of the fingers.

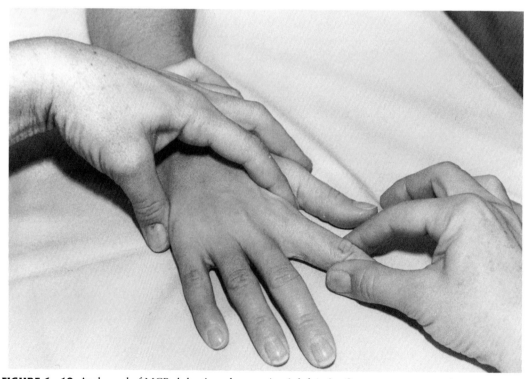

FIGURE 6–19. At the end of MCP abduction, the examiner's left index finger presses against the subject's second metacarpal and prevents radial deviation at the wrist. With her right index finger and thumb holding the distal end of the proximal phalanx, the examiner maintains the subject's second MCP joint in abduction. The examiner is careful to avoid both lifting up and pressing down on the subject's second proximal phalanx.

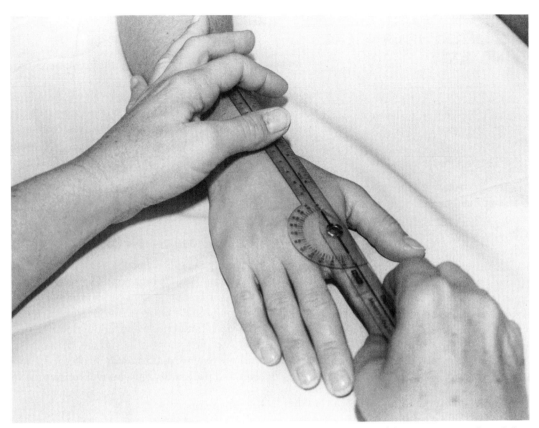

FIGURE 6 – 20. In the starting position for MCP abduction, the proximal arm of the goniometer is aligned along the dorsal midline of the subject's second metacarpal. The distal goniometer arm is aligned over the dorsal midline of the subject's second proximal phalanx.

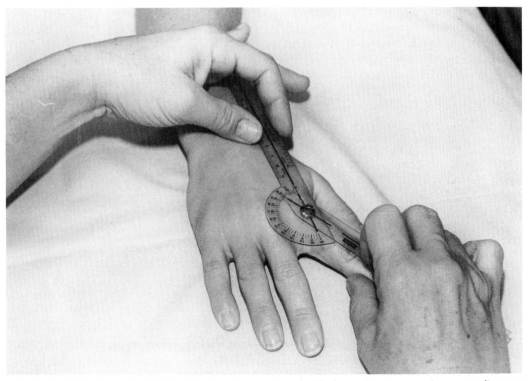

FIGURE 6 – 21. At the end of MCP abduction, the examiner holds the goniometer arms in correct alignment.

TESTING PROCEDURES: PROXIMAL INTERPHALANGEAL JOINTS (FINGERS)

FLEXION

Motion occurs in the sagittal plane around a medial-lateral axis.

Recommended Testing Position

Position the subject sitting, with the forearm in 0 degrees of supination and pronation. The wrist is positioned in 0 degrees of flexion, extension, and radial and ulnar deviation. The MCP joint is positioned in 0 degrees of flexion, extension, abduction, and adduction. The forearm and hand rest on a supporting surface. (If the wrist and MCP joints are positioned in full flexion, tension in the extensor digitorum communis, extensor indicis, or extensor digiti minimi muscles will restrict the motion. If the MCP joint is positioned in full extension, tension in the lumbricalis and interosseus muscles will restrict the motion.)

Stabilization

Stabilize the proximal phalanx to prevent motion of the wrist and MCP joint (Fig. 6–22).

Normal End-Feel

Usually the end-feel is hard because of contact between the palmar aspect of the middle phalanx and the proximal phalanx. In some individuals the end-feel may be soft because of compression of soft tissue between the palmar aspect of the middle and proximal phalanges. In other individuals the end-feel may be firm because of tension in the dorsal joint capsule and the collateral ligaments.

Goniometer Alignment

See Figures 6–23 and 6–24.

1. Center the fulcrum of the goniometer over the dorsal aspect of the PIP joint.
2. Align the proximal arm over the dorsal midline of the proximal phalanx.
3. Align the distal arm over the dorsal midline of the middle phalanx.

EXTENSION

Motion occurs in the sagittal plane around a medial-lateral axis.

Recommended Testing Position

Position the subject sitting, with the forearm in 0 degrees of supination and pronation. The wrist is positioned in 0 degrees of flexion, extension, and radial and ulnar deviation. The MCP joint is positioned in 0 degrees of flexion, extension, abduction, and adduction. The forearm and hand rest on a supporting surface. (If the MCP joint and wrist are extended, tension in the flexor digitorum superficialis and profundus muscles will restrict the motion.)

Stabilization

The stabilization is the same as for PIP flexion of the fingers.

Normal End-Feel

The end-feel is firm because of tension in the palmar joint capsule and palmar fibrocartilaginous plate (palmar ligament).

Goniometer Alignment

Alignment is the same as for PIP flexion of the fingers.

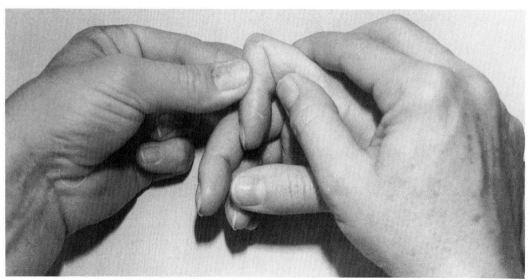

FIGURE 6–22. At the end of PIP flexion the examiner stabilizes the subject's second proximal phalanx with her right thumb and index finger. The examiner uses her left thumb and index finger to maintain the subject's PIP joint in full flexion.

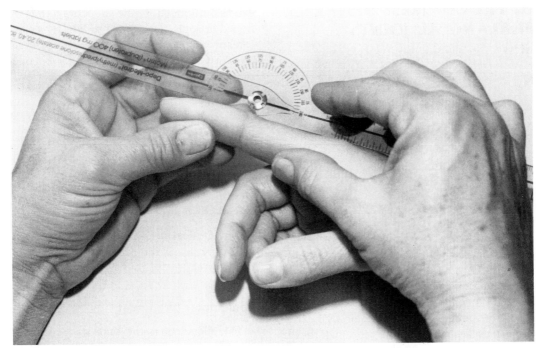

FIGURE 6–23. In the starting position for PIP joint flexion, the subject's hand and forearm rest on the supporting surface. The examiner's right hand holds the proximal arm of the goniometer along the dorsal midline of the subject's second proximal phalanx and maintains the subject's MCP joint in a neutral position relative to flexion and extension. The examiner's left thumb supports the subject's middle phalanx.

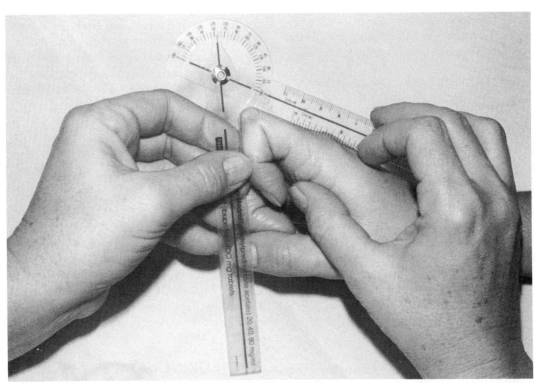

FIGURE 6–24. At the end of PIP flexion, the examiner's right thumb continues to stabilize the subject's MCP joint. The examiner's left thumb is used to hold the distal goniometer arm in alignment over the dorsal midline of the subject's middle phalanx. The fulcrum of the goniometer lies distal and superior to the PIP joint axis.

TESTING PROCEDURES: DISTAL INTERPHALANGEAL JOINTS (FINGERS)

FLEXION

Motion occurs in the sagittal plane around a medial-lateral axis.

Recommended Testing Position

Position the subject sitting, with the forearm in 0 degrees of supination and pronation. The wrist is positioned in 0 degrees of flexion, extension, and radial and ulnar deviation. The MCP joint is positioned in 0 degrees of flexion, extension, abduction, and adduction. The PIP joint is positioned in approximately 70 to 90 degrees of flexion. The forearm and hand rest on a supporting surface. (If the wrist and the MCP and PIP joints are fully flexed, tension in the extensor digitorum communis, extensor indicis, or extensor digiti minimi muscles may restrict the motion. If the PIP joint is extended, tension in the oblique retinacular ligament may restrict the motion even more.)

Stabilization

Stabilize the middle phalanx to prevent further flexion or extension of the wrist and the MCP and PIP joints.

Normal End-Feel

The end-feel is firm because of tension in the dorsal joint capsule, the collateral ligaments, and the oblique retinacular ligament.

Goniometer Alignment

1. Center the fulcrum of the goniometer over the dorsal aspect of the DIP joint.
2. Align the proximal arm over the dorsal midline of the middle phalanx.
3. Align the distal arm over the dorsal midline of the distal phalanx.

EXTENSION

Motion occurs in the sagittal plane around a medial-lateral axis.

Recommended Testing Position

Position the subject sitting, with the forearm in 0 degrees of supination and pronation. The wrist is positioned in 0 degrees of flexion, extension, and radial and ulnar deviation. The MCP joint is positioned in 0 degrees of flexion, extension, abduction, and adduction. The PIP joint is positioned in approximately 70 to 90 degrees of flexion. The forearm and hand rest on a supporting surface. (If the PIP joint, MCP joint, and wrist are fully extended, tension in the flexor digitorum profundus muscle may restrict the motion.)

Stabilization

Stabilize the middle phalanx to prevent extension of the wrist and the MCP and PIP joints.

Normal End-Feel

The end-feel is firm because of tension in the palmar joint capsule and the palmar fibrocartilaginous plate (palmar ligament).

Goniometer Alignment

The alignment is the same as for DIP flexion of the fingers.

CARPOMETACARPAL JOINT (THUMB)

STRUCTURE

The carpometacarpal (CMC) joint is the articulation between the trapezium and the base of the first metacarpal. The saddle-shaped portion of the trapezium is concave in the sagittal plane and convex in the frontal plane. The base of the first metacarpal has a reciprocal shape that conforms to that of the trapezium. The joint capsule is thick but lax and is reinforced by radial, ulnar, volar, and dorsal ligaments.

OSTEOKINEMATICS

The CMC is a saddle joint with 2 degrees of freedom: flexion-extension in the frontal plane and abduction-adduction in the sagittal plane. The joint also permits some axial rotation. This rotation allows the thumb to move into a position for contact with the fingers during opposition. The sequence of motions that combine with rotation and result in opposition is as follows: abduction, flexion, and adduction. Reposition is the movement that returns the thumb to the starting position.

ARTHROKINEMATICS

The convex portion of the first metacarpal base slides on the concave portion of the trapezium in a direction opposite to the shaft of the metacarpal to produce abduction-adduction. The base of the first metacarpal slides dorsally in abduction and volarly in adduction. The concave portion of the first metacarpal slides on the convex portion of the trapezium in the same direction as the metacarpal shaft to produce flexion-extension. During flexion the base of the metacarpal slides in an ulnar direction. During extension it slides in a radial direction.

CAPSULAR PATTERN

The capsular pattern is a limitation of abduction.[4]

CARPOMETACARPAL RANGE OF MOTION

The AMA *Guides*[6] give the average ROM in opposition as 8 cm. See Table 6–6 for other ROM values.

METACARPOPHALANGEAL AND INTERPHALANGEAL JOINTS (THUMB)

STRUCTURE

The MCP joint of the thumb is the articulation between the convex head of the first metacarpal and the concave base of the first phalanx. The joint is reinforced by a joint capsule, collateral ligaments, and by two sesamoid bones on its volar surface.

The interphalangeal (IP) joint of the thumb is identical in structure to the IP joints of the fingers.

OSTEOKINEMATICS

The MCP joint is a condyloid joint with 2 degrees of freedom. The motions permitted are flexion-extension and a minimal amount of abduction-adduction. Motions at this joint are more restricted than at the MCP joints of the fingers.

The IP joint is a synovial hinge joint with 1 degree of freedom: flexion-extension in the sagittal plane.

ARTHROKINEMATICS

At the MCP joint the concave base of the first phalanx glides on the convex head of the first metacarpal in the same direction as the shaft. The base of the proximal phalanx moves volarly in flexion and dorsally in extension.

At the IP joint the concave base of the distal phalanx glides on the convex head of the proximal phalanx in the same direction as the shaft of the bone. The base of the distal phalanx moves volarly in flexion and dorsally in extension.

CAPSULAR PATTERN

The capsular pattern for the MCP joint is a restriction of motion in all directions, but flexion is more limited than extension.

The capsular pattern for the IP joint is equal limitation of flexion and extension.

METACARPOPHALANGEAL AND INTERPHALANGEAL RANGE OF MOTION

According to Hertling and Kessler,[27] MCP flexion ranges from 5 to 100 degrees, with an average of 75 degrees (see Table 6–6 for ROM from various sources).

Effects of Age and Gender

Please refer to the section entitled "Effects of Age and Gender" under "Finger Range of Motion."

TESTING PROCEDURES: CARPOMETACARPAL JOINT (THUMB)

FLEXION

Motion occurs in the frontal plane around an anterior-posterior axis when the subject is in the anatomical position.

Recommended Testing Position

Position the subject sitting, with the forearm in full supination. The wrist is positioned in 0 degrees of flexion, extension, and radial and ulnar deviation. The CMC joint of the thumb is in 0 degrees of abduction and adduction. The MCP and IP joints of the thumb are positioned in 0 degrees of flexion and extension. The forearm and hand rest on a supporting surface. (If the MCP and IP joints of the thumb are positioned in full flexion, tension in the extensor pollicis longus muscle may restrict the motion.)

Stabilization

Stabilize the carpal bones to prevent wrist motions (Fig. 6–25).

Normal End-Feel

The end-feel may be soft because of contact between muscle bulk of the thenar eminence and the palm of the hand, or it may be firm because of tension in the dorsal joint capsule and the extensor pollicis brevis and abductor pollicis brevis muscles.

Goniometer Alignment

See Figures 6–26 and 6–27.

1. Center the fulcrum of the goniometer over the palmar aspect of the first CMC joint.
2. Align the proximal arm with the ventral midline of the radius using the ventral surface of the radial head and radial styloid process for reference.
3. Align the distal arm with the ventral midline of the first metacarpal.

In the starting positions for both flexion and extension, the goniometer may indicate 15 to 20 degrees rather than 0 degrees. The starting-position degrees should be subtracted from the degrees indicated at the end of the ROM. A measurement that begins at 20 degrees and ends at 50 degrees should be recorded as 0 to 30 degrees.

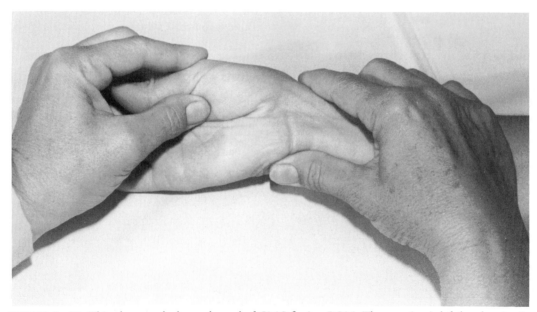

FIGURE 6–25. This photograph shows the end of CMC flexion ROM. The examiner's left hand maintains flexion by pulling medially on the subject's right first metacarpal. The examiner's right hand grasps the subject's carpal bones to prevent both ulnar deviation and palmar flexion of the wrist.

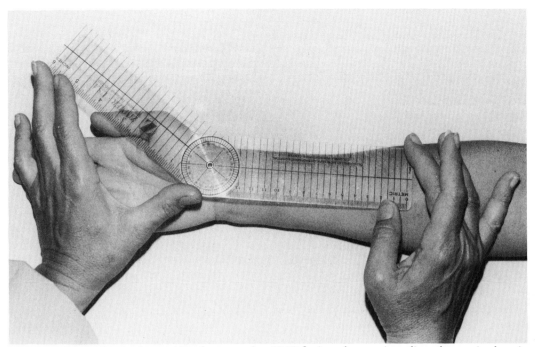

FIGURE 6-26. In the starting position for measuring CMC flexion, the examiner aligns the proximal goniometer arm so that it is parallel with the radius and aligns the distal arm with the subject's first metacarpal. Note that in the starting position the goniometer does not read 0 degrees.

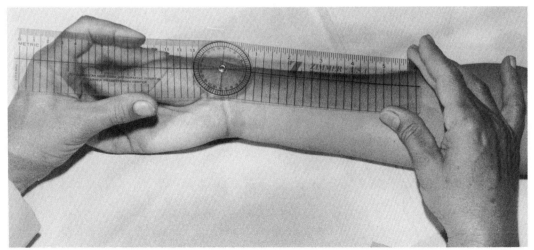

FIGURE 6-27. At the end of the flexion ROM, the examiner's left hand maintains both flexion and alignment of the distal goniometer arm parallel to the radius.

EXTENSION

Motion occurs in the frontal plane around an anterior-posterior axis when the subject is in the anatomical position.

Recommended Testing Position and Stabilization

The testing position and stabilization are the same as for flexion of the CMC joint of the thumb (Fig. 6–28).

Normal End-Feel

The end-feel is firm because of tension in the anterior joint capsule and the flexor pollicis brevis, adductor pollicis, opponens pollicis, and first dorsal interosseus muscles.

Goniometer Alignment

The alignment is the same as for flexion of the CMC joint of the thumb (Figs. 6–29 and 6–30).

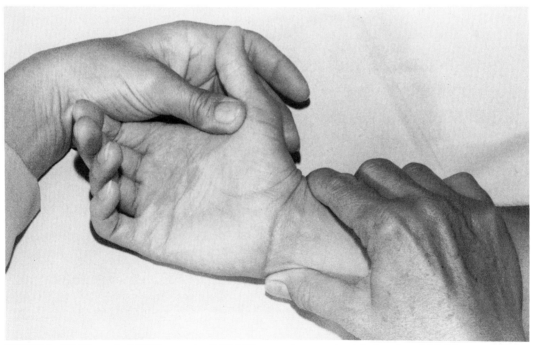

FIGURE 6–28. The end of CMC extension ROM. The examiner uses her left thumb and third finger to pull the metacarpal laterally into extension while placing her right hand on the subject's carpal bones to prevent both radial deviation and palmar flexion.

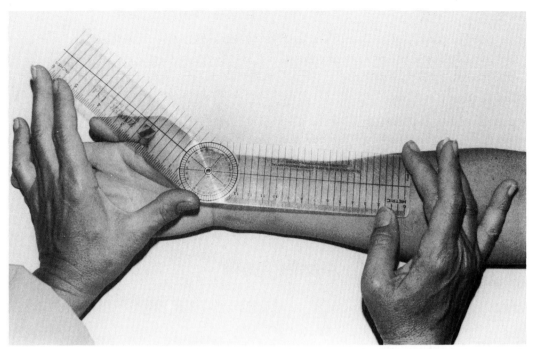

FIGURE 6–29. In the starting position for measuring CMC extension, goniometer alignment is the same as for measuring CMC flexion.

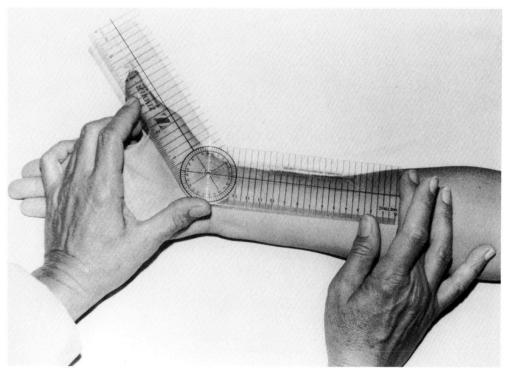

FIGURE 6–30. At the end of CMC extension, the examiner's left hand keeps the distal goniometer aligned with the subject's first metacarpal and also holds the subject's thumb in extension. The examiner's right hand keeps the proximal goniometer aligned with the subject's radius.

ABDUCTION

Motion occurs in the sagittal plane around a medial-lateral axis when the subject is in the anatomical position.

Recommended Testing Position

Position the subject sitting, with the forearm midway between supination and pronation. The wrist is positioned in 0 degrees of flexion, extension, and radial and ulnar deviation. The CMC, MCP, and IP joints of the thumb are positioned in 0 degrees of flexion and extension. The forearm and hand rest on a supporting surface.

Stabilization

Stabilize the carpal bones and the second metacarpal to prevent wrist motions (Fig. 6–31).

Normal End-Feel

The end-feel is firm because of tension in the fascia and skin of the web space between the thumb and index finger. Tension in the adductor pollicis and first dorsal interosseus muscles also contributes to the firm end-feel.

Goniometer Alignment

See Figures 6–32 and 6–33.

1. Center the fulcrum of the goniometer over the lateral aspect of the radial styloid process.
2. Align the proximal arm with the lateral midline of the second metacarpal using the center of the second MCP joint for reference.
3. Align the distal arm with the lateral midline of the first metacarpal using the center of the first MCP joint for reference.

ADDUCTION

Motion occurs in the sagittal plane around a medial-lateral axis when the subject is in the anatomical position. Adduction is the return to the zero starting position from a position of maximal abduction.

Recommended Testing Position, Stabilization, and Goniometer Alignment

The testing position, stabilization, and alignment are the same as for abduction of the CMC joint of the thumb.

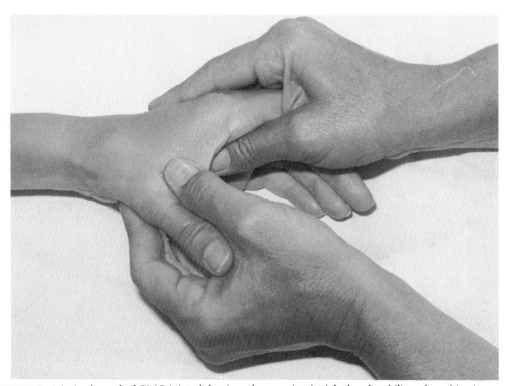

FIGURE 6–31. At the end of CMC joint abduction, the examiner's right hand stabilizes the subject's second metacarpal. With her left thumb and index finger, the examiner grasps the subject's first metacarpal just proximal to the MCP joint to maintain abduction.

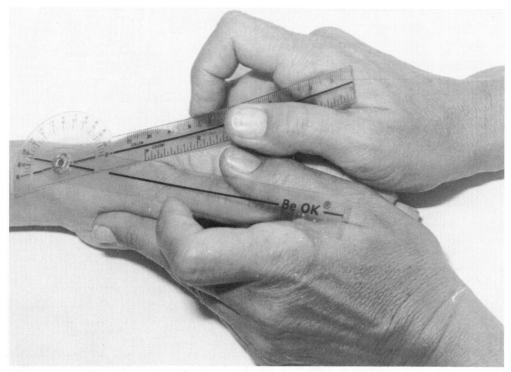

FIGURE 6 – 32. In the starting position for CMC abduction, the subject's first and second metacarpals are separated slightly; therefore, when the arms of the goniometer are aligned with the first and second metacarpals, the goniometer will not be at 0 degrees.

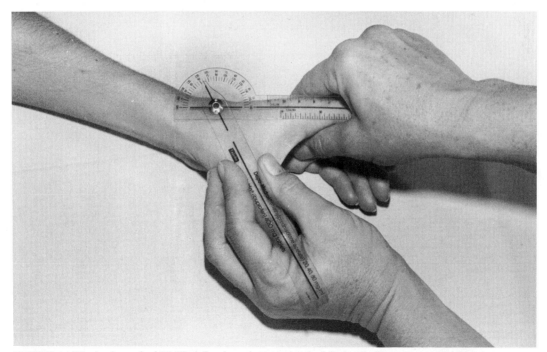

FIGURE 6 – 33. At the end of CMC abduction, the examiner's right hand aligns the proximal goniometer arm with the subject's second metacarpal and at the same time provides stabilization. The examiner's left hand, which is maintaining the alignment of the distal goniometer arm, also maintains abduction.

OPPOSITION

Motion is a combination of abduction, flexion, medial-axial rotation (pronation), and adduction.

Recommended Testing Position

Position the subject sitting, with the forearm in full supination. The wrist is in 0 degrees of flexion, extension, and radial and ulnar deviation. The IP joints of the thumb and little finger are positioned in 0 degrees of flexion and ex-tension. The forearm and hand rest on a supporting surface.

Stabilization

Stabilize the fifth metacarpal to prevent wrist motions (Fig. 6–34).

Normal End-Feel

The end-feel may be soft because of contact between the muscle bulk of the thenar eminence and the palm, or it may

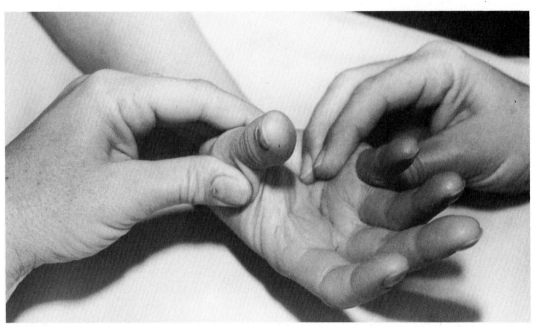

FIGURE 6–34. At the end of the ROM in opposition, the examiner's left hand grasps the subject's thumb at the level of the MCP joint. The examiner is able to maintain the thumb in opposition by exerting pressure on the first metacarpal with her left thumb. The examiner's right hand maintains the subject's fifth metacarpal and proximal phalanx in opposition. (This subject's hand does not have full ROM.)

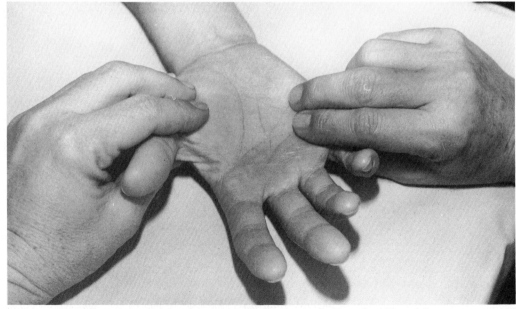

FIGURE 6–35. In the starting position for opposition, the examiner grasps the fifth and first metacarpals. The subject's hand is supported by the table.

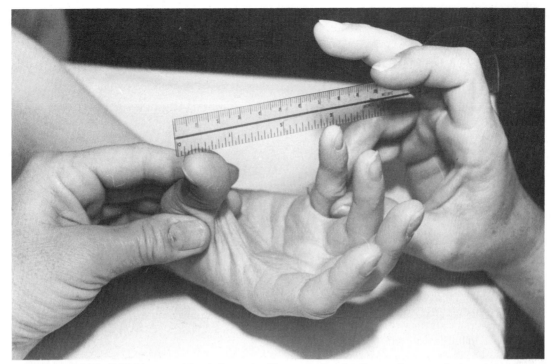

FIGURE 6–36. The ROM in opposition is determined by measuring the distance between the lateral tips of the subject's thumb and fifth digit. The examiner is using the arm of a half-circle plastic goniometer measure, but any ruler or tape measure would do. The photograph does not show the complete ROM of opposition because we wanted to demonstrate clearly how the ROM is measured. When full ROM in opposition is reached, the tips of the fifth finger and thumb are touching.

be firm because of tension in the joint capsule, extensor pollicis brevis muscle, and transverse metacarpal ligament (affecting the fifth finger).

Goniometer Alignment

The goniometer is not commonly used to measure the range of opposition (Fig. 6–35). Instead, often a ruler is used to measure the distance between the tip of the thumb and the tip of the fifth finger (Fig. 6–36). Alternatively, a ruler may be used to measure the distance between the tip of the thumb and the base (MCP joint) of the fifth finger. The AMA *Guides to the Evaluation of Permanent Impairment*[6] recommends using the distance from the flexion crease of the thumb IP joint to the distal palmar crease directly over the third (middle finger) MCP joint (Fig. 6–37).

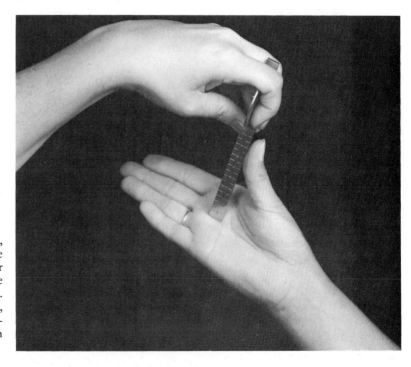

FIGURE 6–37. To measure thumb IP opposition, the examiner uses a centimeter ruler to find the longest possible distance between the distal palmar crease directly over the MCP joint of the middle finger and the flexion crease of the thumb IP joint. The distance is approximately 8 cm. (From Stanley, BG and Tribuzi, SM: Concepts in Hand Rehabilitation. FA Davis, Philadelphia, 1992, p. 546, with permission.)

TESTING PROCEDURES: METACARPOPHALANGEAL JOINT (THUMB)

FLEXION

Motion occurs in the frontal plane around an anterior-posterior axis when the subject is in the anatomical position.

Recommended Testing Position

Position the subject sitting, with the forearm in full supination. The wrist is in 0 degrees of flexion, extension, and radial and ulnar deviation. The CMC joint of the thumb is positioned in 0 degrees of flexion, extension, abduction, adduction, and opposition. The IP joint of the thumb is in 0 degrees of flexion and extension. The forearm and hand rest on a supporting surface. (If the wrist and IP joint of the thumb are positioned in full flexion, tension in the extensor pollicis longus muscle will restrict the motion.)

Stabilization

Stabilize the first metacarpal to prevent wrist motion and flexion and opposition of the CMC joint of the thumb (Fig. 6–38).

Normal End-Feel

The end-feel may be hard because of contact between the palmar aspect of the proximal phalanx and the first metacarpal, or it may be firm because of tension in the dorsal joint capsule, the collateral ligaments, and the extensor pollicis brevis muscle.

Goniometer Alignment

See Figures 6–39 and 6–40.

1. Center the fulcrum of the goniometer over the dorsal aspect of the MCP joint.
2. Align the proximal arm over the dorsal midline of the metacarpal.
3. Align the distal arm with the dorsal midline of the proximal phalanx.

EXTENSION

Motion occurs in the frontal plane around an anterior-posterior axis when the subject is in the anatomical position.

Recommended Testing Position

Position the subject sitting, with the forearm in full supination. The wrist is in 0 degrees of flexion, extension, and radial and ulnar deviation. The CMC joint of the thumb is positioned in 0 degrees of flexion, extension, abduction, adduction, and opposition. The IP joint of the thumb is in 0 degrees of flexion and extension. The forearm and hand rest on a supporting surface. (If the IP joint of the thumb is positioned in full extension, tension in the flexor pollicis longus muscle may restrict the motion.)

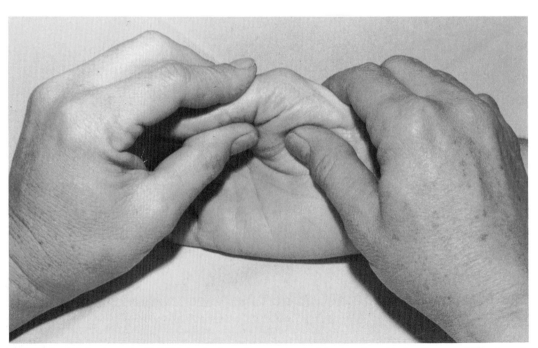

FIGURE 6–38. At the end of MCP joint flexion, the examiner's right thumb and index finger stabilize the subject's first metacarpal. The examiner's left index finger maintains the subject's MCP joint in flexion through pressure on the subject's proximal phalanx. The examiner's left thumb helps to prevent flexion at the subject's IP joint.

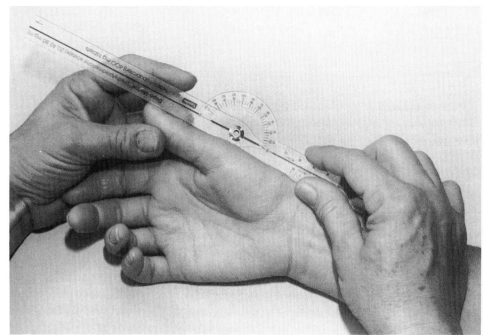

FIGURE 6–39. In the starting position for MCP flexion, the fulcrum of the goniometer is centered over the dorsal aspect of the MCP joint. The distal goniometer arm is aligned along the dorsal midline of the proximal phalanx. The examiner's left hand holds the distal goniometer arm in alignment and maintains the IP joint in extension. The proximal goniometer is aligned along the dorsal midline of the subject's first metacarpal.

Stabilization

Stabilize the first metacarpal to prevent motion at the wrist and CMC joint of the thumb.

Normal End-Feel

The end-feel is firm because of tension in the palmar joint capsule, palmar fibrocartilaginous plate (palmar liga-

ment), intersesamoid ligament, and flexor pollicis brevis muscle.

Goniometer Alignment

The alignment is the same as for flexion of the MCP joint of the thumb.

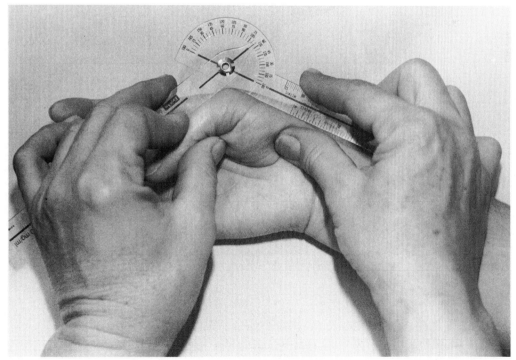

FIGURE 6–40. At the end of MCP flexion, the examiner's left hand stabilizes the subject's IP joint and maintains alignment of the distal arm of the goniometer. The examiner uses her right hand to stabilize the subject's first metacarpal and to keep the proximal arm of the goniometer in correct alignment.

TESTING PROCEDURES: INTERPHALANGEAL JOINT (THUMB)

FLEXION

Motion occurs in the frontal plane around an anterior-posterior axis when the subject is in the anatomical position.

Recommended Testing Position

Position the subject sitting, with the forearm in full supination. The wrist is in 0 degrees of flexion, extension, and radial and ulnar deviation. The CMC joint is positioned in 0 degrees of flexion, extension, abduction, adduction, and opposition. The MCP joint of the thumb is in 0 degrees of flexion and extension. The forearm and hand rest on a supporting surface. (If the wrist and MCP joint of the thumb are flexed, tension in the extensor pollicis longus muscle may restrict the motion. If the MCP joint of the thumb is fully extended, tension in the first palmar interossei, the abductor pollicis brevis, and the oblique fibers of the adductor pollicis may restrict the motion through their insertion into the extensor hood mechanism.)

Stabilization

Stabilize the proximal phalanx to prevent flexion or extension of the MCP joint (Fig. 6–41).

Normal End-Feel

Usually the end-feel is firm because of tension in the collateral ligaments and the dorsal joint capsule. In some individuals, the end-feel may be hard because of contact between the palmar aspect of the distal phalanx, the fibrocartilaginous plate, and the proximal phalanx.

Goniometer Alignment

See Figures 6–42 and 6–43.

1. Center the fulcrum of the goniometer over the dorsal surface of the IP joint.
2. Align the proximal arm with the dorsal aspect of the proximal phalanx.
3. Align the distal arm with the dorsal midline of the distal phalanx.

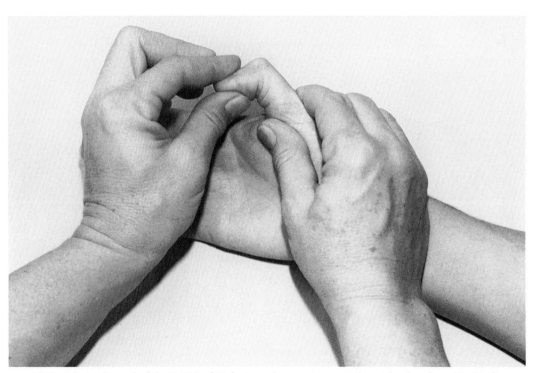

FIGURE 6–41. At the end of the ROM of IP flexion, the examiner uses her right thumb and index finger to maintain the subject's MCP joint in 0 degrees of flexion. The examiner's right hand also keeps the subject's CMC joint in 0 degrees of abduction and opposition. The examiner uses her left thumb and index finger to maintain the subject's IP joint in flexion.

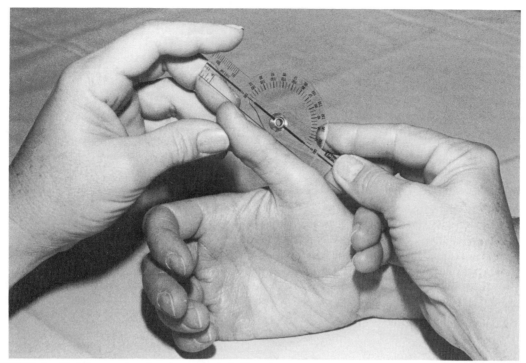

FIGURE 6–42. The examiner is using a plastic half-circle goniometer with the arms cut short. The proximal goniometer arm is aligned on the dorsal midline of the subject's first proximal phalanx. The distal goniometer arm is aligned along the subject's first distal phalanx.

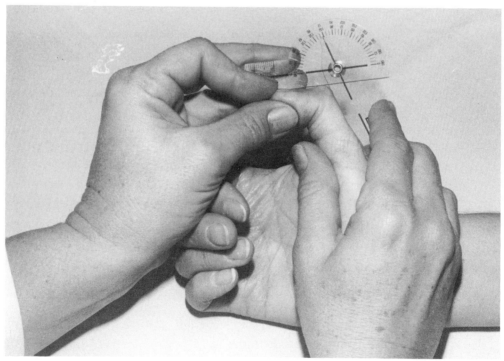

FIGURE 6–43. At the end of the flexion ROM, the examiner's right hand stabilizes the subject's CMC and MCP joints and holds the shortened proximal goniometer arm in alignment. The examiner's left hand holds the distal goniometer arm in alignment and maintains the IP joint in flexion through pressure on the subject's distal phalanx. The fulcrum of the goniometer lies distal and superior to the IP joint.

EXTENSION

Motion occurs in the frontal plane around an anterior-posterior axis when the subject is in the anatomical position.

Recommended Testing Position

Position the subject sitting, with the forearm in full supination. The wrist is in 0 degrees of flexion, extension, and radial and ulnar deviation. The CMC joint of the thumb is positioned in 0 degrees of flexion, extension, abduction, adduction, and opposition. The MCP joint of the thumb is in 0 degrees of flexion and extension. The forearm and hand rest on a supporting surface. (If the wrist and MCP joint of the thumb are extended, tension in the flexor pollicis longus muscle may restrict the motion.)

Stabilization

The stabilization is the same as for flexion of the IP joint of the thumb.

Normal End-Feel

The end-feel is firm because of tension in the palmar joint capsule and the palmar fibrocartilaginous plate (palmar ligament).

Goniometer Alignment

The alignment is the same as for flexion of the IP joint of the thumb.

REFERENCES

1. Linscheid, RL: Kinematic considerations of the wrist. Clin Orthop 202:27, 1986.
2. Norkin, CC and Levangie, PK: Joint Structure and Function: A Comprehensive Analysis, ed 2. FA Davis, Philadelphia, 1992.
3. Kisner, C and Colby, LA: Therapeutic Exercise: Foundations and Techniques. FA Davis, Philadelphia, 1985.
4. Cyriax, JH and Cyriax, PJ: Illustrated Manual of Orthopaedic Medicine. Butterworths, London, 1983.
5. American Academy of Orthopaedic Surgeons: Joint Motion: Methods of Measuring and Recording. AAOS, Chicago, 1965.
6. American Medical Association: Guides to the Evaluation of Permanent Impairment, ed 3. AMA, Chicago, 1988.
7. Boone, DC and Azen, SP: Normal range of motion in male subjects. J Bone Joint Surg Am 61:756, 1979.
8. Brumfield, RH and Champoux, JA: A biomechanical study of normal functional wrist motion. Clin Orthop 187:23, 1984.
9. Wanatabe, H, et al: The range of joint motions of the extremities in healthy Japanese people: The difference according to age. Cited in Walker, JM: Musculoskeletal development: A review. Phys Ther 71:878, 1991.
10. Boone, DC: Techniques of measurement of joint motion. (Unpublished supplement to Boone, DC and Azen, SP: Normal range of motion in male subjects. J Bone Joint Surg Am 61:756, 1979.)
11. Walker, JM, et al: Active mobility of the extremities in older subjects. Phys Ther 64:919, 1984.
12. Hewitt, D: The range of active motion at the wrist of women. J Bone Joint Surg Br 26:775, 1928.
13. Allander, E, et al: Normal range of joint movements in shoulder, hip, wrist and thumb with special reference to side: A comparison between two populations. Int J Epidemiol 3:253, 1974.
14. Cobe, HM: The range of active motion of the wrist of white adults. J Bone Joint Surg Br 26:763, 1928.
15. Hellebrandt, FA, Duvall, EN, and Moore, ML: The measurement of joint motion. Part III: Reliability of goniometry. Physical Therapy Review 29:302, 1949.
16. Low, JL: The reliability of joint measurement. Physiotherapy 62:227, 1976.
17. Boone, DC, et al: Reliability of goniometric measurements. Phys Ther 58:1355, 1978.
18. Bird, HA and Stowe, J: The wrist. Clinics in Rheumatic Disease 8:559, 1982.
19. Solgaard, S, et al: Reproducibility of goniometry of the wrist. Scand J Rehabil Med 18:5, 1986.
20. Horger, MM: The reliability of goniometric measurements of active and passive wrist motions. Am J Occup Ther 44:342, 1990.
21. La Stayo, PC and Wheeler, DL: Reliability of passive wrist flexion and extension measurements: A multicenter study. Phys Ther 74:162, 1994.
22. Stanley, BG and Tribuzi, SM: Concepts in Hand Rehabilitation. FA Davis, Philadelphia, 1992.
23. Beighton, P, Solomon, L, and Soskolne, CL: Articular mobility in an African population. Ann Rheum Dis 32:23, 1973.
24. Fairbank, JCT, Pynsett, PB, and Phillips, H: Quantitative measurements of joint mobility in adolescents. Ann Rheum Dis 43:288, 1984.
25. Hamilton, GF and Lachenbruch, PA: Reliability of goniometers in assessing finger joint angle. Phys Ther 49:465, 1969.
26. Bear-Lehman, J and Abreu, BC: Evaluating the hand: Issues in reliability and validity. Phys Ther 69:1025, 1989.
27. Hertling, D and Kessler, RM: Management of Common Musculoskeletal Disorders, ed 2. JB Lippincott, Philadelphia, 1993.

Lower-Extremity Testing

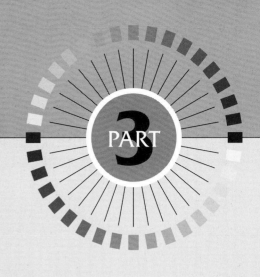

PART 3

OBJECTIVES

On completion of Part 3, the reader will be able to:

1. Identify:
   the appropriate planes and axes for each lower-extremity joint motion
   the structures that limit the end of the ROM at each lower-extremity joint
   the expected normal end-feel

2. Describe:
   the recommended testing positions used for each lower-extremity joint motion
   goniometer alignment
   capsular pattern of limitation
   ROM necessary for functional activities

3. Explain:
   how age and gender may affect the ROM
   how sources of error in measurement may affect testing results

4. Perform a goniometric evaluation of any lower-extremity joint including:

a clear explanation of the testing procedure
positioning of the subject in recommended testing position
adequate stabilization of the proximal joint component
correct determination of the end of the ROM
correct identification of the end-feel
palpation of the correct bony landmarks
accurate alignment of the goniometer
correct reading and recording

5. Plan goniometric evaluations of the hip, knee, ankle, and foot that are organized by body position

6. Assess the intratester and intertester reliability of goniometric evaluations of the lower-extremity joints

The recommended testing positions, stabilization techniques, normal end-feels, and goniometer alignment for the joints of the lower extremities are presented in Chapters 7 to 9. The goniometric evaluation should follow the 12-step sequence that was presented in Exercise 5 in Chapter 2.

7

The Hip

STRUCTURE

The hip joint, or coxa, links the lower extremity with the trunk. The proximal joint surface is the acetabulum, which is formed superiorly by the ileum, posteroinferiorly by the ischium, and anteroinferiorly by the pubis. The concave acetabulum faces laterally, inferiorly, and anteriorly and is deepened by a fibrocartilaginous acetabular labrum. The distal joint surface is the convex head of the femur. The joint is enclosed by a strong, thick capsule, which is reinforced by the iliofemoral, ischiofemoral, and pubofemoral ligaments.

OSTEOKINEMATICS

The hip is a synovial ball-and-socket joint with 3 degrees of freedom. The motions permitted at the joint are flexion-extension in the sagittal plane around a medial-lateral axis, abduction-adduction in the frontal plane around an anterior-posterior axis, and medial and lateral rotation in the transverse plane around a vertical or longitudinal axis.[1] The axis of motion goes through the center of the femoral head.[2]

ARTHROKINEMATICS

In an open kinematic (non–weight-bearing) chain, the convex femoral head slides on the concave acetabulum in a direction opposite to the movement of the shaft of the bone. In flexion, the femoral head slides posteriorly and inferiorly on the acetabulum, whereas in extension, the fem-

oral head slides anteriorly and superiorly. In medial rotation, the femoral head slides posteriorly on the acetabulum. In lateral rotation, the femoral head slides anteriorly. In abduction, the femoral head slides inferiorly. In adduction, the femoral head slides superiorly.[2]

CAPSULAR PATTERN

The capsular pattern is characterized by a marked restriction of medial rotation accompanied by limitations in flexion and abduction. A slight limitation may be present in extension, but no limitation is present in either lateral rotation or adduction.[3]

RANGE OF MOTION

Table 7–1 shows hip ROM values from various sources. The age, gender, and number of subjects measured to obtain values reported for the AAOS and the AMA in Table 7–1 are unknown. Boone and Azen[6] measured active ROM on male subjects using a universal goniometer. Roach and Miles[7] also measured active ROM using a universal goniometer, but their measurements were obtained from both males and females.

In Table 7–1, large differences in mean values are evident among the different sources for hip flexion, extension, and both medial and lateral rotation. The AMA value of 100 degrees for hip flexion differs from mean values from the other sources by more than one standard deviation. This difference may be the result of differences in the methods used for testing or differences in the age or gender

Table 7–1 **HIP MOTION: MEAN VALUES IN DEGREES FROM SELECTED SOURCES**

Motion	AMERICAN ACADEMY OF ORTHOPAEDIC SURGEONS[4]	AMERICAN MEDICAL ASSOCIATION[5]	BOONE AND AZEN[6] 18 MO–54 YR (N = 109)		ROACH AND MILES[7] 25–74 YR (N = 1683)	
			Mean	Standard Deviation	Mean	Standard Deviation
Flexion	120.0	100.0	122.3	6.1	121.0	13.0
Extension	30.0	30.0	9.8	6.8	19.0	8.0
Abduction	45.0	40.0	45.9	9.3	42.0	11.0
Adduction	30.0	20.0	26.9	4.1		
Medial rotation	45.0	40.0*	47.3	6.0	32.0	8.0
Lateral rotation	45.0	50.0*	47.2	6.3	32.0	9.0

Values from Roach and Miles[7] reprinted from Physical Therapy with the permission of the American Physical Therapy Association.
*Measurements taken in the supine position.

of the population tested. The fact that the mean values from the study by Boone and Azen[6] for hip extension differ by more than two standard deviations from AMA and AAOS values, and by one standard deviation from the values obtained by Roach and Miles,[7] is most likely attributable to differences in the ages of the populations tested. Boone and Azen[6] included a much younger age range in their measurements than did Roach and Miles.[7] Therefore, the mean values could have been skewed toward the values for the youngest age groups, which are much lower than the adult values (see Table 7–3). Differences in rotation values between those of Roach and Miles and those of the other sources are not easily explained but may be caused either by differences in measurement techniques or by age or gender differences in the population tested. All sources have general agreement on the values for hip abduction.

In a recent study, Ellison et al.[8] used both a universal goniometer and a fluid-filled inclinometer to measure passive hip ROM in 100 healthy subjects (25 males and 75 females 20 to 41 years of age) and 50 patients with low back pain. These authors found that both groups demonstrated three different patterns of PROM in rotation at the hip. In pattern 1, medial and lateral rotation (both right and left extremities) were equal within 10 degrees. In pattern 2, the total medial rotation (sum of left and right extremities) was greater than the total lateral rotation (sum of left and right extremities). In pattern 3, the total lateral rotation was greater than the total medial rotation. Pattern 2 was the most common pattern demonstrated by 41 of the healthy subjects (5 male and 36 female). A greater proportion of the patients than of the healthy subjects demonstrated pattern 3, in which the total lateral rotation was greater than the total medial rotation.

FUNCTIONAL RANGE OF MOTION

Table 7–2 shows the hip flexion ROM necessary for selected functional activities as reported in several sources. An adequate ROM at the hip is important in meeting mobility demands such as walking, stairclimbing, and performing many activities of daily living that require sitting and bending. According to the values in the *Observational Gait Analysis Handbook*, published by the Rancho Los Amigos Medical Center,[10] the following ROMs are required for level walking: 0 to 30 degrees of hip flexion, 0 to 10 degrees of hip extension, and 0 to 5 degrees of abduction, adduction, and medial and lateral rotation.

Livingston et al.[9] studied stair ascent and descent on stairs of different dimensions using 15 female subjects be-

Table 7–2 **HIP FLEXION RANGE OF MOTION REQUIRED FOR FUNCTIONAL ACTIVITIES: MEAN VALUES IN DEGREES FROM SELECTED SOURCES**

Activity	LIVINGSTON ET AL.[9] (N = 6)	RANCHO LOS AMIGOS MEDICAL CENTER[10]	MCFAYDEN AND WINTER[11]	
			Mean	Standard Deviation
Walking on level surfaces	0–30	0–30	0–44	4.5
Ascending stairs	1–0–66		0–60	
Descending stairs	1–0–45		0–66	0.1

tween 19 and 26 years of age. This population employed 0 to 1 degree of hip extension and 0 to 66 degrees of hip flexion for ascending stairs, and 0 to 1 degree of hip extension and 0 to 45 degrees of hip flexion for descending stairs. McFayden and Winter[11] also studied stairclimbing; however, these authors used eight repeated trials of one subject. In their study the subject used 0 to 60 degrees of hip flexion to ascend stairs and 0 to 66 degrees of hip flexion to descend stairs.

Sitting requires at least 90 degrees of hip flexion with the knee flexed. Additional flexion ROM is necessary for tying shoes and putting on pants.

EFFECTS OF AGE AND GENDER

Table 7–3 shows hip ROM values for newborns and children up to 5 years of age as reported in five studies. All values presented in Table 7–3 were obtained with a universal goniometer. Passive ROM was measured in each study, with the exception of the study by Boone,[16] in which active ROM was measured. Males and females were included in each study except for the study by Boone,[16] which included only male subjects. The infants in the study by Waugh et al.[12] included 18 males and 22 females. All of these infants met the following criteria: gestational age of at least 37 weeks, birth weight of at least 2500 g (5.5 lb) and an Apgar score of at least 8 at 5 minutes. Drews et al.[13] measured 26 males and 28 females who were considered full term (38 to 42 weeks), had a birth weight between 2000 and 4999 g, and had no pathology involving the lower extremities. Phelps et al.[15] measured 44 males and 44 females who had a gestational age between 37 and 42 weeks, an uncomplicated delivery, cephalad presentation, no history of hip trauma, and no observed abnormalities involving the hip.

In Table 7–3, the most notable effect of age is on hip extension ROM. Newborns and infants are unable to extend the hip from full flexion to the neutral position (returning to 0 degrees from flexion). Waugh et al.[12] found that all 40 infants tested lacked complete hip extension, with limitations ranging from 21.7 to 68.3 degrees. Phelps et al.[15] found that 100 percent of the 9- and 12-month-old infants tested ($N = 50$) had some degree of hip extension limitation. At 18 months, 89 percent had limitations, and at 24 months, 72 percent had limitations. The term "physiological limitation of motion" has been used by both Waugh et al.[12] and Walker[17] to describe this normal limitation of motion in infants. According to Walker, movement into extension evolves without the need for intervention and should not be considered pathological in newborns and infants. Usually a return from flexion to the neutral position is attained by 2 years of age. Extension (hyperextension) ROM approaching adult values usually is attained by early adolescence.

Another effect of age is noted by comparing ROM values for hip lateral and medial rotation in newborns and young

children in Table 7–3, with ROM values for older children and adults in Table 7–4. Hip lateral rotation values are larger for the infants and young children than for the adults. Also, in newborns and infants, the ROM values for lateral rotation exceed the values for medial rotation, whereas in children and adults, the medial rotation values are either the same as or exceed the values for lateral rotation.[8] The difference between ROM values presented in Table 7–3 and the values presented in Table 7–4 demonstrates the need for using age-appropriate norms whenever possible in making clinical judgments regarding children's ROM.

The values in Table 7–4 were obtained from measurements of active ROM using a universal goniometer. The subjects in the study by Boone[16] were males, whereas the subjects in the study by Roach and Miles[7] were both female and male.

The ROM values for all motions of the hip presented in Table 7–4 for the 6- to 12-year-olds do not appear to be substantially different from the ROM values for the 13- to 19-year-old group. Also, very little difference (less than one standard deviation) is evident between the ROM values for hip flexion and hip abduction in the 6- to 12-year-old group and the values for the 60- to 74-year-old group. The ROM values for medial and lateral rotation for the youngest groups reported by Boone[16] are two or more standard deviations greater than for the 60- to 74-year-old group reported by Roach and Miles.[7] Roach and Miles[7] have suggested that differences in AROM that represent less than 10 percent of the arc of motion are of little clinical significance. According to these authors, any substantial loss of mobility between 25 and 74 years of age should be viewed as abnormal and not attributable to aging.

Other authors who have investigated age or gender effects at the hip include Allander et al.,[18] Walker et al.,[19] Boone et al.,[20] and James and Parker.[21] Allander et al.[18] measured the ROM of different joints (shoulder, hip, wrist, and thumb MCP) in a population of 517 females and 203 males between 33 and 70 years of age. These authors found that older groups had significantly less hip rotation ROM than younger groups.

Walker et al.[19] measured 28 active motions (including all hip motions) in 30 women and 30 men ranging from 60 to 84 years of age. Although Walker et al. found no differences in hip ROM between the 60- to 69-year-old group and the 75- to 84-year-old group, both age groups demonstrated a reduced ability to attain a neutral starting position for hip flexion. The mean starting position for both groups for measurements of flexion ROM was 11 degrees instead of 0 degrees. The mean ROM values obtained for both age groups for hip rotation, abduction, and adduction were 14 to 25 degrees less than the average values published by the AAOS. This finding provides strong support for the use of age-appropriate norms.

Boone et al.[20] found significant differences for most hip motions when gender comparisons were made for three age

Table 7 – 3 EFFECTS OF AGE ON HIP MOTION IN NEWBORNS AND CHILDREN AGE 6 HR – 5 YR: MEAN VALUES IN DEGREES

	WAUGH ET AL.[12] 6–65 HR (N=40)		DREWS ET AL.[13] 12 HR–6 D (N=54)		WANATABE ET AL.[14] 4 WK (N=62)	4–8 MO (N=54)	PHELPS ET AL.[15] 9 MO (N=25)		18 MO (N=18)		BOONE[16] 1–5 YR (N=19)	
Motion	Mean	Standard Deviation	Mean	Standard Deviation	Mean	Mean	Mean	Standard Deviation	Mean	Standard Deviation	Mean	Standard Deviation
Flexion					138.0	136.0					123.2‡	5.8
Extension*	46.3	8.2†	28.3‡	6.0	12.0	4.0	10.0§	2.6	4.0§	3.2	0.8§	3.4§
Abduction			55.5†	9.5	51.0	55.0	59.0†	7.3	59.0†	5.4	59.3†	7.6
Adduction			6.4†	3.9							30.5†	4.4
Medial rotation			79.8†	9.3	24.0	39.0	41.0§	7.8	45.0§	7.6	55.0¶	5.0
Lateral rotation			113.7†	10.4	66.0	66.0	56.0§	6.6	52.0§	8.8	56.1¶	5.0

*All values in this row represent the magnitude of the limitation from 0 degrees of hip extension (neutral position).
†Tested in the supine position.
‡Tested in the side-lying position with the opposite hip maximally flexed.
§Tested in the prone position.
¶Tested in the sitting position.

Table 7 – 4 EFFECTS OF AGE ON HIP MOTION IN INDIVIDUALS AGE 6 – 74 YR OF AGE MEAN VALUES IN DEGREES

	BOONE[16] 6–12 YR (N=17)		13–19 YR (N=17)		ROACH AND MILES[7]* 25–39 YR (N=433)		40–59 YR (N=727)		60–74 YR (N=523)	
Motion	Mean	Standard Deviation	Mean	Standard Deviation	Mean	Standard Deviation	Mean	Standard Deviation	Mean	Standard Deviation
Flexion	124.4	5.9	122.6	5.2	122.0	12.0	120.0	14.0	118.0	13.0
Extension	10.4	7.5	11.6	5.0	22.0	8.0	18.0	7.0	17.0	8.0
Abduction	48.1	6.3	46.8	6.0	44.0	11.0	42.0	11.0	39.0	12.0
Adduction	27.6	3.8	26.3	2.9						
Medial rotation	48.4	4.8	47.1	5.2	33.0	7.0	31.0	8.0	30.0	7.0
Lateral rotation	47.5	3.2	47.4	5.2	34.0	8.0	32.0	8.0	29.0	9.0

*Values from Roach and Miles[7] reprinted from Physical Therapy with the permission of the American Physical Therapy Association.

groupings of males and females 1 to 69 years of age. Female children (1 to 9 years), young adult females (21 to 29 years) and older adult females (61 to 69 years) had significantly more hip flexion than their male counterparts. However, female children and young adult females had less hip adduction and outward rotation than males in comparison groups. Both young adult and older adult females had less hip extension ROM than males. Allander et al.[18] found that in five of eight age groups tested, females had a greater amount of hip rotation than males. Walker et al.[19] found that 30 females 60 to 84 years of age had 14 degrees more ROM in hip medial rotation than their male counterparts. In contrast to Walker et al., Phelps et al.[15] found no gender differences in hip rotation in 86 infants and young children (9 to 24 months).

James and Parker[21] measured active and passive ROM at the hip, knee, and ankle in 80 healthy men and women ranging from 70 to 92 years of age. Measurements of hip abduction ROM were taken with a universal goniometer. All other measurements were taken with a Leighton flexometer. Systematic decreases in both active and passive ROM were found from 70 to 92 years of age. Passive ROM was greater than active ROM for all joint motions tested, with the largest differences occurring in hip flexion with the knee flexed. Hip abduction decreased the most with age and was 33.4 percent less in the oldest group of men and women (85 to 92 years) compared with the youngest group (70 to 74 years). Medial and lateral rotation also decreased considerably, but the decrease was not as great as in abduction. In contrast, hip flexion with the knee either extended or flexed was least affected by age, with a significant reduction occurring only after 85 years of age. Women were significantly more mobile than men in 7 of the 10 motions tested.

RELIABILITY AND VALIDITY

Studies of the reliability of hip measurements have included both active and passive motion and different types of measuring instruments. Therefore, comparisons among studies are difficult. Boone et al.[22] and Clapper and Wolf[23] investigated the reliability of measurements of active ROM. Ekstrand et al.,[24] Pandya et al.,[25] and Ellison et al.[8] studied passive motion.

Boone et al.[22] conducted a study in which four physical therapists used a universal goniometer to measure active ROM of three upper-extremity and three lower-extremity motions in 12 male volunteers 26 to 54 years of age. One of the motions tested was hip abduction. Three measurements were taken by each tester at each of four sessions scheduled on a weekly basis for 4 weeks. Intratester reliability for hip abduction was $r = 0.75$, with a total stan-

dard deviation between measurements taken by the same testers of 4 degrees. Intertester reliability for hip abduction was $r = 0.55$, with a total standard deviation between measurements taken by different testers of 5.2 degrees.

Clapper and Wolf[23] compared the reliability of the Orthoranger (Orthotronics, Daytona Beach, FL), an electronic computerized pendulum goniometer, with the universal goniometer in a study of active hip motion involving 10 males and 10 females between the ages of 23 and 40 years. The authors found that the universal goniometer showed significantly less variation within sessions than the Orthoranger, except for measurements of hip adduction and lateral rotation. The authors concluded that the universal goniometer was a more reliable instrument than the Orthoranger. The poor relationship between the Orthoranger and the universal goniometer for hip adduction and abduction ROM values demonstrated that the two instruments could not be used interchangeably.

Ekstrand et al.[24] measured the passive ROM of hip flexion, extension, and abduction in 22 healthy men 20 to 30 years of age. They used a specially constructed goniometer to measure hip abduction and a flexometer to measure hip flexion and extension in two testing series. In the first series, the testing procedures were not controlled. In the second series, procedures were standardized and anatomical landmarks were indicated. The intratester coefficient of variation was lower than the intertester coefficient of variation for both series. Standardization of procedures improved reliability considerably. The intertester coefficient of variation was significantly lower in the second series than in the first series when the procedures were not standardized.

In a study by Pandya et al.,[25] five physical therapists using universal goniometers measured passive joint motions in the upper and lower extremities, including hip extension in 105 children and adolescents 1 to 20 years of age with Duchenne muscular dystrophy. Intratester reliability was high for all measurements; the ICC ranged from 0.81 to 0.94. The intratester reliability for measurements of hip extension was good (ICC = 0.85). The overall ICC for intertester reliability for all measurements ranged from 0.25 to 0.91. Intertester reliability for measurements of hip extension was fair (ICC = 0.74). The results indicated the need for the same examiner to take measurements for long-term follow-up and to assess the results of therapeutic intervention.

Ellison et al.[8] compared passive ROM measurements of hip rotation taken with an inclinometer and a universal goniometer and found no significant differences between the means. Both instruments were found to be reliable, but the authors preferred the inclinometer because it was easier to use.

TESTING PROCEDURES

FLEXION

Motion occurs in the sagittal plane around a medial-lateral axis.

Recommended Testing Position

Position the subject supine, with the hip in 0 degrees of abduction, adduction, and rotation. Initially the knee is extended, but as the range of hip flexion is completed, the knee is allowed to flex. If the knee is kept in extension, tension in the hamstring muscles will restrict the motion.

Stabilization

Stabilize the pelvis to prevent rotation or posterior tilting (Fig. 7–1).

Normal End-Feel

The end-feel is usually soft because of contact between the muscle bulk of the anterior thigh and the lower abdomen. However, the end-feel may be firm because of tension in the posterior joint capsule and the gluteus maximus muscle.

Goniometer Alignment

See Figures 7–2 and 7–3.

1. Center the fulcrum of the goniometer over the lateral aspect of the hip joint using the greater trochanter of the femur for reference.
2. Align the proximal arm with the lateral midline of the pelvis.
3. Align the distal arm with the lateral midline of the femur using the lateral epicondyle for reference.

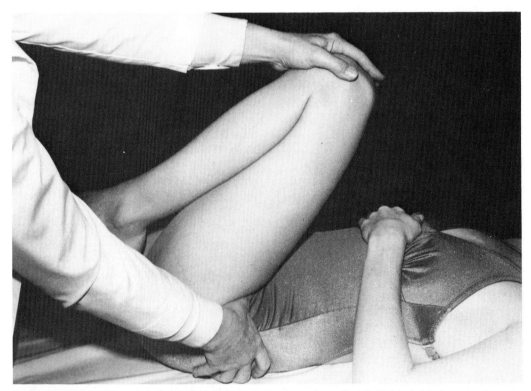

FIGURE 7–1. This photograph shows the left lower extremity at the end of the ROM in hip flexion. The examiner's left hand holds the hip in flexion by pushing on the distal femur. Stress on the knee joint is avoided, and the subject's knee is allowed to flex passively. Another hand placement that may be more comfortable for the subject is with the examiner's hand on the posterior surface of the distal femur. The end of the ROM occurs when the muscle bulk of the anterior thigh contacts the lower abdomen or when motion of the femur causes posterior tilting of the pelvis. The placement of the examiner's hand on the pelvis allows her to detect any pelvic motion.

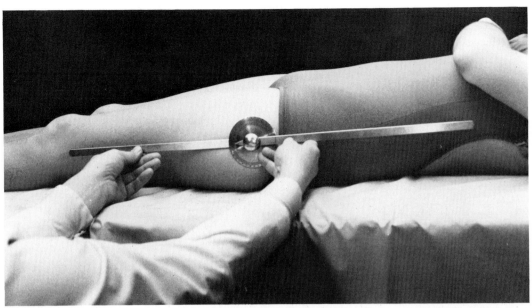

FIGURE 7–2. At the beginning of the ROM, the proximal arm of the goniometer is aligned along the lateral midline of the subject's pelvis. The fulcrum is centered over the greater trochanter, and the distal arm is aligned with the lateral midline of the femur using the femoral epicondyle for reference.

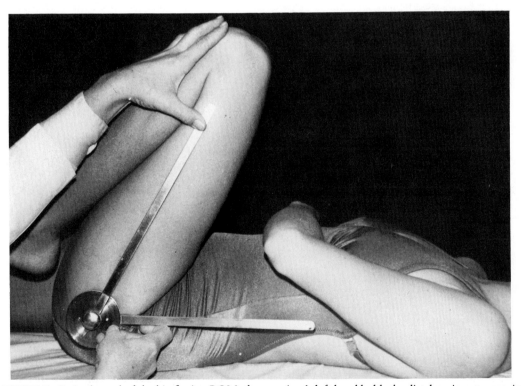

FIGURE 7–3. At the end of the hip flexion ROM, the examiner's left hand holds the distal goniometer arm in alignment and maintains the hip in flexion. The examiner's right hand holds the proximal goniometer arm aligned with the lateral midline of the subject's pelvis.

EXTENSION

Motion occurs in a sagittal plane around a medial-lateral axis.

Recommended Testing Position

Position the subject prone, with the hip in 0 degrees of abduction, adduction, and rotation. The knee is extended. If the knee is flexed, tension in the rectus femoris muscle will restrict the motion. No pillow is placed under the head.

Stabilization

Stabilize the pelvis to prevent rotation or anterior tilting (Fig. 7–4).

Normal End-Feel

The end-feel is firm because of tension in the anterior joint capsule, iliofemoral ligament, and to a lesser extent, the ischiofemoral and pubofemoral ligaments. On occasion, tension in various muscles that flex the hip, such as the iliopsoas, sartorius, tensor fasciae latae, gracilis, and adductor longus, may contribute to the firm end-feel.

Goniometer Alignment

The alignment is the same as for measuring hip flexion (Figs. 7–5 and 7–6).

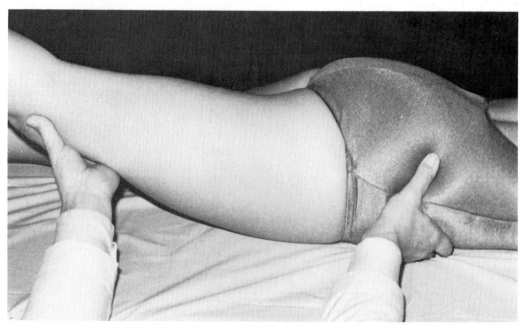

FIGURE 7–4. The subject's right lower extremity at the end of hip extension ROM. The examiner's left hand supports the distal femur and maintains the hip in extension while her right hand grasps the pelvis at the level of the anterior superior iliac spine. The end of the ROM occurs when movement of the femur produces anterior tilting of the pelvis. Because the examiner's right hand is on the subject's pelvis, the examiner is able to detect pelvic tilting.

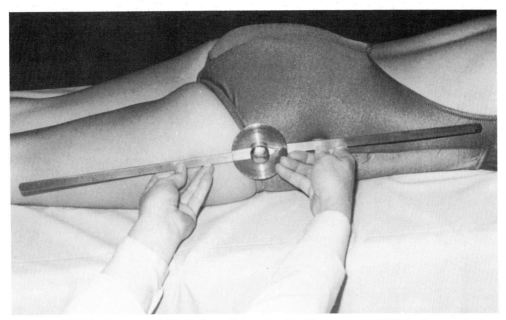

FIGURE 7–5. In the prone starting position for measuring hip extension ROM, the proximal goniometer arm is aligned with the lateral midline of the subject's pelvis. Using the lateral femoral epicondyle as a landmark, the examiner aligns the distal arm along the lateral midline of the thigh. She aligns the fulcrum over the greater trochanter.

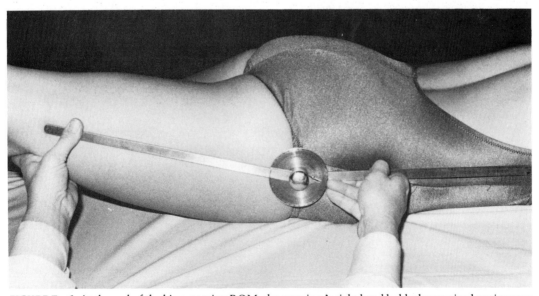

FIGURE 7–6. At the end of the hip extension ROM, the examiner's right hand holds the proximal goniometer arm in correct alignment. The examiner's left hand supports the subject's femur and keeps the distal goniometer arm in correct alignment.

ABDUCTION

Motion occurs in the frontal plane around an anterior-posterior axis.

Recommended Testing Position

Position the subject supine, with the hip in 0 degrees of flexion, extension, and rotation. The knee is extended.

Stabilization

Stabilize the pelvis to prevent rotation and lateral tilting (Fig. 7–7).

Normal End-Feel

The end-feel is firm because of tension in the inferior (medial) joint capsule, pubofemoral ligament, ischiofe-moral ligament, and inferior band of the iliofemoral ligament. Tension in the adductor magnus, adductor longus, adductor brevis, pectineus, and gracilis muscles may contribute to the firm end-feel.

Goniometer Alignment

See Figures 7–8 and 7–9.

1. Center the fulcrum of the goniometer over the anterior superior iliac spine (ASIS) of the extremity being measured.
2. Align the proximal arm with an imaginary horizontal line extending from one ASIS to the other ASIS.
3. Align the distal arm with the anterior midline of the femur using the midline of the patella for reference.

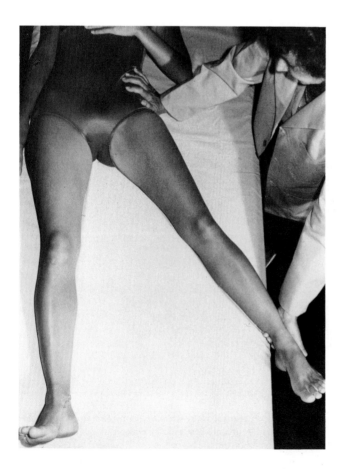

FIGURE 7–7. The left lower extremity at the end of the hip abduction ROM. The examiner uses her left hand to pull the subject's leg into abduction. The examiner's grip on the ankle is designed to prevent lateral rotation of the hip. The end of the ROM occurs when lateral motion of the extremity causes lateral tilting of the pelvis and lateral spinal flexion. The pelvic motion is detected by the examiner's right hand.

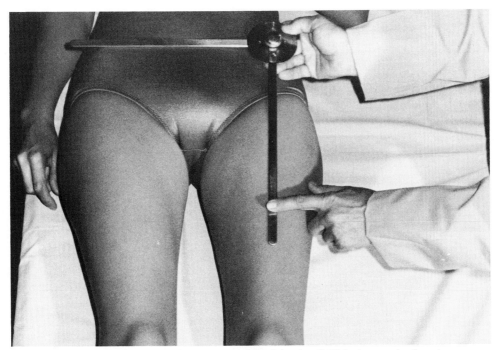

FIGURE 7–8. In the starting position for measuring hip abduction ROM, the proximal goniometer arm is aligned with the subject's anterior superior iliac spines. The distal arm is aligned with the midline of the patella. Although the goniometer is at 90 degrees, this is the 0-degree starting position. Therefore, the examiner must transpose her reading from 90 degrees to 0 degrees. For example, an actual reading of 90–120 degrees on the goniometer is recorded as 0–30 degrees.

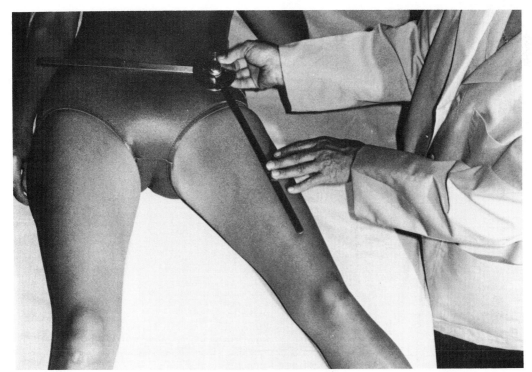

FIGURE 7–9. At the end of the hip abduction ROM, the distal goniometer arm is aligned with the midline of the patella, and the proximal arm is aligned with the anterior superior iliac spines.

ADDUCTION

Motion occurs in a frontal plane around an anterior-posterior axis.

Recommended Testing Position

The testing position is similar to the position used for measuring hip abduction. However, the contralateral hip is abducted to allow the hip being measured to complete its full range of adduction.

Stabilization

Stabilization is the same as for measuring hip abduction (Fig. 7–10).

Normal End-Feel

The end-feel is firm because of tension in the superior (lateral) joint capsule and the superior band of the iliofemoral ligament. Tension in the gluteus medius and minimus and the tensor fasciae latae muscles may also contribute to the firm end-feel.

Goniometer Alignment

Use the same alignment as that used for hip abduction, and see Figures 7–11 and 7–12.

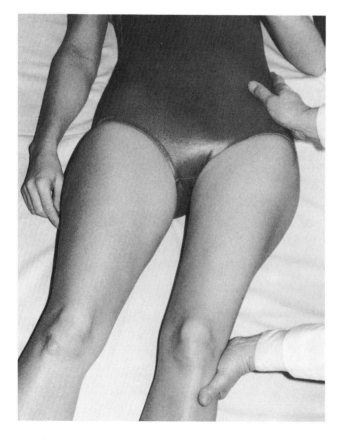

FIGURE 7–10. The subject's left lower extremity at the end of the hip adduction ROM. With her left hand, the examiner maintains the hip in adduction, and with her right hand she grasps the subject's pelvis. The end of the ROM occurs when further adduction of the extremity causes the subject's pelvis to tilt laterally; the examiner will be able to detect the lateral tilt through her hand on the subject's pelvis.

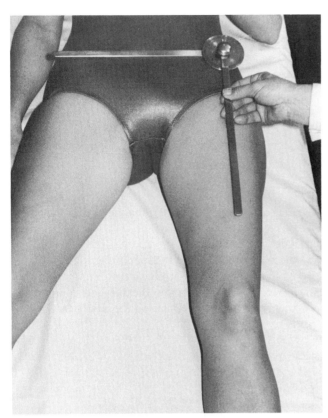

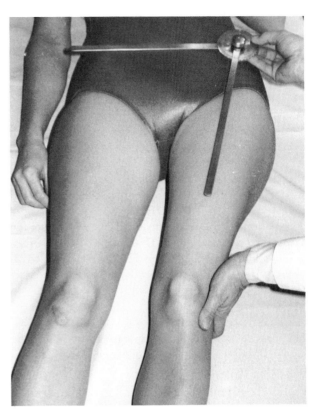

FIGURE 7 – 11. In the starting position for measuring left hip adduction, the subject's right lower extremity has been abducted to allow adequate space for adduction of the left lower extremity. The proximal goniometer arm is aligned with the subject's anterior superior iliac spines, and the distal arm is aligned along the anterior midline of the femur. This alignment places the goniometer at 90 degrees. Therefore, when the examiner records the measurement, she will transpose the reading so that 90 degrees is equivalent to 0 degrees. For example, an actual reading of 90 – 60 degrees is recorded as 0 – 30 degrees.

FIGURE 7 – 12. At the end of the hip adduction ROM, the examiner's right hand holds the goniometer body over the subject's anterior superior iliac spine. The examiner is able to prevent hip rotation by maintaining a firm grasp at the subject's knee.

MEDIAL (INTERNAL) ROTATION

Motion occurs in a transverse plane around a vertical axis when the subject is in anatomical position.

Recommended Testing Position

Position the subject sitting on a supporting surface, with the knees flexed to 90 degrees over the edge of the surface. The hip is in 0 degrees of abduction and adduction and in 90 degrees of flexion. A towel roll is placed under the distal end of the femur to maintain the femur in a horizontal plane.

As an alternative, measurements may be taken with the subject either supine or prone. The hip is in 0 degrees of abduction, adduction, and flexion. The knee is flexed to 90 degrees.

Stabilization

Stabilize the distal end of the femur to prevent adduction or further flexion of the hip. Avoid rotations and lateral tilting of the pelvis (Fig. 7–13).

Normal End-Feel

The end-feel is firm because of tension in the posterior joint capsule and the ischiofemoral ligament. Tension in the following muscles may also contribute to the firm end-feel: piriformis, obturatorii internus and externus, gemelli superior and inferior, quadratus femoris, the posterior fibers of the gluteus medius, and the gluteus maximus.

Goniometer Alignment

See Figures 7–14 and 7–15.

1. Center the fulcrum of the goniometer over the anterior aspect of the patella.
2. Align the proximal arm so that it is perpendicular to the floor or parallel to the supporting surface.
3. Align the distal arm with the anterior midline of the lower leg, using the crest of the tibia and a point midway between the two malleoli for reference.

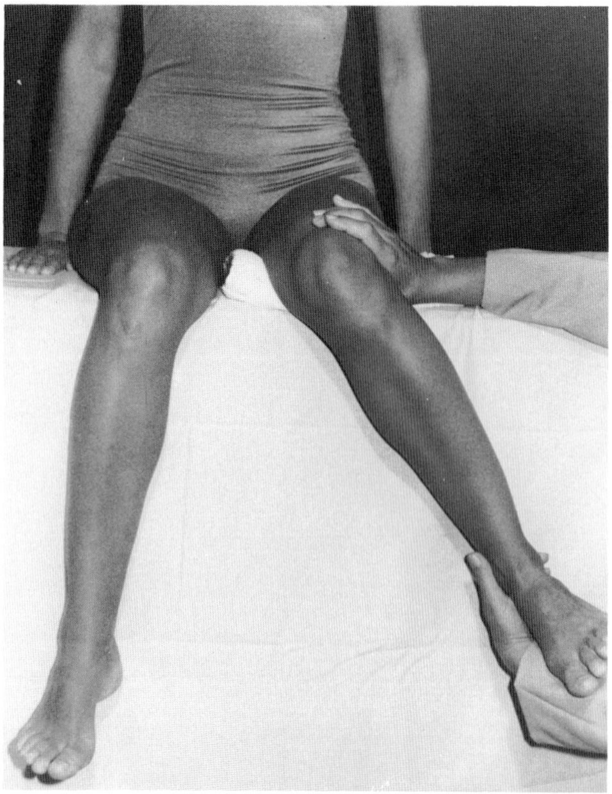

FIGURE 7–13. The left lower extremity at the end of the ROM of hip medial rotation. The examiner's right hand is placed on the subject's distal femur to prevent hip flexion and adduction.

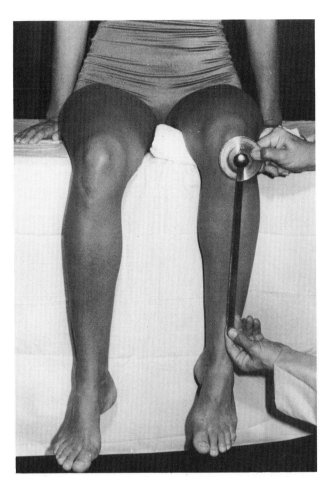

FIGURE 7 – 14. In the starting position for measuring hip rotation, the fulcrum of the goniometer is placed over the patella. Both arms of the instrument are together.

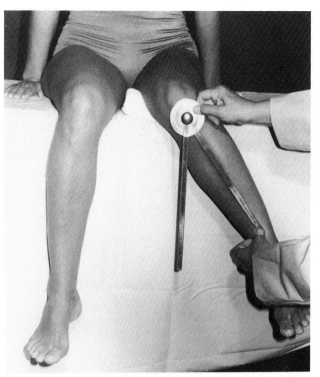

FIGURE 7 – 15. At the end of hip medial rotation, the proximal goniometer arm hangs freely so that it is perpendicular to the floor. The distal goniometer arm is aligned along the crest of the tibia.

LATERAL (EXTERNAL) ROTATION

Motion occurs in a transverse plane around a longitudinal axis when the subject is in anatomical position.

Recommended Testing Position

The testing position is similar to the position used to measure medial rotation of the hip. However, the contralateral knee may need to be flexed to allow the hip being measured to complete its full range of lateral rotation.

As an alternative, measurements may be taken with the subject either supine or prone as in the position used to measure medial rotation of the hip.

Stabilization

Stabilize the distal end of the femur to prevent abduction or further flexion of the hip. Avoid rotations and lateral tilting of the pelvis (Fig. 7–16).

Normal End-Feel

The end-feel is firm because of tension in the anterior joint capsule, iliofemoral ligament, and pubofemoral ligament. Tension in the anterior portion of the gluteus medius, gluteus minimus, adductor magnus and longus, pectineus, and piriformis muscles also may contribute to the firm end-feel.

Goniometer Alignment

The alignment is the same as for measuring medial rotation of the hip (Figs. 7–17 and 7–18).

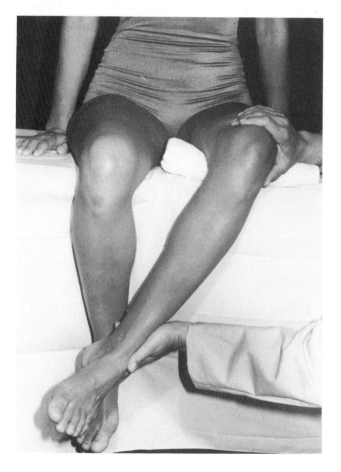

FIGURE 7–16. The left lower extremity is at the end of the ROM of hip lateral rotation. The examiner places her right hand on the subject's distal femur to prevent both hip flexion and hip abduction. The subject assists with stabilization by placing her hands on the supporting surface and shifting her weight over her left hip. The subject flexes her right knee to allow the left lower extremity to complete the ROM.

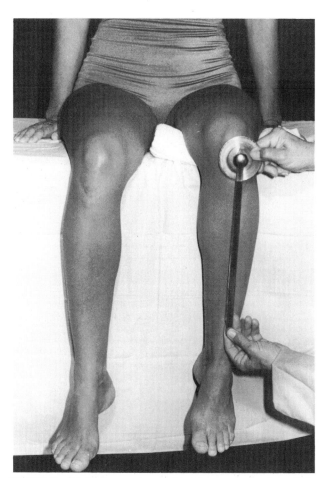

FIGURE 7 – 17. In the starting position for measuring lateral hip rotation, goniometer alignment is the same as that for measuring medial hip rotation.

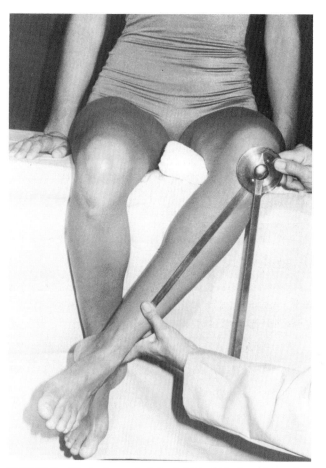

FIGURE 7 – 18. At the end of the ROM of hip lateral rotation, the examiner uses her left hand to support the subject's leg and to maintain alignment of the distal goniometer arm. When the examiner holds the goniometer body, the freely moving proximal arm hangs so that it is perpendicular to the floor.

REFERENCES

1. Norkin, CC and Levangie, PK: Joint Structure and Function: A Comprehensive Analysis, ed 2. FA Davis, Philadelphia, 1992.
2. Palmer, ML and Epley, M: Clinical Assessment Procedures in Physical Therapy. JB Lippincott, Philadelphia, 1990.
3. Cyriax, JH and Cyriax, PJ: Illustrated Manual of Orthopaedic Medicine. Butterworths, London, 1983.
4. American Academy of Orthopaedic Surgeons: Joint Motion: Method of Measuring and Recording. AAOS, Chicago, 1965.
5. American Medical Association: Guides to The Evaluation of Permanent Impairment, ed 3. AMA, Chicago, 1990.
6. Boone, DC and Azen, SP: Normal range of motion of joints in male subjects. J Bone Joint Surg Am 61:756, 1979.
7. Roach, KE and Miles, TP: Normal hip and knee active range of motion: The relationship to age. Phys Ther 71:656, 1991.
8. Ellison, JB, Rose, SJ, and Sahrman, SA: Patterns of hip rotation: A comparison between healthy subjects and patients with low back pain. Phys Ther 70:537, 1990.
9. Livingston, LA, Stevenson, JM, and Olney, SJ: Stairclimbing kinematics on stairs of differing dimensions. Arch Phys Med Rehabil 72:398, 1991.
10. Professional Staff Association, Rancho Los Amigos Medical Center: Observational Gait Analysis Handbook. Ranchos Los Amigos Medical Center, Downey, CA, 1989.
11. McFayden, BJ and Winter, DA: An integrated biomechanical analysis of normal stair ascent and descent. J Biomech 21:733, 1988.
12. Waugh, KG, et al: Measurement of selected hip, knee and ankle joint motions in newborns. Phys Ther 63:1616, 1983.
13. Drews, JE, Vraciu, JK, and Pellino, G: Range of motion of the joints of the lower extremities of newborns. Physical and Occupational Therapy in Pediatrics 4:49, 1984.
14. Wanatabe, H, et al: The range of joint motions of the extremities in healthy Japanese people: The difference according to age. Cited in Walker, JM: Musculoskeletal development: A review. Phys Ther 71:878, 1991.
15. Phelps, E, Smith, LJ, and Hallum, A: Normal range of hip motion of infants between nine and 24 months of age. Dev Med Child Neurol 27:785, 1985.
16. Boone, DC: Techniques of measurement of joint motion. (Unpublished supplement to Boone, DC and Azen, SP: Normal range of motion in male subjects. J Bone Joint Surg Am 61:756, 1979.)
17. Walker, JM: Musculoskeletal development: A review. Phys Ther 71:878, 1991.
18. Allander, E, et al: Normal range of joint movements in shoulder, hip, wrist and thumb with special reference to side: A comparison between two populations. Int J Epidemiol 3:253, 1974.
19. Walker, JM, et al: Active mobility of the extremities in older subjects. Phys Ther 64:919, 1984.
20. Boone, DC, Walker, JM, and Perry, J: Age and sex differences in lower extremity joint motion. Presented at National Conference, American Physical Therapy Association, Washington, DC, 1981.
21. James, B and Parker, AW: Active and passive mobility of lower limb joints in elderly men and women. Am J Phys Med Rehabil 68:162, 1989.
22. Boone, DC, et al: Reliability of goniometric measurements. Phys Ther 58:1355, 1978.
23. Clapper, MP and Wolf, SL: Comparison of the reliability of the Orthoranger and the standard goniometer for assessing active lower extremity range of motion. Phys Ther 68:214, 1988.
24. Ekstrand, J, et al: Lower extremity goniometric measurements: A study to determine their reliability. Arch Phys Med Rehabil 63:171, 1982.
25. Pandya, S, et al: Reliability of goniometric measurements in patients with Duchenne muscular dystrophy. Phys Ther 65:1339, 1985.

8

The Knee

STRUCTURE

The knee is composed of two distinct articulations enclosed within a single joint capsule: the tibiofemoral joint and the patellofemoral joint. The tibiofemoral joint links the femur and the tibia. The proximal joint surfaces are the convex medial and lateral condyles of the distal femur. The longer medial condyle is separated posteriorly and inferiorly from the lateral condyle by a deep groove called the intercondylar notch. The condyles are separated anteriorly by a shallow area of bone called the femoral patellar surface. The distal articulating surfaces are the two concave medial and lateral condyles on the proximal end of the tibia. The condylar surfaces are shallow, and the larger medial condyle is separated from the lateral condyle by two bony spines called the intercondylar tubercles. Two joint discs called menisci are attached to the articulating surfaces on the tibial condyles. The articulating surfaces of the patellofemoral joint are the posterior surface of the patella and the femoral patellar surface.

The joint capsule that encloses both joints is large, loose, and reinforced by tendons and expansions from the surrounding muscles and ligaments. The quadriceps tendon, the patellar ligament, and expansions from the extensor muscles provide anterior stability. The lateral and medial collateral ligaments, the iliotibial band, and the pes anserinus help to provide medial-lateral stability, and the knee flexors help to provide posterior stability. In addition, the tibiofemoral joint is reinforced by the anterior and posterior cruciate ligaments, which are located within the joint.

OSTEOKINEMATICS

The tibiofemoral joint is a double condyloid joint with 2 degrees of freedom. Flexion-extension occurs in the sagittal plane around a medial-lateral axis; rotation occurs in the transverse plane around a vertical (longitudinal) axis.[1] The incongruence and asymmetry of the tibiofemoral joint surfaces combined with muscle activity and ligamentous restraints produce an automatic rotation. This automatic rotation occurs primarily at the extreme of extension as motion stops on the shorter lateral condyle but continues on the longer medial condylar surface. During the last portion of the active extension ROM, automatic rotation produces what is referred to as either the screw-home mechanism or locking of the knee. To begin flexion, the knee must be unlocked by rotation in the opposite direction. For example, during non–weight-bearing active knee extension, lateral rotation of the tibia occurs during the last 10 to 15 degrees of extension to "lock" the knee. To "unlock" the knee that is "locked" in full extension, the tibia rotates medially. This rotation is not under voluntary control and should not be confused with the voluntary rotation movement possible at the joint.

The passive ROM in flexion is generally considered to be between 130 and 140 degrees. Hyperextension of 5 to 10 degrees is considered to be within normal limits.[2] The greatest range of knee rotation is at 90 degree of flexion, at which point about 45 degrees of lateral and 15 degrees of medial rotation are possible.

ARTHROKINEMATICS

The incongruence of the tibiofemoral joint and the fact that the femoral articulating surfaces are larger than the tibial articulating surfaces dictates that, when the femoral condyles are moving on the tibial condyles (in a weight-bearing situation), the femoral condyles must roll and slide to remain on the tibia. In weight-bearing flexion, the femoral condyles roll posteriorly and slide anteriorly. The menisci follow the roll of the condyles by distorting posteriorly in flexion. In extension, the femoral condyles roll anteriorly and slide posteriorly.[1] In the last portion of extension, motion stops at the lateral femoral condyle, but sliding continues on the medial femoral condyle to produce locking of the knee.

In non–weight-bearing active motion, the concave tibial articulating surfaces slide on the convex femoral condyles in the same direction as the movement of the shaft of the tibia. The tibial condyles slide posteriorly on the femoral condyles during flexion. During extension from full flexion, the tibial condyles slide anteriorly on the femoral condyles.

The patella slides superiorly in extension and inferiorly in flexion. Some patellar rotation and tilting accompany the sliding during flexion and extension.[1]

CAPSULAR PATTERN

The capsular pattern at the knee is characterized by a greater limitation of flexion than of extension and no restriction of rotations.[3,4]

RANGE OF MOTION

Table 8–1 provides knee ROM values from selected sources. The number and gender of the subjects measured to obtain values reported for the AAOS and the AMA in Table 8–1 are unknown. Boone and Azen[7] measured active ROM on male subjects using a universal goniometer. Roach and Miles[8] also measured active ROM using a uni-

versal goniometer, but their measurements were obtained from both males and females.

FUNCTIONAL RANGE OF MOTION

Table 8–2 provides knee ROM values required for various functional activities. The mean values presented from Jevsevar et al.[9] were obtained from laboratory measurements of both knees of 11 healthy subjects (six males and five females) ranging from 26 to 88 years of age. Among the activities measured (stair ascent and descent, gait, and rising from a chair), stair ascent required the greatest range of knee motion. Comparisons between the ROM of the healthy group of subjects and a group of postarthroplasty patients, who had been discharged from physical therapy services as fully rehabilitated, demonstrated that the post-patient population had significantly less knee ROM in all activities than the healthy subjects. The authors suggested that an increase in hip ROM may compensate for the decreased amount of knee ROM in the postarthroplasty group and that rehabilitation discharge criteria may need to be reassessed.

Livingston et al.[10] obtained their values from 15 healthy women ranging in age from 19 to 26 years. Data were collected by means of a high-speed camera. Three testing staircases (designated a, b, and c) were used with the following step heights and tread depths, respectively: (a: 20 cm, 21 cm; b: 20.3 cm, 30.5 cm; c: 12.7 cm, 41.9 cm). Maximum knee flexion values for staircases (a) and (b) were significantly different from values obtained for staircase (c). Shorter subjects used greater maximum knee flexion ranges (92 to 105 degrees) in comparison with taller subjects (83 to 96 degrees).

McFayden and Winter[11] obtained their values from eight trials by one subject. Stair dimensions were 22 cm for stair height and 28 cm for the stair tread. The Rancho Los Amigos Medical Center's[12] values for knee motion in gait are presented in Table 8–2 because these values are used as norms by many physical therapists. However, information about the population from which the values were derived was not supplied by the authors.

Table 8–1 **KNEE MOTION: MEAN VALUES IN DEGREES FROM SELECTED SOURCES**

Motion	AMERICAN ACADEMY OF ORTHOPAEDIC SURGEONS[5]	AMERICAN MEDICAL ASSOCIATION[6]	BOONE AND AZEN[7] 18 MO–54 YR (*N* = 109)		ROACH AND MILES[8] 25–74 YR (*N* = 1683)	
			Mean	Standard Deviation	Mean	Standard Deviation
Beginning position flexion			1.6	2.7		
Flexion	135	150	142.5	5.4	132.0	10.0
Hyperextension	10					

Table 8-2 **KNEE FLEXION RANGE OF MOTION NECESSARY FOR FUNCTIONAL ACTIVITIES: MEAN VALUES IN DEGREES FROM SELECTED SOURCES**

Motion (flexion)	JEVSEVAR ET AL.[9]		LIVINGSTON ET AL.[10]	McFAYDEN AND WINTER[11]	RANCHO LOS AMIGOS MEDICAL CENTER[12]	LAUBENTHAL ET AL.[13]	
	Mean Range	Standard Deviation	Mean Range	Mean Range	Mean Range	Mean Range	Standard Deviation
Walk on level surfaces	0–63.1	7.7			0–60.0		
Ascend stairs	0–92.9	9.4	2–105.0	10–100.0		9–83.0	8.4
Descend stairs	0–86.9	5.7	1–107.0	20–100.0			
Rise from chair	0–90.1	9.8					
Sit in chair						0–93.0	10.3
Tie shoes	0–106.0	9.3					

Laubenthal et al.[13] used an electrogoniometric method to measure knee motion in three planes (sagittal, coronal, and transverse) in 30 normal men with a mean age of 25 years.

EFFECTS OF AGE AND GENDER

Table 8-3 provides knee ROM values for newborns and children. The mean values and ranges presented in Table 8-3 from Waugh et al.,[14] Drews et al.,[15] and Wanatabe et al.[16] were derived from passive ROM measurements using a universal goniometer. The values presented from the study by Boone[17] were derived from measurements of active ROM in males using a universal goniometer. The infants in the study by Waugh et al.[14] included 18 males and 22 females. All infants met the following criteria: gestational age of at least 37 weeks, birth weight of at least 2500 g (5.5 lb), and an Apgar score of at least 8 at 5 minutes. Drews et al.[15] included 26 male and 28 female infants who were considered full term (38 to 42 weeks), had a birth weight between 2000 and 4999 g, and had no pathology involving the lower extremities.

Waugh et al.[14] and Drews et al.[15] found that newborns lacked approximately 15 to 20 degrees of knee extension (return from flexion to the zero starting position). These findings agree with the findings of Wanatabe et al.[16] who found that newborns lacked 14 degrees of knee extension. The 2-year-olds in the Wanatabe study had a complete ROM in extension (return from flexion to the neutral position) and up to 5 degrees of hyperextension. This finding is similar to the mean of 5.4 degrees of hyperextension for the group of 1- to 5-year-olds noted by Boone.[17]

Table 8-4 provides knee ROM values for adolescents and adults. The mean values presented in Table 8-4 were derived from measurements of active ROM using a universal goniometer. The mean values obtained by Boone[17] are from male subjects, whereas the values obtained by Roach and Miles[8] are from both males and females. A comparison of the knee extension mean values for the 13- to 19-year-olds in Table 8-4 with the extension values for the 1- to 5-year-olds in Table 8-3 shows that the 13- to 19-year-old group does not have any hyperextension. Values presented for the oldest groups (40 to 74 years of age) compared with the values for the youngest group show that the oldest groups have smaller mean values of flexion. However, with a standard deviation of 11 in the oldest groups, the difference between the youngest and oldest groups is not more than one standard deviation. Also, one should be aware that the values are derived from different investigators. Roach and Miles,[8] in their study that included knee motion

Table 8-3 **EFFECTS OF AGE ON KNEE MOTION: MEAN VALUES IN DEGREES FOR NEWBORNS AND CHILDREN AGE 6 HR–12 YR**

Motion	WAUGH ET AL.[14] 6–65 HR (N = 40)		DREWS ET AL.[15] 12 HR–6 DAYS (N = 54)		WANATABE ET AL.[16] 0–2 YR (N = 109)	BOONE[17] 1–5 YR (N = 19)		6–12 YR (N = 17)	
	Mean	Standard Deviation	Mean	Standard Deviation	Range of Means	Mean	Standard Deviation	Mean	Standard Deviation
Flexion					148–159	141.7	6.2	147.1	3.5
Extension	−15.3*	9.9	−20.4*	6.7		5.4†	3.1	0.4	0.9

*The minus sign indicates a limitation in extension (return to 0° from flexion).
†Indicates hyperextension.

Table 8–4 **EFFECTS OF AGE ON KNEE MOTION IN INDIVIDUALS AGE 13–74 YR: MEAN VALUES IN DEGREES FROM SELECTED SOURCES**

| Motion | BOONE[17] | | | | | | ROACH AND MILES[8] | | | |
| | 13–19 YR (N = 17) | | 20–29 YR (N = 19) | | 40–54 YR (N = 19) | | 40–59 YR (N = 727) | | 60–74 YR (N = 523) | |
	Mean	Standard Deviation	Mean	Standard Deviation	Mean	Standard Deviation	Mean	Standard Deviation	Mean	Standard Deviation
Flexion	142.9	3.7	140.2	5.2	142.6	5.6	132.0	11.0	131.0	11.0
Extension	0.0	0.0	0.4	0.9	1.6	2.4				

Values from Roach and Miles[8] reprinted from Physical Therapy with the permission of the American Physical Therapy Association.

in 1683 males and females 25 to 74 years of age, concluded that, at least up to 74 years of age, any substantial loss (greater than 10 percent of the arc of motion) in joint mobility should be viewed as abnormal and not attributable to the aging process. These authors found that the values they obtained were considerably smaller than the average values published by the AMA (see Table 8–1).

Beighton et al.,[18] in a study of joint laxity in 1081 males and females, found that females had more laxity than males at any age. These authors used more than 10 degrees of knee hyperextension as one of their criteria. They found that joint laxity decreased rapidly throughout childhood in both genders and decreased at a slower rate during adulthood.

Walker et al.[19] included the knee in a study of active ROM of the extremity joints in 30 men and 30 women ranging in age from 60 to 84 years. The men and women in the study were selected from recreational centers. No differences were found in knee ROM between the group of 60- to 69-year-olds and a group composed of 75- to 84-year-olds. However, average values indicated that the subjects had a limitation in extension (were unable to attain a neutral 0-degree starting position). This finding was similar to their findings for the hip, elbow, and first MTP joints. The 2-degree mean extension limitation found at the knee was much smaller than the limitation found at the hip joint.

Mollinger and Steffan,[20] in a study of knee ROM among 112 nursing home residents with an average age of 83 years, found that only 14 subjects were able to reach full passive knee extension. Thirty-seven subjects had between 1 and 5 degrees of limitation in extension bilaterally, and 14 had 6 to 10 degrees of limitation. The remainder had over 10 degrees of limitation in extension.

RELIABILITY AND VALIDITY

Reliability studies of active and passive range of knee motion have been conducted in healthy subjects, by Boone et al.,[21] Gogia et al.,[22] Rheault et al.,[23] and Enwemeka,[24] and in patient populations, by Rothstein et al.,[25] Watkins et al.,[26] and Pandya et al.[27] Boone et al.,[21] in a study in which

four testers using universal goniometers measured active ROM in knee flexion and extension on 12 subjects at four weekly sessions, found that intratester reliability was higher than intertester reliability. The total intratester standard deviation for measurements at the knee was 4 degrees, whereas the intertester standard deviation was 5.9 degrees. The authors recommended that when more than one tester measures the range of knee motion, changes in ROM should exceed 6 degrees to show that a real change has occurred.

Gogia et al.[22] studied the reliability and validity of joint angle measurements using a universal goniometer. Two physical therapists measured knee joint angles between 0 and 120 degrees of flexion on 30 volunteers (13 women and 17 men) between 20 and 60 years of age. These measurements were immediately followed by radiographs. Intertester reliability was high, with average correlation coefficients of 0.98 (r) and 0.99 (ICC). The correlation coefficients for validity also were high, ranging from 0.97 to 0.98 (r) and from 0.98 to 0.99 (ICC). The authors concluded that goniometric measurements were both reliable and valid.

Rheault et al.[23] investigated intertester reliability and concurrent validity of the universal goniometer and a fluid-based goniometer, using two testers who measured the active range of knee motion of 20 healthy subjects with a mean age of 24.8 years. These investigators found good intertester reliability for the universal goniometer ($r = 0.87$), and for the fluid-based goniometer ($r = 0.83$) for measurements of knee flexion. However, significant differences were found between the instruments for each tester. Therefore the authors concluded that although the universal and fluid-based goniometers each appeared to have good reliability and validity, they should not be used interchangeably in the clinical setting.

Enwemeka[24] compared the measurements of six knee joint positions (0, 15, 30, 45, 60, and 90 degrees) taken with a universal goniometer with radiographs of bone angle measurements. The measurements were taken on 10 healthy adult volunteers (four women and six men) between 21 and 35 years of age. The mean differences ranged from 0.52 to 3.81 degrees between goniometric and radiographic measurements taken between 30 and 90 degrees of flexion. However, the mean differences were higher (4.59 degrees) between goniometric and radiographic measurements of the angles between 0 and 15 degrees.

Rothstein et al.,[25] investigated intratester, intertester, and interdevice reliability in a study involving 24 patients referred for physical therapy. Intratester reliability for passive ROM measurements for flexion and extension was high. Intertester reliability also was high among the 12 testers for passive ROM measurements for flexion, but was relatively poor for knee extension measurements. Intertester reliability was not improved by repeated measurements, but was improved when testers used the same patient positioning. Interdevice reliability was high for all measurements. Neither the composition of the universal goniometer (metal or plastic) nor the size (large or small) had a significant effect on the measurements.

Watkins et al.[26] compared passive ROM measurements at the knee using a universal goniometer and visual estimates made by 14 physical therapists on 43 patients. These authors found that intratester reliability using the universal goniometer was high for both knee flexion (ICC = 0.99) and extension (ICC = 0.98). Intertester reliability for goniometric measurements also was high (ICC = 0.90) for knee flexion and good (ICC = 0.86) for knee extension. Intratester and intertester reliability were lower for visual estimation than for goniometric measurement. The authors suggested that therapists should not substitute visual estimates for goniometric measurements when assessing a patient's range of knee motion because of the additional error that is introduced using visual estimation. A patient's diagnosis did not appear to affect reliability except in the case of below-knee amputees. However, the small number of amputees in the patient sample prevented the authors from making any conclusions about reliability in this type of patient.

Pandya et al.[27] studied intratester and intertester reliability of knee extension passive ROM measurements in 150 children 1 to 20 years of age with a diagnosis of Duchenne muscular dystrophy. Intratester reliability using the universal goniometer was high (ICC = 0.93), but intertester reliability was only fair (ICC = 0.73).

TESTING PROCEDURES

FLEXION

Motion occurs in the sagittal plane around a medial-lateral axis.

Recommended Testing Position

The subject should be placed in the supine position with the knee in extension. Initially the hip is in 0 degrees of extension, abduction, and adduction, but as the knee begins to flex, the hip also flexes. If the rectus femoris muscle does not appear to be limiting the ROM, the subject may be placed in the prone position to obtain better stabilization.

Stabilization

Stabilize the femur to prevent rotation, abduction, and adduction of the hip (Fig. 8–1).

Normal End-Feel

Usually the end-feel is soft because of contact between the muscle bulk of the posterior calf and thigh or between the heel and the buttocks. The end-feel may be firm because of tension in the vastus medialis, vastus lateralis, and vastus intermedialis muscles.

Goniometer Alignment

See Figures 8–2 and 8–3.

1. Center the fulcrum of the goniometer over the lateral epicondyle of the femur.
2. Align the proximal arm with the lateral midline of the femur, using the greater trochanter for reference.
3. Align the distal arm with the lateral midline of the fibula, using the lateral malleolus and fibular head for reference.

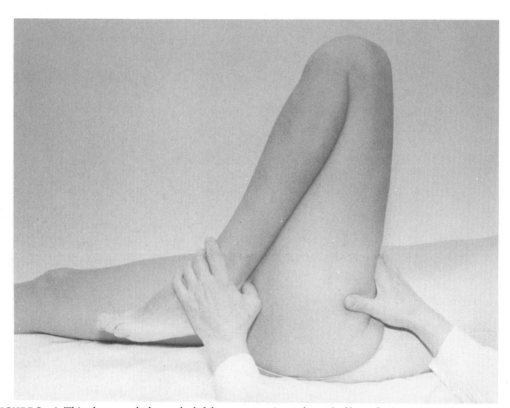

FIGURE 8–1. This photograph shows the left lower extremity at the end of knee flexion ROM. The examiner's right hand moves the subject's left thigh to approximately 90 degrees of hip flexion and then stabilizes the femur to prevent further flexion. The examiner's left hand guides the subject's lower leg through full knee flexion ROM. Usually, the amount and degree of compressibility of soft tissue present on the posterior surfaces of the lower extremity determine the extent of the flexion ROM.

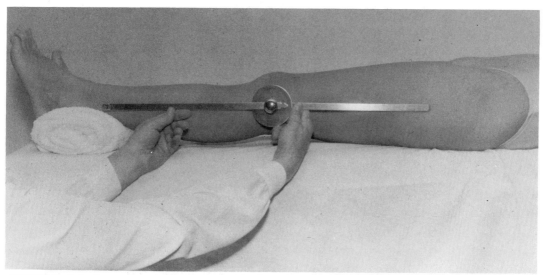

FIGURE 8–2. In the starting position for measuring knee flexion ROM, the subject is supine. A towel is placed under the ankle to allow the knee to extend fully. The examiner either kneels or sits on a stool in order to align and read the goniometer at eye level.

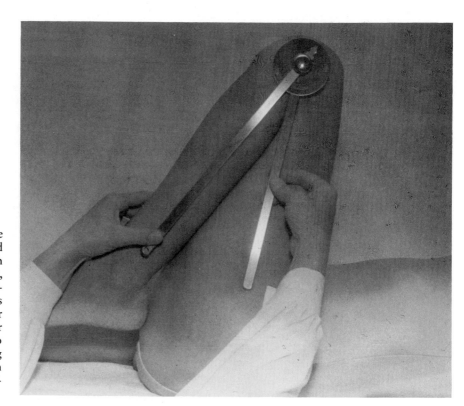

FIGURE 8–3. At the end of the knee flexion ROM, the examiner's right hand aligns the proximal goniometer arm with the lateral midline of the subject's thigh, using the greater trochanter as a reference point. The subject's upper thigh is exposed so that the greater trochanter may be palpated. The examiner uses her left hand to maintain knee flexion and to keep the distal goniometer aligned along the lateral midline of the lower leg, with the lateral malleolus and head of the fibula as reference points.

Alternative Testing Position

The subject is placed in the prone position, with the hip in 0 degrees of abduction, adduction, flexion, extension, and rotation. The foot is over the edge of the supporting surface.

Stabilization

Stabilize the femur to prevent rotation, abduction, adduction, flexion, or extension at the hip (Fig. 8–4).

Normal End-Feel

Usually the end-feel is soft because of contact between the muscle bulk of the posterior calf and thigh or between the heel and the buttocks. The end-feel may be firm because of tension in the rectus femoris muscle.

Goniometer Alignment

The alignment is the same as was described previously for the supine position (Figs. 8–5 and 8–6).

EXTENSION

Motion occurs in the sagittal plane around a medial-lateral axis.

Recommended Testing Position and Goniometer Alignment

The testing position and alignment are the same as for measuring knee flexion.

Stabilization

Stabilize the femur to prevent rotation, abduction, and adduction of the hip.

Normal End-Feel

The end-feel is firm because of tension in the posterior joint capsule, the oblique and arcuate popliteal ligaments, the collateral ligaments, and the anterior and posterior cruciate ligaments.

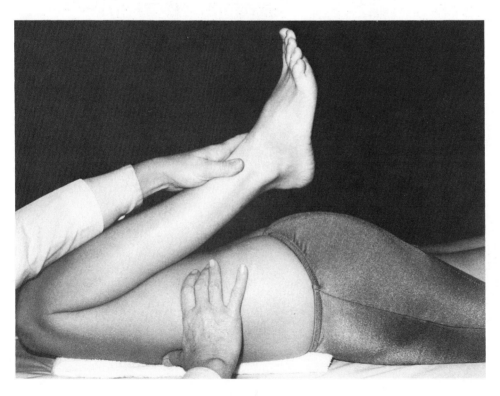

FIGURE 8–4. The right lower extremity at the end of knee flexion ROM in the alternative testing position. The examiner's right hand is on the proximal rather than the distal femur, so that the posterior surfaces of the distal thigh can make contact without interference. This alternative, prone-testing position allows for more stability than the supine position, but knee flexion ROM is often limited by the length of the rectus femoris muscle as well as contact between posterior thigh and lower leg.

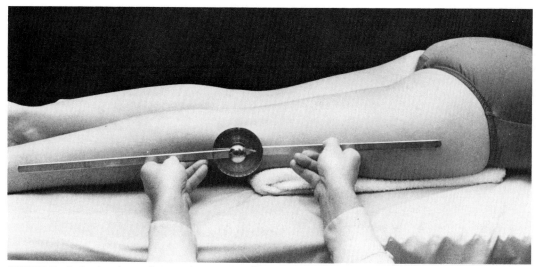

FIGURE 8-5. In the alternative starting position for measuring knee flexion ROM, the subject is prone. A towel is placed under the thigh, and the foot is off the supporting surface to allow the knee to extend fully.

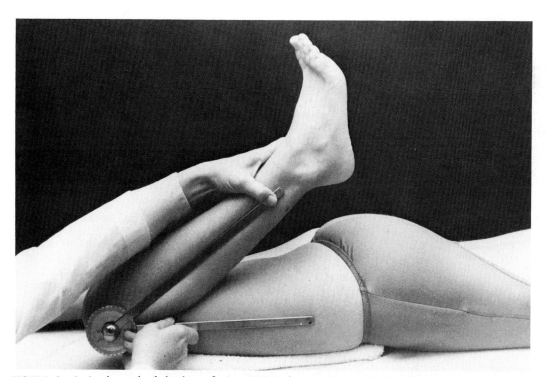

FIGURE 8-6. At the end of the knee flexion ROM, the examiner's right hand aligns the proximal goniometer arm with the lateral midline of the subject's thigh, using the greater trochanter as a reference point. The examiner uses her left hand to maintain knee flexion and to keep the distal goniometer arm aligned along the lateral midline of the lower leg.

REFERENCES

1. Norkin, CC and Levangie, PK: Joint Structure and Function: A Comprehensive Analysis, ed 2. FA Davis, Philadelphia, 1992.
2. Williams, PL and Warwick, R (eds): Gray's Anatomy, ed 37. WB Saunders, Philadelphia, 1985.
3. Kaltenborn, FM: Mobilization of the Extremity Joints. Olaf Norlis Bokhandel, Oslo, 1980.
4. Cyriax, JH and Cyriax, PJ: Illustrated Manual of Orthopaedic Medicine. Butterworths, London, 1983.
5. American Academy of Orthopaedic Surgeons: Joint Motion: Method of Measuring and Recording. AAOS, Chicago, 1965.
6. American Medical Association: Guides to the Evaluation of Permanent Impairment, ed 3 (revised). AMA, Chicago, 1990.
7. Boone, DC and Azen, SP: Normal range of motion of joints in male subjects. J Bone Joint Surg Am 61:756, 1979.
8. Roach, KE and Miles, TP: Normal hip and knee active range of motion: The relationship to age. Phys Ther 71:656, 1991.
9. Jevsevar, DS, et al: Knee kinematics and kinetics during locomotor activities of daily living in subjects with knee arthroplasty and in healthy control subjects. Phys Ther 73:229, 1993.
10. Livingston, LA, Stevenson, JM, and Olney, SJ: Stairclimbing kinematics on stairs of differing dimensions. Arch Phys Med Rehabil 72:398, 1991.
11. McFayden, BJ and Winter, DA: An integrated biomechanical analysis of normal stair ascent and descent. J Biomech 21:733, 1988.
12. Professional Staff Association, Rancho Los Amigos Medical Center: Observational Gait Analysis Handbook. Ranchos Los Amigos Medical Center, Downey, CA, 1989.
13. Laubenthal, KN, Smidt, GL, and Kettlekamp, DB: A quantitative analysis of knee motion during activities of daily living. Phys Ther 52:34, 1972.
14. Waugh, KG, et al: Measurement of selected hip, knee, and ankle joint motions in newborns. Phys Ther 63:1616, 1983.
15. Drews, JE, Vraciu, JK, and Pellino, G: Range of motion of the lower extremities of newborns. Physical and Occupational Therapy in Pediatrics 4:49, 1984.
16. Wanatabe, H, et al: The range of joint motions of the extremities in healthy Japanese people: The difference according to age. Cited in Walker, JM: Musculoskeletal development: A review. Phys Ther 71:878, 1991.
17. Boone, DC: Techniques of measurement of joint motion. (Unpublished supplement to Boone, DC and Azen, SP: Normal range of motion in male subjects. J Bone Joint Surg Am 61:756, 1979.)
18. Beighton, P, Solomon, L, and Soskolne, CL: Articular mobility in an African population. Ann Rheum Dis 32:23, 1973.
19. Walker, JM, et al: Active mobility of the extremities in older subjects. Phys Ther 64:919, 1984.
20. Mollinger, LA and Steffan, TM: Knee flexion contractures in institutionalized elderly: Prevalence, severity, stability and related variables. Phys Ther 73:437, 1993.
21. Boone, DC, et al: Reliability of goniometric measurements. Phys Ther 58:1355, 1978.
22. Gogia, PP, et al: Reliability and validity of goniometric measurements at the knee. Phys Ther 67:192, 1987.
23. Rheault, W, et al: Intertester reliability and concurrent validity of fluid-based and universal goniometers for active knee flexion. Phys Ther 68:1676, 1988.
24. Enwemeka, CS: Radiographic verification of knee goniometry. Scand J Rehabil Med 18:47, 1986.
25. Rothstein, JM, Miller, PJ, and Roettger, RF: Goniometric reliability in a clinical setting. Phys Ther 63:1611, 1983.
26. Watkins, MA, et al: Reliability of goniometric measurements and visual estimates of knee range of motion obtained in a clinical setting. Phys Ther 71:90, 1991.
27. Pandya, S, et al: Reliability of goniometric measurements in patients with Duchenne muscular dystrophy. Phys Ther 65:1339, 1985.

9

The Ankle and Foot

PROXIMAL AND DISTAL TIBIOFIBULAR AND TALOCRURAL JOINTS

STRUCTURE

The proximal tibiofibular joint is formed by a slightly convex tibial facet and a slightly concave fibular facet, and is surrounded by a joint capsule that is reinforced by anterior and posterior ligaments. The distal tibiofibular joint is formed by a fibrous union between a concave facet on the lateral aspect of the distal tibia and a convex facet on the distal fibula. The distal joint does not have a joint capsule but is supported by anterior and posterior ligaments and the crural interosseous tibiofibular ligament. Both joints are supported by the interosseous membrane, which is located between the tibia and the fibula.

The talocrural joint comprises the articulations between the talus and the distal tibia and fibula. The proximal joint surface is composed of the concave surfaces of the distal tibia and the tibial and fibular malleoli. The distal joint surface is the convex dome of the talus. The joint capsule is thin and weak anteriorly and posteriorly, and the joint is reinforced by medial and lateral ligaments. The deltoid ligament provides medial support, and the anterior and posterior talofibular ligaments and calcaneofibular ligament provide lateral support for the capsule and joint.

OSTEOKINEMATICS

The proximal and distal tibiofibular joints are anatomically distinct from the talocrural joint but function to serve the ankle. The proximal joint is a plane synovial joint that allows a small amount of superior and inferior sliding of the fibula on the tibia and a slight amount of rotation. The distal joint is a syndesmosis, or fibrous union.

The talocrural joint is a synovial hinge joint with 1 degree of freedom. The motions available are dorsiflexion and plantar flexion. These motions occur around an oblique axis and thus do not occur purely in the sagittal plane. The motions cross three planes and therefore are considered to be triplanar. Dorsiflexion of the ankle brings the foot up and slightly laterally, whereas plantar flexion brings the foot down and medially. The ankle is considered to be in the 0-degree neutral position when the foot is at a right angle to the tibia.

ARTHROKINEMATICS

During dorsiflexion of the ankle, the talus glides posteriorly, and the fibula moves proximally and laterally away from the tibia. During plantar flexion, the talus slides anteriorly, and the fibula moves distally, slightly anteriorly, and toward the tibia.

CAPSULAR PATTERN

The pattern is a greater limitation in plantar flexion than in dorsiflexion if the plantar flexor muscles are not shortened.[2]

SUBTALAR JOINT

STRUCTURE

The subtalar (talocalcaneal) joint is composed of posterior, anterior, and middle articulations between the talus and the calcaneus. The posterior articulation, which is the largest, is composed of a concave facet on the inferior surface of the talus and a convex facet on the body of the calcaneus. The anterior and middle articulations are formed by two convex facets on the talus and two concave facets on the calcaneus. The anterior and middle articulations share a joint capsule with the talonavicular joint; the posterior articulation has its own capsule. The subtalar joint is reinforced by anterior, posterior, lateral, and medial talocalcaneal ligaments and the interosseus talocalcaneal ligament.

OSTEOKINEMATICS

The subtalar joint is considered to be a plane synovial joint with 1 degree of freedom. The motions permitted at the joint are inversion and eversion, which occur around an oblique axis. These motions are composite motions consisting of abduction-adduction, flexion-extension, and supination-pronation. In non–weight-bearing inversion, the calcaneus adducts around an anterior-posterior axis, supinates around a longitudinal axis, and plantar flexes around a medial-lateral axis. In eversion, the calcaneus abducts, pronates, and dorsiflexes.

ARTHROKINEMATICS

The alternating convex and concave facets limit mobility and create a twisting motion of the calcaneus on the talus. In inversion of the foot, the calcaneus slides laterally on a fixed talus. In eversion, the calcaneus slides medially on the talus.[3]

CAPSULAR PATTERN

The capsular pattern consists of a greater limitation in inversion than in eversion.[2]

TRANSVERSE TARSAL (MIDTARSAL) JOINT

STRUCTURE

The transverse tarsal, or midtarsal, joint is a compound joint formed by the talonavicular and calcaneocuboid joints. The talonavicular joint is composed of the large convex head of the talus and the concave posterior portion of the navicular bone. The concavity is enlarged by the plantar calcaneonavicular ligament (spring ligament). The joint shares a capsule with the anterior and middle portions of the subtalar joint and is reinforced by the spring, bifurcate, and dorsal talonavicular ligaments.

The calcaneocuboid joint is composed of the shallow convex-concave surfaces on the anterior calcaneus and the convex-concave surfaces on the posterior cuboid. The joint is enclosed in a capsule that is reinforced by the bifurcate (calcaneocuboid), dorsal calcaneocuboid, plantar calcaneocuboid, and long plantar ligaments.

OSTEOKINEMATICS

The joint is considered to have two axes, one longitudinal and one oblique. Motions around both axes are triplanar and consist of inversion and eversion. The transverse tarsal joint is the transitional link between the hindfoot and forefoot.

ARTHROKINEMATICS

The concave navicular slides medially and dorsally on the convex talus in inversion. The navicular slides laterally and toward the plantar surface on the talus in eversion.

TARSOMETATARSAL JOINTS

STRUCTURE

The five tarsometatarsal (TMT) joints link the distal tarsals with the bases of the five metatarsals. The concave base of the first metatarsal articulates with the convex surface of the medial cuneiform. The bases of the second and third metatarsals articulate with the mortise formed by the intermedial cuneiform and the sides of the medial and lateral cuneiforms. The base of the third metatarsal articulates with the lateral cuneiform, and the bases of the fourth and fifth metatarsals articulate with the cuboid. The first joint has its own capsule, whereas the second and third and the fourth and fifth joints share capsules. Each joint is reinforced by numerous dorsal, plantar, and interosseous ligaments.

OSTEOKINEMATICS

The TMT joints are plane synovial joints that permit gliding motions, including flexion-extension, a minimal amount of abduction-adduction, and rotation. The type and amount of motion vary at each joint. For example, at the third TMT joint, the predominant motion is flexion-extension. The combination of motions at the various joints contributes to the hollowing and flattening of the foot, which helps the foot conform to a supporting surface.

ARTHROKINEMATICS

The distal joint surfaces glide in the same direction as the shafts of the metatarsals.

METATARSOPHALANGEAL JOINTS

STRUCTURE

The five MTP joints are formed proximally by the convex heads of the five metatarsals and distally by the concave bases of the proximal phalanges. The first MTP joint has two sesamoid bones, which lie in two grooves on the plantar surface of the distal metatarsal. The four lesser toes are interconnected on the plantar surface by the deep transverse metatarsal ligament. The plantar aponeurosis helps to provide stability and limits extension.

OSTEOKINEMATICS

The five MTP joints are condyloid synovial joints with 2 degrees of freedom, permitting flexion-extension and abduction-adduction. The axis for flexion-extension is oblique and is referred to as the metatarsal break. The ROM in extension is greater than in flexion, but the total ROM varies according to the relative lengths of the metatarsals and weight-bearing status.

ARTHROKINEMATICS

In flexion, the bases of the phalanges slide in a plantar direction on the heads of the metatarsals. In abduction, the concave bases of the phalanges slide on the convex heads of the metatarsals in a lateral direction away from the second toe. In adduction, the bases of the phalanges slide in a medial direction toward the second toe.

CAPSULAR PATTERN

The pattern at the first MTP joint is greater limitation in extension than in flexion. At the other joints (second to fifth), the limitation is variable.[2]

INTERPHALANGEAL JOINTS

STRUCTURE

The structure of the IP joints is identical to the structure of the IP joints of the fingers. Each IP joint is composed of the concave base of a distal phalanx and the convex head of a proximal phalanx.

OSTEOKINEMATICS

The IP joints are synovial hinge joints with 1 degree of freedom. The motions permitted are flexion and extension in the sagittal plane. Each joint is enclosed in a capsule and reinforced with collateral ligaments.

ARTHROKINEMATICS

The concave base of the distal phalanx slides on the convex head of the proximal phalanx in the same direction as the shaft of the distal bone. The concave base slides toward the plantar surface of the foot during flexion and toward the dorsum of the foot during extension.

RANGE OF MOTION

Tables 9–1 and 9–2 provide ankle and the ROM values from various sources. The age, gender, and number of the subjects who were measured to obtain values reported for the AAOS and the AMA in Tables 9–1 and 9–2 are unknown. Boone and Azen[6] measured active ROM on male subjects using a universal goniometer.

FUNCTIONAL RANGE OF MOTION

Table 9–3 provides ankle ROM values for functional locomotor activities. Livingston et al.[8] derived their mean values using cinematography and computer analysis. Subjects were 15 physically active women ranging from 19 to 26 years of age. Fifteen trials of stair ascent and descent were made on each of three test staircases.

Table 9–1 **ANKLE MOTION: MEAN VALUES IN DEGREES FROM SELECTED SOURCES**

| Motion | AMERICAN ACADEMY OF ORTHOPAEDIC SURGEONS[4] | AMERICAN MEDICAL ASSOCIATION[5] | BOONE AND AZEN[6] 1–54 YR ($N = 109$) | |
			Mean	Standard Deviation
Dorsiflexion	20.0	20.0	12.6	4.4
Plantar flexion	50.0	40.0	56.2	6.1
Forefoot inversion	35.0	30.0*	36.8†	4.5
Forefoot eversion	15.0	20.0*	20.7†	5.0
Hindfoot inversion	5.0			
Hindfoot eversion	5.0			

*Values represent visual estimation of arc of motion.
†Forefoot measurement only.

Table 9–2 **TOE MOTION: MEAN VALUES IN DEGREES FROM SELECTED SOURCES**

Joint	EXTENSION AMERICAN MEDICAL ASSOCIATION[5]	EXTENSION AMERICAN ACADEMY OF ORTHOPAEDIC SURGEONS[4]	FLEXION AMERICAN MEDICAL ASSOCIATION[5]	FLEXION AMERICAN ACADEMY OF ORTHOPAEDIC SURGEONS[4]
MTP1	50.0	70.0	30.0	45.0
2	40.0	40.0	30.0	40.0
3	30.0	40.0	20.0	40.0
4	20.0	40.0	10.0	40.0
5	10.0	40.0	10.0	40.0
IP1			30.0	90.0
PIP2–5				35.0
DIP2–5	30.0			60.0

EFFECTS OF AGE AND GENDER

Table 9–4 presents the effects of age on ankle motion in newborns and children. All values presented in Table 9–4 were obtained with a universal goniometer. Passive ROM was measured in each study, with the exception of the study by Boone,[14] in which active ROM was measured. Males and females were included in each study except for the study by Boone, which included only male subjects. The infants in the study by Waugh et al.[12] included 18 males and 22 females. All infants met the following criteria: gestational age of at least 37 weeks, birth weight of at least 2500 g (5.5 lb), and an Apgar score of at least 8 at 5 minutes.

The most noticeable effect of age on ankle ROM is that newborn, infant, and young children have a greater amount of dorsiflexion than adults (see Tables 9–1 and 9–4). The mean values for dorsiflexion in the youngest age groups are more than double the values published by the AAOS and AMA as average values for adults. Also, it is evident from Tables 9–4 and 9–5 that newborns (6 to 72 hours old) have

less plantar flexion than adults. However, the plantar flexion values reach average adult values within the first few weeks of life. According to Walker,[15] the persistence in infants of less than normal adult values for plantar flexion may indicate pathology.

Table 9–5 presents the effects of age on ankle motion in individuals 13 to 69 years of age. A universal goniometer was used to obtain the active ROM measurements in Table 9–5. The subjects in the study by Boone[14] were males, whereas the subjects in the study by Boone et al.[16] were both males and females. The dorsiflexion values in the oldest group are smaller than the values for the younger groups, but the difference constitutes less than one standard deviation. The values for plantar flexion in the oldest group are more than one standard deviation less than the values for the youngest group.

The only gender differences noted by Boone et al.[16] were that females in the 1- to 9-year-old and 61- to 69-year-old groups had significantly more ROM in plantar flexion than males in the same age groups. Two other studies found that women had more plantar flexion than men. Bell and Ho-

Table 9–3 RANGE OF ANKLE MOTION NECESSARY FOR FUNCTIONAL LOCOMOTOR ACTIVITIES: VALUES IN DEGREES

	Gait Level Surfaces	Stair Ascent	Stair Descent
Dorsiflexion	0–10 (Murray[7]) 0–15 (Rancho Los Amigos Medical Center[9]) 0–15 (Ostrosky et al.[11])	14–27 (Livingston et al.[8]) 15–25 (McFayden and Winter[10])	20–35 (Livingston et al.[8])
Plantar flexion	15–30 (Murray[7]) 0–20 (Rancho Los Amigos Medical Center[9]) 0–31 (Ostrosky et al.[11])	23–30 (Livingston et al.[8]) 15–25 (McFayden and Winter[10])	20–30 (Livingston et al.[8])

shizaki[17] studied 17 joint motions in 124 females and 66 males ranging in age from 18 to 88 years. These authors found that females between 17 and 30 years of age had a greater ROM in both dorsiflexion and plantar flexion than males in the same age groups. Walker et al.[18] studied active ROM in 30 men and 30 women ranging in age from 60 to 84 years. In their study, women had 11 degrees more ROM in ankle plantar flexion than men. Also, both men and women had less flexion ROM of the first MTP joint (mean of 6 degrees) than values reported by the AMA and AAOS.

RELIABILITY AND VALIDITY

Reliability studies involving one or more motions at the ankle have been conducted on healthy subjects by Boone et al.,[19] Clapper and Wolf,[20] and Bohannon et al.,[21] and on patient populations by Elveru et al.[22] and Youdas et al.[23] Also, the following authors have investigated motions of the subtalar joint and the subtalar joint neutral position: Elveru et al.,[24] Elveru et al.,[22] Bailey et al.,[25] Lattanza et al.,[26] and Picciano et al.[27]

As with findings at other joints, intratester reliability has

been found to be greater than intertester reliability for ROM measurements at the ankle and foot using the universal goniometer. In the study by Boone et al.,[19] intratester reliability for selected motions at the ankle was found to be higher than values obtained for hip and wrist motions but lower than values obtained for selected motions at the shoulder, elbow, and knee.

Clapper and Wolf,[20] in a study involving 10 females and 10 males with mean ages of 30 years and 28.3 years, respectively, found that both the universal goniometer and the Orthoranger (Orthotronics, Daytona Beach, FL) were reliable instruments but that the ICCs were higher for the universal goniometer. The ICC for measurements of active dorsiflexion for the universal goniometer was 0.92, in comparison with 0.80 for the Orthoranger. The ICC for the goniometer for plantar flexion was 0.96, whereas the ICC for the Orthoranger was 0.93. Considering the fact that the Orthoranger, a type of pendulum goniometer, costs considerably more than a universal goniometer, the authors concluded that the additional cost involved in purchasing an Orthoranger to measure ROM could not be justified.

Bohannon et al.,[21] in a study involving 11 males and 11 females 21 to 43 years of age, investigated the passive ROM

Table 9–4 EFFECTS OF AGE ON ANKLE MOTION: MEAN VALUES IN NEWBORNS AND CHILDREN AGE 6–12 YR

	WAUGH ET AL.[12]		WANATABE ET AL.[13]			BOONE[14]			
	6–72 HR (N = 40)		2–4 WK (N = 57)	4–8 MO (N = 54)	2 YR (N = 57)	1–5 YR (N = 19)		6–12 YR (N = 17)	
Motion	Mean	Standard Deviation	Mean Range			Mean	Standard Deviation	Mean	Standard Deviation
Dorsiflexion	58.9	7.9	0–53.0	0–51.0	0–41.0	14.5	5.0	13.8	4.4
Plantar flexion	25.7	6.3	0–58.0	0–60.0	0–62.0	59.7	5.4	59.6	4.7

Table 9–5 **EFFECTS OF AGE ON ACTIVE ANKLE MOTION: MEAN VALUES IN DEGREES FOR INDIVIDUALS 13–69 YR OF AGE**

| | BOONE[14] | | | | | | | | BOONE ET AL.[16] | |
| | 13–19 YR (N = 17) | | 20–29 YR (N = 19) | | 30–39 YR (N = 18) | | 40–54 YR (N = 19) | | 61–69 YR (N = 10) | |
Motion	Mean	Standard Deviation	Mean	Standard Deviation	Mean	Standard Deviation	Mean	Standard Deviation	Mean	Standard Deviation
Dorsiflexion	10.6	3.7	12.1	3.4	12.2	4.3	12.4	4.7	8.2	4.6
Plantar flexion	55.5	5.7	55.4	3.6	54.6	6.0	52.9	7.6	46.2	7.7

for ankle dorsiflexion using different goniometer alignments. In one alignment, the arms of the goniometer were aligned with the fibula and the heel. The second alignment used the fibula and a line parallel to the fifth metatarsal. These authors found that passive ROM measurements for dorsiflexion differed significantly according to which landmarks were used.

Elveru et al.[22] employed 12 physical therapists using universal goniometers to measure the passive ROM in inversion and eversion on 43 patients with either neurological or orthopedic problems. The authors found that the ICCs for intratester reliability for inversion and eversion were 0.74 and 0.75, respectively. Intertester reliability was poor for dorsiflexion, and patient diagnosis affected the reliability of dorsiflexion measurements. Sources of error were identified as variable amounts of force being exerted by the therapist, resistance to movement in neurological patients, and difficulties in maintaining the foot and ankle in the desired position while holding the goniometer.

Youdas et al.[23] examined intratester and intertester reliability for active ROM in dorsiflexion and plantar flexion using a universal goniometer and visual estimation. Ten physical therapists measured ROM on 38 patients with orthopedic problems. The authors concluded that considerable measurement error exists when two or more therapists make either repeated goniometric or visual estimates of the ankle ROM on the same patient. The authors suggested that a single therapist should use a goniometer when making repeated measurements of ankle ROM.

The subtalar joint neutral position, which has been the subject of numerous studies, is not the same as the zero starting position for the subtalar joint used in this book and many others, including those of the AAOS,[4] the AMA,[5] Clarkson and Gilewich,[28] and Palmer and Epler.[29] The subtalar joint neutral position under investigation is defined as one in which the calcaneus will invert twice as many degrees as it will evert. According to Elveru et al.,[24] this position can be found when the head of the talus either cannot

be palpated or is equally extended at the medial and lateral borders of the talonavicular joint. This is the position usually used in casting for foot orthotics, but it also has been used for measurement of joint motion. We have not elected to use the subtalar neutral position as defined by Elveru et al., because according to the following studies, use of the position adds error to ROM measurements.

Bailey et al.[25] used tomography to study the subtalar joint neutral position in 2 female and 13 male volunteers 20 to 30 years of age. These authors found that the neutral subtalar joint position was quite variable in relation to the total ROM, and that it was not always found at one third of the total ROM from the maximally everted position. Furthermore, the neutral position varied not only from subject to subject but also between the right and left sides of each subject.

Elveru et al.[24] proposed a method for measuring the subtalar joint neutral position and the passive ROM. The authors described the necessary palpation and the testing position for the foot and lower extremities. Elveru et al.[22] found that referencing passive ROM measurements for inversion and eversion to the subtalar joint neutral position consistently reduced reliability.

Lattanza et al.[26] measured subtalar joint eversion in weight bearing and non–weight bearing on 15 female and 2 male subjects. Measurements of subtalar joint eversion in a weight-bearing posture were found to be significantly greater than in a non–weight-bearing posture. The ROM in weight bearing was 5 to 16 degrees with a mean of 10.4 degrees, whereas the range of eversion in non–weight bearing ranged from 3 to 10 degrees with a mean of 6.6 degrees. The authors advocated measurement in both positions.

Picciano et al.[27] conducted a study to determine the intratester and intertester reliability of measurements of open- and closed-chain subtalar joint neutral positions. Both ankles of 15 volunteer subjects, with a mean age of 27.06 years, were measured by two inexperienced physical therapy students. The students had a 2-hour training session prior to data collection using a universal goniometer. The method of taking measurements was based on the work of Elveru et al.[22,24] Intratester reliability of open-chain measurements of the subtalar joint neutral position was ICC = 0.27 for one tester and ICC = 0.06 for the other tester. Intertester reliability was 0.00. Intratester and intertester reliability also were poor for closed–kinematic-chain measurements. Picciano et al.[27] concluded that subtalar joint neutral measurements taken by inexperienced testers are unreliable, and recommended that clinicians determine their own reliability for these measurements.

TESTING PROCEDURES: TALOCRURAL JOINT

DORSIFLEXION

Motion occurs in the sagittal plane around a medial-lateral axis.

Recommended Testing Position

Position the subject sitting or supine, with knee flexed at least 30 degrees. The foot is positioned in 0 degrees of inversion and eversion.

Stabilization

Stabilize the tibia and fibula to prevent knee motion and hip rotation (Fig. 9–1).

Normal End-Feel

The end-feel is firm because of tension in the posterior joint capsule, the Achilles tendon, the posterior portion of the deltoid ligament, the posterior talofibular ligament, and the calcaneofibular ligament.

Goniometer Alignment

See Figures 9–2 and 9–3.

1. Center the fulcrum of the goniometer over the lateral aspect of the lateral malleolus.
2. Align the proximal arm with the lateral midline of the fibula, using the head of the fibula for reference.
3. Align the distal arm parallel to the lateral aspect of the fifth metatarsal. Although it is usually easier to palpate and align the distal arm parallel to the fifth metatarsal, as an alternative, the distal arm can be aligned parallel to the inferior aspect of the calcaneus. However, if the alternative landmark is used, the total ROM in the sagittal plane (dorsiflexion plus plantar flexion) may be similar to the total ROM of the preferred technique, but the separate ROM values for dorsiflexion and plantar flexion will differ considerably.

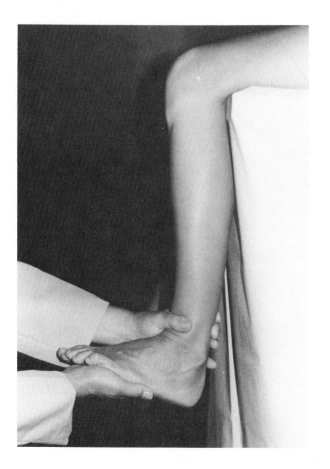

FIGURE 9–1. This photograph shows the left ankle at the end of the dorsiflexion ROM. The examiner holds the distal portion of the lower leg with her left hand to prevent knee motion. The examiner's right hand pushes upward on the plantar surface of the subject's foot to produce dorsiflexion. The examiner avoids pushing on the toes. A considerable amount of upward force is necessary to overcome the tension in the Achilles tendon. Often, comparing the active and passive ranges of motion helps to determine the amount of upward force necessary to complete the passive ROM in dorsiflexion for a particular individual. If this position is awkward for the examiner, the subject may be positioned in supine with the knee flexed to 30 degrees and supported by a pillow.

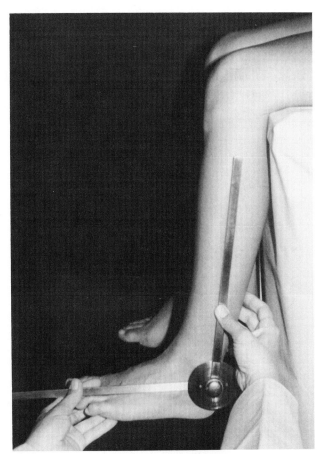

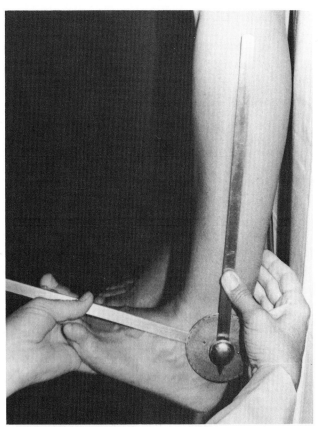

FIGURE 9 – 2. In the starting position for measuring dorsiflexion ROM, the examiner aligns the proximal arm of the goniometer with the lateral midline of the lower leg, using the head of the fibula as a reference point. The examiner aligns the distal goniometer arm parallel to the fifth metatarsal. The ankle is positioned so that the goniometer is at 90 degrees. However, this goniometer reading is transposed and recorded as 0 degrees. The examiner sits on a stool or kneels in order to align and read the goniometer at eye level.

FIGURE 9 – 3. At the end of dorsiflexion, the examiner's right hand aligns the proximal goniometer arm, while the examiner's left hand maintains dorsiflexion and alignment of the distal goniometer arm.

PLANTAR FLEXION

Motion occurs in the sagittal plane around a medial-lateral axis.

Recommended Testing Position

The testing position and alignment are the same as for ankle dorsiflexion.

Stabilization

Stabilize the tibia and fibula to prevent knee flexion and hip rotation (Fig. 9–4).

Normal End-Feel

Usually the end-feel is firm because of tension in the anterior joint capsule; the anterior portion of the deltoid ligament; the anterior talofibular ligament; and the tibialis anterior, extensor hallucis longus, and extensor digitorum longus muscles. The end-feel may be hard because of contact between the posterior tubercles of the talus and the posterior margin of the tibia.

Goniometer Alignment

The alignment is the same as for ankle dorsiflexion (Figs. 9–5 and 9–6).

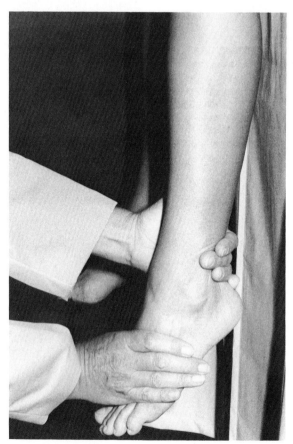

FIGURE 9–4. This photograph shows the left ankle at the end of the plantar flexion ROM. The examiner holds the subject's lower leg to prevent knee flexion. The examiner's right hand pushes downward on the dorsum of the subject's foot to produce plantar flexion. The examiner exerts no force on the subject's toes and is careful to avoid pushing the ankle into inversion or eversion.

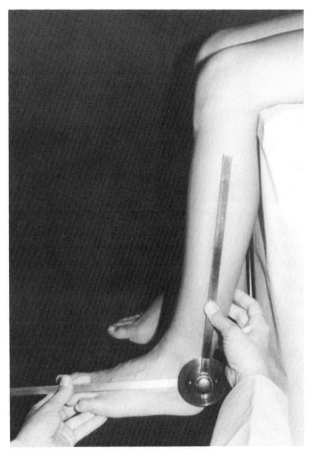

FIGURE 9–5. The starting position and goniometer alignment for measuring plantar flexion ROM are the same as those for measuring dorsiflexion ROM.

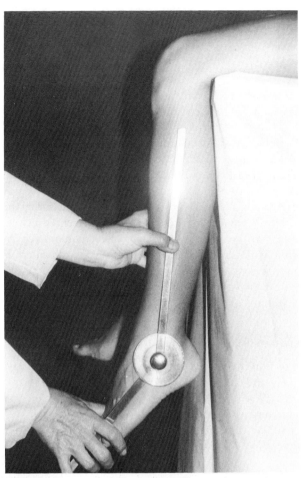

FIGURE 9–6. At the end of plantar flexion, the examiner uses her right hand to maintain plantar flexion and to align the distal goniometer arm. The examiner grasps the dorsum and sides of the foot to avoid exerting pressure on the toes.

TESTING PROCEDURES: TARSAL JOINTS

INVERSION

This motion is a combination of supination, adduction, and plantar flexion occurring in varying degrees at the subtalar, transverse tarsal (talocalcaneonavicular and calcaneocuboid), cuboideonavicular, cuneonavicular, intercuneiform, cuneocuboid, TMT, and intermetatarsal joints. The functional ability of the foot to adapt to the ground and to absorb contact forces depends on the combined movement in all of these joints. A method of measuring the combined movements at these joints is presented below. Because of the uniaxial limitations of the goniometer, inversion is measured in the frontal plane around an anterior-posterior axis. Methods for measuring inversion of the hindfoot, and of the midfoot and forefoot, are included in the sections on the subtalar and transverse tarsal joints.

Recommended Testing Position

Position the subject sitting, with the knee flexed to 90 degrees and the lower leg over the edge of the supporting surface. The hip is in 0 degrees of rotation, adduction, and abduction. Alternatively, it is possible to position the subject supine with the foot over the edge of the supporting surface.

Stabilization

Stabilize the tibia and fibula to prevent medial rotation and extension of the knee and lateral rotation and abduction of the hip (Fig. 9–7).

Normal End-Feel

The end-feel is firm because of tension in the joint capsules; the anterior and posterior talofibular ligament; the calcaneofibular ligament; the anterior, posterior, lateral, and interosseous talocalcaneal ligaments; the dorsal calcaneal ligaments; the dorsal calcaneocuboid ligament; the dorsal talonavicular ligament; the lateral band of the bifurcate ligament; the transverse metatarsal ligament; various dorsal, plantar, and interosseous ligaments of the cuboideonavicular, cuneonavicular, intercuneiform, cuneocuboid, TMT, and intermetatarsal joints; and the peroneus longus and brevis muscles.

Goniometer Alignment

See Figures 9–8 and 9–9.

1. Center the fulcrum of the goniometer over the anterior aspect of the ankle midway between the malleoli.
2. Align the proximal arm of the goniometer with the anterior midline of the lower leg, using the tibial tuberosity for reference.
3. Align the distal arm with the anterior midline of the second metatarsal.

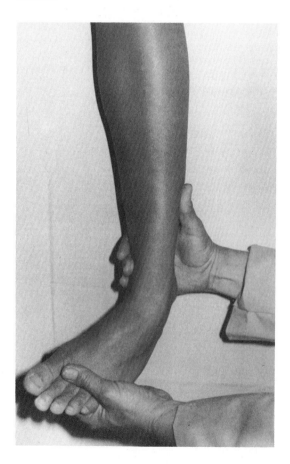

FIGURE 9–7. This photograph shows the left foot and ankle at the end of the inversion ROM. The examiner's right hand grasps the subject's distal lower leg to prevent both knee and hip motion. The examiner's left hand maintains inversion. Because inversion includes supination, adduction, and plantar flexion, the subject's ankle moves in these three directions.

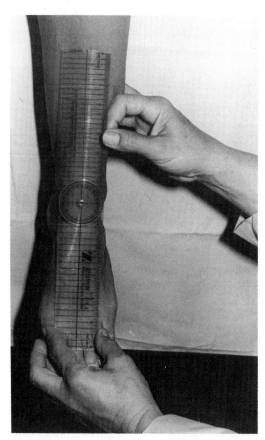

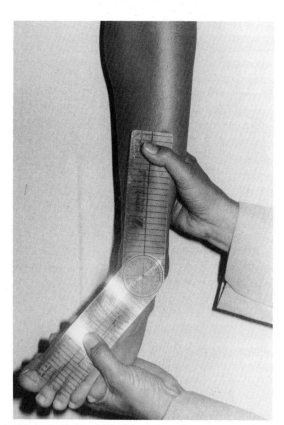

FIGURE 9–9. At the end of the ROM, the examiner uses her left hand to maintain inversion and to align the distal goniometer arm.

FIGURE 9–8. In the starting position for measuring inversion ROM, the body of the plastic full-circle goniometer is positioned midway between the two malleoli. The flexibility of the plastic goniometer makes this instrument easier to use for measuring inversion than a metal goniometer. The examiner aligns the proximal goniometer arm with the anterior midline of the tibia and the distal arm with the second metatarsal.

EVERSION

This motion is a combination of pronation, abduction, and dorsiflexion occurring in varying degrees at the subtalar, transverse tarsal (talocalcaneonavicular and calcaneocuboid), cuboideonavicular, cuneonavicular, intercuneiform, cuneocuboid, and TMT and intermetatarsal joints. The functional ability of the foot to adapt to the ground and to absorb contact forces depends on the combined movement of all of these joints. A method for measuring the combined movements at these joints is presented below. Because of the uniaxial limitations of the goniometer, this motion is measured in the frontal plane around an anterior-posterior axis. Methods for measuring eversion isolated to the hindfoot, and to the midfoot and forefoot, are included in the sections on the subtalar and transverse tarsal joints.

Recommended Testing Position

The testing position is the same as for measuring inversion of the foot.

Stabilization

Stabilize the tibia and fibula to prevent lateral rotation and flexion of the knee and medial rotation and adduction of the hip (Fig. 9–10).

Normal End-Feel

The end-feel may be hard because of contact between the calcaneus and the floor of the sinus tarsi. In some cases the end-feel may be firm because of tension in the joint capsules; the deltoid ligament; the medial talocalcaneal ligament; the plantar calcaneonavicular and calcaneocuboid ligaments; the dorsal talonavicular ligament; the medial band of the bifurcated ligament; the transverse metatarsal ligament; various dorsal, plantar, and interosseous ligaments of the cuboideonavicular, cuneonavicular, intercuneiform, cuneocuboid, TMT, and intermetatarsal joints; and the tibialis posterior muscle.

Goniometer Alignment

The alignment is the same as for measuring inversion of the foot (Figs. 9–11 and 9–12).

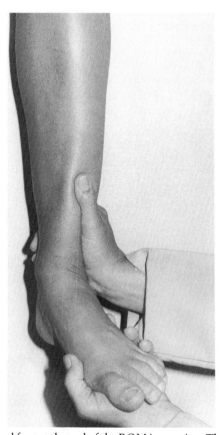

FIGURE 9 – 10. The left ankle and foot at the end of the ROM in eversion. The examiner uses her right hand on the subject's distal lower leg to prevent both knee flexion and lateral rotation. The examiner's left hand is maintaining eversion.

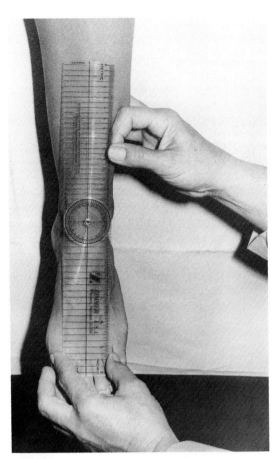

FIGURE 9–11. In the starting position for measuring eversion ROM, goniometer alignment is the same as for measuring inversion ROM.

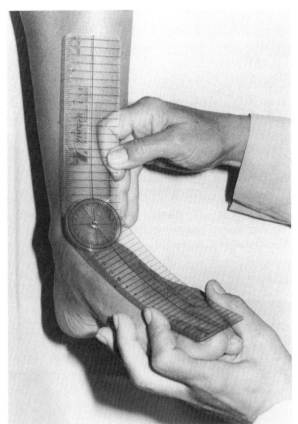

FIGURE 9–12. At the end of the eversion ROM, the examiner's left hand maintains eversion and keeps the distal goniometer arm aligned with the subject's second metatarsal. The examiner's right hand maintains the alignment of the proximal goniometer arm with the anterior midline of the tibia. Because eversion includes pronation, abduction, and dorsiflexion, the subject's foot is moved in these three directions.

TESTING PROCEDURES: SUBTALAR JOINT (HINDFOOT)

INVERSION

Motion is a combination of supination, adduction, and plantar flexion. Because of the uniaxial limitations of the goniometer, this motion is measured in the frontal plane around an anterior-posterior axis.

Recommended Testing Position

Position the subject prone, with the hip in 0 degrees of flexion, extension, abduction, adduction, and rotation. The knee is in 0 degrees of flexion and extension. The foot is placed over the edge of the supporting surface.

Stabilization

Stabilize the tibia and fibula to prevent hip and knee motion (Fig. 9–13).

Normal End-Feel

The end-feel is firm because of tension in the lateral joint capsule, the anterior and posterior talofibular ligaments, the calcaneofibular ligament, and the lateral, posterior, anterior, and interosseous talocalcaneal ligaments.

Goniometer Alignment

See Figures 9–14 and 9–15.

1. Center the fulcrum of the goniometer over the posterior aspect of the ankle midway between the malleoli.
2. Align the proximal arm with the posterior midline of the lower leg.
3. Align the distal arm with the posterior midline of the calcaneus.

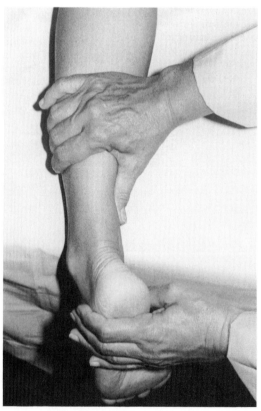

FIGURE 9–13. The left lower extremity at the end of the subtalar inversion ROM. The subject is in the prone position with her left foot and ankle placed over the edge of the supporting surface. The examiner is stabilizing the lower leg to prevent medial knee rotation and hip adduction. The examiner's left hand pulls the subject's calcaneus medially to produce subtalar inversion. The examiner avoids pushing on the forefoot.

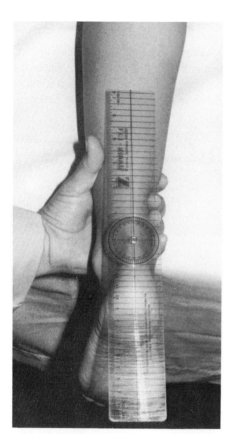

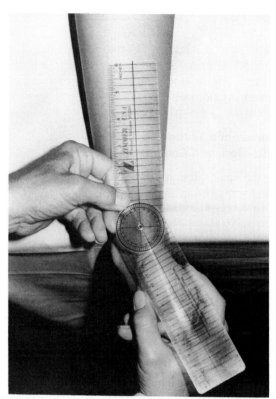

FIGURE 9 – 14. In the starting position for measuring subtalar inversion ROM, the goniometer body is centered midway between the two malleoli. The proximal goniometer arm is aligned along the midline of the posterior lower leg. The distal arm is aligned with the posterior midline of the calcaneus. Normally, the examiner's right hand would be holding the distal goniometer arm, but for the purpose of this photograph, this is not being done here.

FIGURE 9 – 15. At the end of subtalar inversion, the examiner's right hand maintains inversion and keeps the distal goniometer arm in alignment. The examiner uses her left hand to maintain alignment of the proximal arm of the goniometer.

EVERSION

Motion is a combination of pronation, abduction, and dorsiflexion. Because of the uniaxial limitations of the goniometer, this motion is measured in the frontal plane around an anterior-posterior axis.

Recommended Testing Position, Stabilization, and Goniometer Alignment

The testing position, stabilization, and alignment are the same as for measuring inversion at the subtalar joint (Figs. 9–16 to 9–18).

Normal End-Feel

The end-feel may be hard because of contact between the calcaneus and the floor of the sinus tarsi, or it may be firm because of tension in the deltoid ligament, the medial talocalcaneal ligament, and the tibialis posterior muscle.

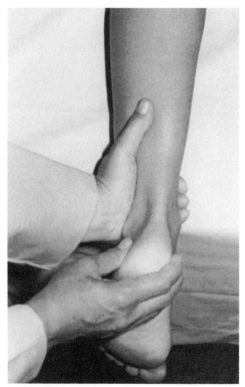

FIGURE 9–16. This photograph shows the left lower extremity at the end of subtalar eversion. One can observe that this subject's eversion ROM is more limited than her subtalar inversion ROM. The examiner stabilizes the subject's distal tibia and fibula to prevent knee lateral rotation and hip abduction. The examiner's right hand maintains subtalar eversion by pulling the calcaneus laterally.

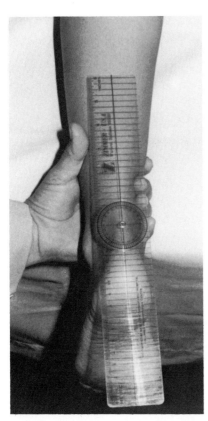

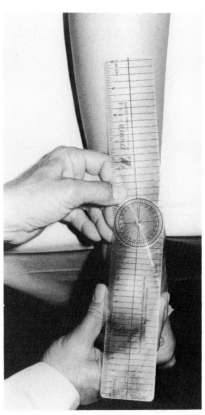

FIGURE 9 – 17. In the starting position for measuring subtalar eversion ROM, the goniometer alignment is the same as for measuring subtalar inversion ROM.

FIGURE 9 – 18. At the end of subtalar eversion, the examiner's right hand maintains eversion and keeps the distal goniometer arm aligned with the midline of the calcaneus. The examiner's left hand maintains alignment of the proximal arm with the midline of the lower leg.

TESTING PROCEDURES: TRANSVERSE TARSAL JOINT

Most of the motion in the midfoot and forefoot occurs at the cuboideonavicular, cuneonavicular, intercuneiform, cuneocuboid, and TMT joints.

INVERSION

Motion is a combination of supination, adduction, and plantar flexion. Because of the uniaxial limitation of the goniometer, this motion is measured in the frontal plane around an anterior-posterior axis.

Recommended Testing Position

The testing position is the same as for measuring inversion at the tarsal joints.

Stabilization

Stabilize the calcaneus and talus to prevent dorsiflexion of the ankle and inversion of the subtalar joint (Fig. 9–19).

Normal End-Feel

The end-feel is firm because of tension in the joint capsules; the dorsal calcaneocuboid ligament; the dorsal tal-onavicular ligament; the lateral band of the bifurcated ligament; the transverse metatarsal ligament; various dorsal, plantar, and interosseous ligaments of the cuboideonavicular, cuneonavicular, intercuneiform, cuneocuboid, TMT, and intermetatarsal joints; and the peroneus longus and brevis muscles.

Goniometer Alignment

See Figures 9–20 and 9–21.

1. Center the fulcrum of the goniometer over the anterior aspect of the ankle slightly distal to a point midway between the malleoli.
2. Align the proximal arm with the anterior midline of the lower leg, using the tibial tuberosity for reference.
3. Align the distal arm with the anterior midline of the second metatarsal.

Alternative Goniometer Alignment

See Figures 9–22 and 9–23.

1. Place the fulcrum of the goniometer at the lateral aspect of the fifth metatarsal head.
2. Align the proximal arm parallel to the anterior midline of the lower leg.
3. Align the distal arm with the plantar aspect of the first through the fifth metatarsal heads.

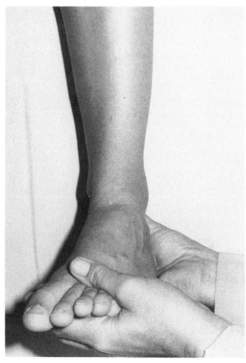

FIGURE 9–19. This photograph shows the left lower extremity at the end of transverse tarsal inversion ROM. The examiner's right hand cups the calcaneus to prevent subtalar inversion. The examiner's left hand pushes the forefoot medially to produce inversion. The examiner's left hand grasps the metatarsals rather than the toes. Notice that the ROM for the transverse tarsal joint is less than the ROM for all of the tarsal joints combined.

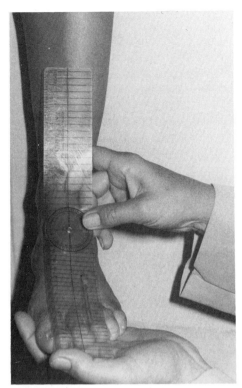

FIGURE 9–20. In the starting position for measuring transverse tarsal inversion, the goniometer alignment is similar to the alignment used for measuring inversion (Fig. 9–8). In Figure 9–8, the body of the goniometer is placed between the two malleoli, whereas when measuring transverse tarsal inversion, the examiner places the goniometer distal to the malleoli on the dorsum of the foot.

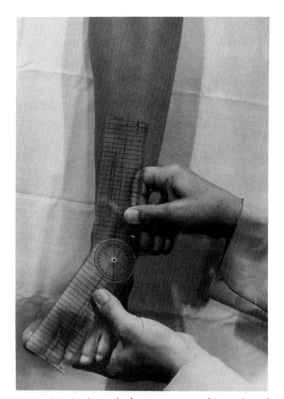

FIGURE 9–21. At the end of transverse tarsal inversion, the examiner's left hand maintains inversion and holds the distal goniometer aligned along the second metatarsal. The examiner's right hand maintains alignment of the proximal goniometer arm.

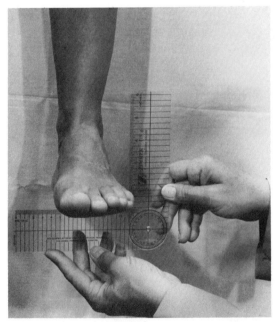

FIGURE 9–22. In the alternative starting position for measuring transverse tarsal inversion ROM, the examiner aligns the proximal goniometer arm so that it is perpendicular to the subject's tibia. The examiner positions the distal goniometer arm across the plantar surface of the foot on a level with the heads of the metatarsals. This goniometer alignment places the goniometer at 90 degrees, which is the zero starting position. The goniometer reading should be transposed and recorded as starting at 0 degrees.

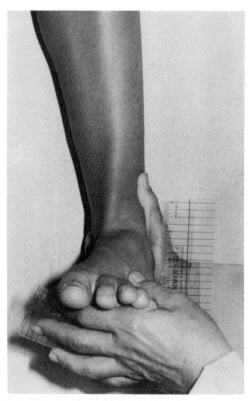

FIGURE 9–23. At the end of the transverse tarsal inversion ROM, the examiner uses her left hand to maintain inversion and to keep the distal goniometer arm aligned.

167

EVERSION

Motion is a combination of pronation, abduction, and dorsiflexion. Because of the uniaxial limitations of the goniometer, this motion is measured in the frontal plane around an anterior-posterior axis.

Recommended Testing Position

The testing position is the same as for measuring eversion at the tarsal joints.

Stabilization

Stabilize the calcaneus and talus to prevent plantar flexion of the ankle and eversion of the subtalar joint (Fig. 9–24).

Normal End-Feel

The end-feel is firm because of tension in the joint capsules; the deltoid ligament; the plantar calcaneonavicular and calcaneocuboid ligaments; the dorsal talonavicular ligament; the medial band of the bifurcated ligament; the transverse metatarsal ligament; various dorsal, plantar, and interosseous ligaments of the cuboideonavicular, cuneonavicular, intercuneiform, cuneocuboid, TMT, and intermetatarsal joints; and the tibialis posterior muscle.

Goniometer Alignment

The alignment is the same as for measuring inversion at the transverse tarsal joint (Figs. 9–25 and 9–26).

Alternative Goniometer Alignment

See Figures 9–27 and 9–28.

1. Place the fulcrum of the goniometer at the medial aspect of the first metatarsal head.
2. Align the proximal arm parallel to the anterior midline of the lower leg.
3. Align the distal arm with the plantar aspect of the first through the fifth metatarsal heads.

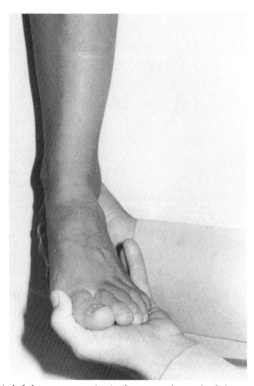

FIGURE 9–24. The subject's left lower extremity is shown at the end of the transverse tarsal eversion ROM. The examiner's right hand is stabilizing the calcaneus to prevent subtalar eversion. As can be seen in the photograph, only a small amount of motion is available at the transverse tarsal joint in this subject.

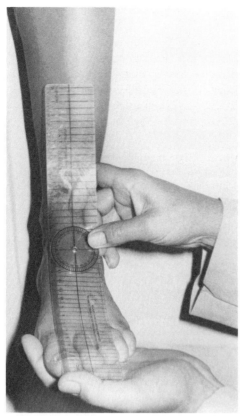

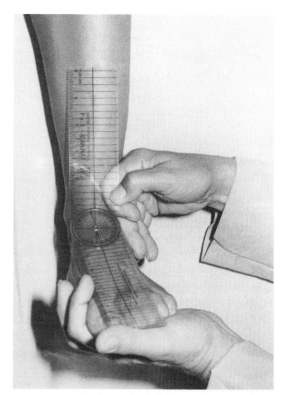

FIGURE 9–25. In the starting position for measuring transverse tarsal eversion ROM, goniometer alignment is the same as that used for measuring transverse tarsal inversion.

FIGURE 9–26. At the end of the transverse tarsal eversion ROM, the examiner's left hand maintains eversion and holds the distal goniometer arm aligned with the second metatarsal.

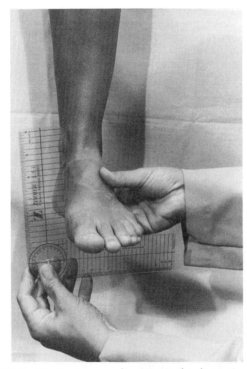

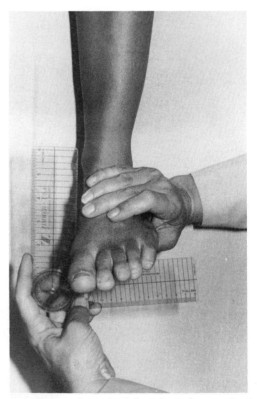

FIGURE 9–27. Goniometer alignment in the alternative starting position for measuring transverse tarsal eversion is similar to that used for measuring transverse tarsal inversion (Fig. 9–22). However, when measuring eversion, the examiner positions the goniometer on the medial rather than on the lateral aspect of the foot.

FIGURE 9–28. At the end of the ROM, the examiner's right hand maintains eversion, while her left hand aligns the goniometer. Because the subject is sitting on a table, the examiner sits on a low stool in order to align and read the goniometer at eye level.

TESTING PROCEDURES: METATARSOPHALANGEAL JOINT

FLEXION

The MTP joint moves in the sagittal plane around a medial-lateral axis.

Recommended Testing Position

Position the subject supine or sitting, with the ankle and foot in 0 degrees of dorsiflexion, plantar flexion, inversion, and eversion. The MTP joint is in 0 degrees of abduction and adduction. The IP joints are positioned in 0 degrees of flexion and extension. (If the ankle is flexed plantarly, and the IP joints of the toe being tested are flexed, tension in the extensor hallucis longus or extensor digitorum longus muscle will restrict the motion.)

Stabilization

Stabilize the metatarsal to prevent plantar flexion of the ankle and inversion or eversion of the foot. Do not hold the MTP joints of the other toes in extension, because tension in the transverse metatarsal ligament will restrict the motion (Fig. 9–29).

Normal End-Feel

The end-feel is firm because of tension in the dorsal joint capsule and the collateral ligaments. Tension in the extensor digitorum brevis muscle may contribute to the firm end-feel.

Goniometer Alignment

See Figures 9–30 and 9–31.

1. Center the fulcrum of the goniometer over the dorsal aspect of the MTP joint.
2. Align the proximal arm over the dorsal midline of the metatarsal.
3. Align the distal arm over the dorsal midline of the proximal phalanx.

Alternative Goniometer Alignment for First MTP Joint

1. Center the fulcrum of the goniometer over the medial aspect of the first MTP joint.
2. Align the proximal arm with the medial midline of the first metatarsal.
3. Align the distal arm with the medial midline of the proximal phalanx of the first toe.

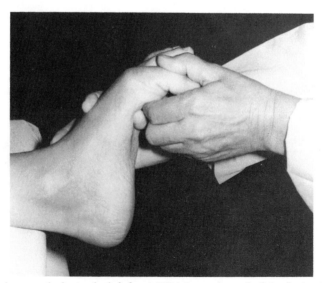

FIGURE 9–29. This photograph shows the left first MTP joint at the end of the flexion ROM. The subject is supine, and in this photograph her foot and ankle are placed over the edge of the supporting surface. However, the subject's foot can rest on the supporting surface. The examiner's right thumb is placed across the metatarsals to prevent plantar flexion. The examiner's left hand maintains the first MTP joint in flexion.

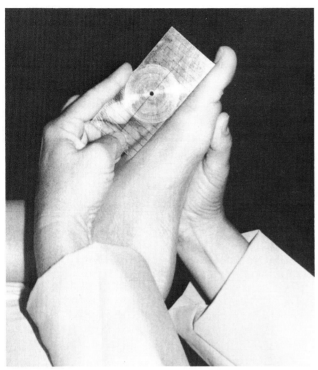

FIGURE 9–30. In the starting position for measuring MTP flexion ROM, the arms of the goniometer are placed on the dorsal surface of the metatarsal and proximal phalanx. The arms of this goniometer have been cut short to accommodate the relative shortness of the proximal and distal joint segments.

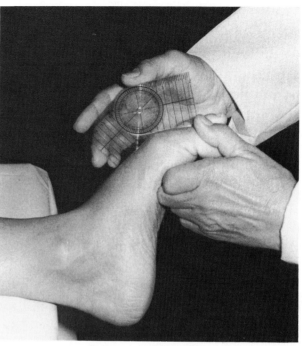

FIGURE 9–31. At the end of the ROM, the examiner's right hand aligns the goniometer, while her left hand maintains MTP flexion.

EXTENSION

Motion occurs in the sagittal plane around a medial-lateral axis.

Recommended Testing Position

The testing position is the same as for measuring flexion of the MTP joint. (If the ankle is dorsiflexed, and the IP joints of the toe being tested are extended, tension in the flexor hallucis longus or flexor digitorum longus muscle will restrict the motion. If the IP joints of the toe being tested are in extreme flexion, tension in the lumbricalis and interosseus muscles may restrict the motion.)

Stabilization

Stabilize the metatarsal to prevent dorsiflexion of the ankle and inversion or eversion of the foot. Do not hold the MTP joints of the other toes in extreme flexion, because tension in the transverse metatarsal ligament will restrict the motion (Fig. 9–32).

Normal End-Feel

The end-feel is firm because of tension in the plantar joint capsule, the plantar pad (plantar fibrocartilaginous plate), and the flexor hallucis brevis, flexor digitorum brevis, and flexor digiti minimi muscles.

Goniometer Alignment

The alignment is the same as for measuring flexion of the MTP joint (Figs. 9–33 and 9–34).

Alternative Goniometer Alignment for First MTP Joint

The alternative alignment is the same as the alternative alignment for measuring flexion of the first MTP joint.

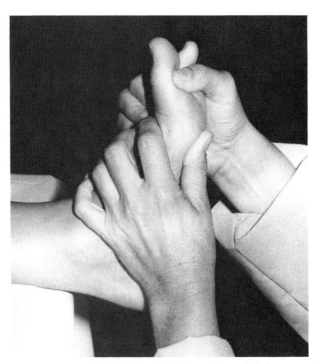

FIGURE 9–32. This photograph shows the left first MTP joint at the end of the extension ROM. The subject's position is the same as that used for measuring MTP flexion ROM. The examiner places her left digits on the dorsum of the subject's foot to prevent dorsiflexion and uses her right thumb to push the proximal phalanx into extension.

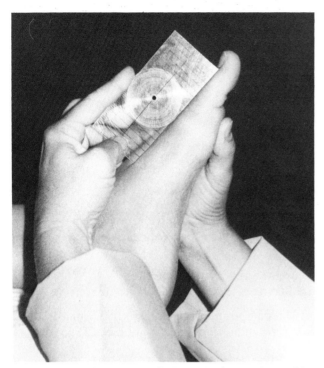

FIGURE 9–33. Goniometer alignment in the starting position for measuring MTP extension ROM is the same as that for measuring MTP flexion ROM.

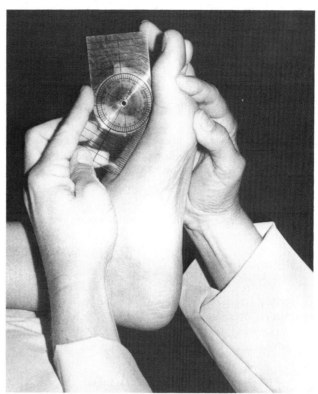

FIGURE 9–34. At the end of MTP extension, the examiner maintains goniometer alignment with her left hand while using her right index finger to maintain extension.

ABDUCTION

Motion occurs in the transverse plane around a vertical axis when the subject is in anatomical position.

Recommended Testing Position

Position the subject supine or sitting, with the foot in 0 degrees of inversion and eversion. The MTP and IP joints are positioned in 0 degrees of flexion and extension.

Stabilization

Stabilize the metatarsal to prevent inversion or eversion of the foot (Fig. 9–35).

Normal End-Feel

The end-feel is firm because of tension in the joint capsule, the collateral ligaments, the fascia of the web space between the toes, and the adductor hallucis and plantar interosseus muscles.

Goniometer Alignment

See Figures 9–36 and 9–37.

1. Center the fulcrum of the goniometer over the dorsal aspect of the MTP joint.
2. Align the proximal arm with the dorsal midline of the metatarsal.
3. Align the distal arm with the dorsal midline of the proximal phalanx.

ADDUCTION

Motion occurs in the transverse plane around a vertical axis when the subject is in anatomical position.

Recommended Testing Position, Stabilization, and Goniometer Alignment

The testing position, stabilization, and alignment are the same as for measuring abduction of the MTP joints.

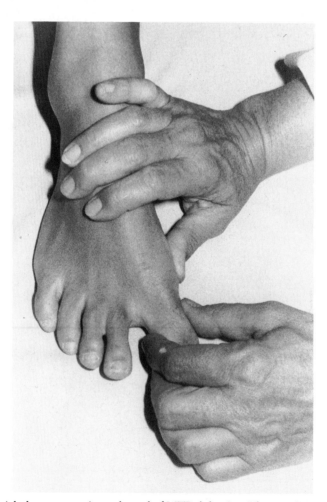

FIGURE 9–35. The right lower extremity at the end of MTP abduction. The examiner uses her right thumb to prevent transverse tarsal inversion while using her left index finger and thumb to pull the proximal phalanx of the toe into abduction.

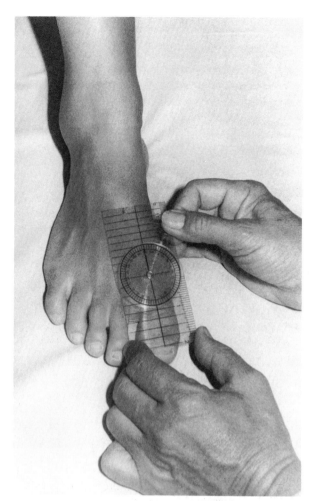

FIGURE 9-36. In the starting position for measuring MTP abduction ROM, the adapted full-circle plastic goniometer is positioned so that the fulcrum is over the MTP joint. The proximal arm is aligned with the first metatarsal, and the distal arm is aligned along the midline of the proximal phalanx.

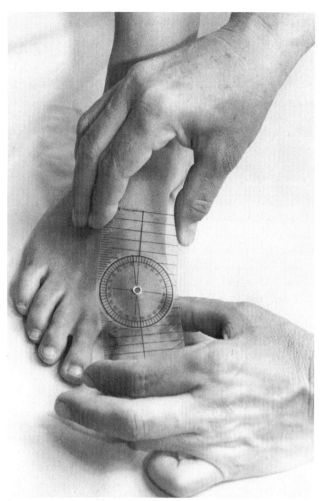

FIGURE 9-37. At the end of MTP abduction, the examiner's right hand maintains alignment of the proximal goniometer arm. The examiner's left hand maintains alignment of the distal goniometer arm while maintaining the MTP in abduction.

TESTING PROCEDURES: PROXIMAL INTERPHALANGEAL JOINT

FLEXION

Motion occurs in the sagittal plane around a medial-lateral axis.

Recommended Testing Position

Position the subject supine or sitting, with the ankle and foot in 0 degrees of dorsiflexion, plantar flexion, inversion, and eversion. The MTP joint is positioned in 0 degrees of flexion, extension, abduction, and adduction. (If the ankle is positioned in plantar flexion, and the MTP joint is flexed, tension in the extensor hallucis longus or extensor digitorum longus muscles will restrict the motion. If the MTP joint is positioned in full extension, tension in the lumbricalis and interosseus muscles may restrict the motion.)

Stabilization

Stabilize the metatarsal and proximal phalanx to prevent dorsiflexion or plantar flexion of the ankle and inversion or eversion of the foot. Avoid flexion and extension of the MTP joint.

Normal End-Feel

The end-feel for flexion of the IP joint of the big toe and the PIP joints of the smaller toes may be soft because of compression of soft tissues between the plantar surfaces of the phalanges. Sometimes the end-feel is firm because of tension in the dorsal joint capsule and the collateral ligaments.

Goniometer Alignment

1. Center the fulcrum of the goniometer over the dorsal aspect of the interphalangeal joint being tested.
2. Align the proximal arm over the dorsal midline of the proximal phalanx.
3. Align the distal arm over the dorsal midline of the phalanx distal to the joint being tested.

EXTENSION

Motion occurs in the sagittal plane around a medial-lateral axis.

Recommended Testing Position, Stabilization, and Goniometer Alignment

The testing position, stabilization, and alignment are the same as for measuring flexion of the PIP joints. (If the ankle is positioned in dorsiflexion, and the MTP joint is extended, tension in the flexor hallucis longus and brevis muscles and flexor digitorum longus and brevis muscles will restrict the motion.)

Normal End-Feel

The end-feel is firm because of tension in the plantar joint capsule and plantar pad (plantar fibrocartilaginous plate).

TESTING PROCEDURES: DISTAL INTERPHALANGEAL JOINT

FLEXION

Motion occurs in the sagittal plane around a medial-lateral axis.

Recommended Testing Position

Position the subject supine or sitting, with the ankle and foot in 0 degrees of dorsiflexion, plantar flexion, inversion, and eversion. The MTP and PIP joints are positioned in 0 degrees of flexion, extension, abduction, and adduction. (If the ankle is positioned in plantar flexion, and the MTP and PIP joints are flexed, tension in the extensor digitorum longus may restrict the motion. If the MTP and PIP joints are held in extreme extension, additional tension in the oblique retinacular ligament will restrict the motion).

Stabilization

Stabilize the metatarsal, proximal, and middle phalanx to prevent dorsiflexion or plantar flexion of the ankle and inversion or eversion of the foot. Avoid flexion and extension of the MTP and PIP joints of the toe being tested.

Normal End-Feel

The end-feel is firm because of tension in the dorsal joint capsule, the collateral ligaments, and the oblique retinacular ligament.

Goniometer Alignment

1. Center the fulcrum of the goniometer over the dorsal aspect of the DIP joint.
2. Align the proximal arm over the dorsal midline of the middle phalanx.

3. Align the distal arm over the dorsal midline of the distal phalanx.

EXTENSION

Motion occurs in the sagittal plane around a medial-lateral axis.

Recommended Testing Position

The testing position is the same as for flexion of the DIP joints of the toes. (If the ankle is positioned in dorsiflexion and the MTP and PIP joints are fully extended, tension in the flexor digitorum longus, lumbricalis, and interosseus muscles will restrict the motion.)

Stabilization

Stabilize the metatarsal, proximal, and middle phalanx to prevent dorsiflexion or plantar flexion of the ankle and inversion or eversion of the foot. Avoid extreme extension of the MTP and PIP joints of the toe being tested.

Normal End-Feel

The end-feel is firm because of tension in the plantar joint capsule and the plantar pad (plantar fibrocartilaginous plate).

Goniometer Alignment

The alignment is the same as for DIP flexion of the toes.

REFERENCES

1. Norkin, CC and Levangie, PK: Joint Structure and Function: A Comprehensive Analysis, ed 2. FA Davis, Philadelphia, 1992.
2. Cyriax, JM and Cyriax, PJ: Illustrated Manual of Orthopaedic Medicine. Butterworths, London, 1983.
3. Kisner, C and Colby, LA: Therapeutic Exercise: Foundations and Techniques, ed 2. FA Davis, Philadelphia, 1992.
4. American Academy of Orthopaedic Surgeons: Joint Motion: Method of Measuring and Recording. AAOS, Chicago, 1965.
5. American Medical Association: Guides to the Evaluation of Permanent Impairment, ed 3 (revised). AMA, Chicago, 1988.
6. Boone, DC and Azen, SP: Normal range of motion of joints in male subjects. J Bone Joint Surg Am 61:756, 1979.
7. Murray, MP: Gait as a total pattern of movement. Am J Phys Med Rehabil 46:290, 1967.
8. Livingston, LA, Stevenson, JM, and Olney, SJ: Stairclimbing kinematics on stairs of differing dimensions. Arch Phys Med Rehabil 72:398, 1991.
9. Professional Staff Association, Rancho Los Amigos Medical Center: Observational Gait Analysis Handbook. Ranchos Los Amigos Medical Center, Downey, CA, 1989.
10. McFayden, BJ and Winter, DA: An integrated biomechanical analysis of normal stair ascent and descent. J Biomech 21:733, 1988.
11. Ostrosky, KM: A comparison of gait characteristics in young and old subjects. Phys Ther 74:637–646, 1994.
12. Waugh, KG, et al: Measurement of selected hip, knee and ankle joint motions in newborns. Phys Ther 63:1616, 1983.
13. Wanatabe, H, et al: The range of joint motion of the extremities in healthy Japanese people: The differences according to age. Cited in Walker, JM: Musculoskeletal development: A review. Phys Ther 71:878, 1991.
14. Boone, DC: Techniques of measurement of joint motion. (Unpublished supplement to Boone, DC and Azen, SP: Normal range of motion in male subjects. J Bone Joint Surg Am 61:756, 1979.
15. Walker, JM: Musculoskeletal development: A review. Phys Ther 71:878, 1991.
16. Boone, DC, Walker, JM, and Perry, J: Age and sex differences in lower extremity joint motion. Presented at the National Conference, American Physical Therapy Association, Washington, DC, 1981.
17. Bell, RD and Hoshizaki, TB: Relationships of age and sex with range of motion of seventeen joint actions in humans. Canadian Journal of Applied Sport Sciences, 6:202, 1981.
18. Walker, JM, et al: Active mobility of the extremities of older subjects. Phys Ther 64:919, 1984.
19. Boone, DC, et al.: Reliability of goniometric measurements. Phys Ther 68:1355, 1978.
20. Clapper, MP and Wolf, SL: Comparison of the reliability of the Orthoranger and the standard goniometer for assessing active lower extremity range of motion. Phys Ther 68:214, 1988.
21. Bohannon, RW, Tiberio, D, and Waters, G: Motion measured from forefoot and hindfoot landmarks during passive ankle dorsiflexion range of motion. Journal of Orthopaedic and Sports Physical Therapy 13:20, 1991.
22. Elveru, RA, Rothstein, J, and Lamb, RL: Goniometric reliability in a clinical setting: Subtalar and ankle joint measurements. Phys Ther 68:672, 1988.
23. Youdas, JW, Bogard, CL, and Suman, VJ: Reliability of goniometric measurements and visual estimates of ankle joint range of motion obtained in a clinical setting (abstract). Phys Ther 72(Suppl):S113, 1992.
24. Elveru, RA, et al: Methods for taking subtalar joint measurements: A clinical report. Phys Ther 68:678, 1988.
25. Bailey, DS, Perillo, JT, and Forman, M: Subtalar joint neutral: A study using tomography. Journal of the American Podiatry Association 74:59, 1984.
26. Lattanza, L, Gray, GW, and Kanter, RM: Closed versus open kinematic chain measurements of subtalar joint eversion: Implications for clinical practice. Journal of Orthopedic and Sports Physical Therapy 9:310, 1988.
27. Picciano, AM, Rowlands, MS, and Worrell, T: Reliability of open and closed kinetic chain subtalar joint neutral positions and navicular drop test. Journal of Orthopedic and Sports Physical Therapy 18:553, 1993.
28. Clarkson, HM and Gilewich, GB: Musculoskeletal Assessment: Joint Range of Motion and Manual Muscle Strength. Williams & Wilkins, Baltimore, 1989.
29. Palmer, ML and Epler, M: Clinical Assessment Procedures in Physical Therapy. JB Lippincott, Philadelphia, 1990.

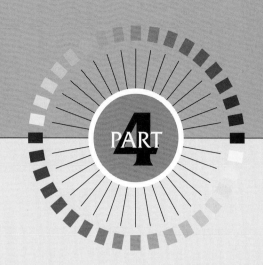

PART 4

Testing of the Spine and Temporo-mandibular Joint

OBJECTIVES

On completion of Part 4, the reader will be able to:

1. Identify:
   the appropriate planes and axes for each spinal motion

2. Describe the recommended testing positions for motions of the spine

3. Explain:
   how age and gender may affect the ROM
   how sources of error in measurement may affect testing results

4. Perform a goniometric evaluation of the cervical, thoracic, and lumbar spines including:
   a clear explanation of the testing procedure
   positioning of the subject in a recommended testing position

adequate stabilization of the proximal joint component
correct determination of the end of the ROM
palpation of the correct bony landmarks
correct alignment of the goniometer
correct reading and recording

5. Perform an evaluation of the cervical, thoracic, and lumbar spine using a tape measure

6. Perform an evaluation of the temporomandibular joint (TMJ) using either a tape measure or a ruler

7. Assess the intratester and intertester reliability of measurements of the spine and TMJ

Chapters 10 to 12 present common clinical techniques for measuring gross motions of the cervical, thoracic, and lumbar spine and the TMJ. Evaluation of the ROM and end-feels of individual facet joints of the spine are not included.

10

The Cervical Spine

ATLANTO-OCCIPITAL AND ATLANTOAXIAL JOINTS

STRUCTURE

The atlanto-occipital joint is composed of the right and left slightly concave superior facets of the atlas (C1) that articulate with the right and left convex occipital condyles of the skull.

The atlantoaxial joint is composed of three separate articulations: the median atlantoaxial and two lateral joints. The median atlantoaxial joint consists of an anterior facet on the dens (the odontoid process of C2) that articulates with a facet on the internal surface of the atlas (C1). The two lateral joints are composed of the right and left superior facets of the axis (C2) that articulate with the right and left slightly convex inferior facets on the atlas (C1).

The atlanto-occipital and atlantoaxial joints are reinforced by the posterior and anterior atlantoaxial ligaments, the transverse ligament, the alar ligaments, and the tectorial membrane.

OSTEOKINEMATICS

The atlanto-occipital joint and the two lateral atlantoaxial joints are plane synovial joints. The motions permitted at the atlanto-occipital joint are flexion-extension in the sagittal plane around a medial-lateral axis and some rotation and lateral flexion. The median atlantoaxial joint is a synovial trochoid (pivot) joint permitting rotation in the transverse plane around a vertical axis.

The motions permitted at the three articulations are flexion-extension, lateral flexion, and rotation.

CAPSULAR PATTERN

The capsular pattern for the atlanto-occipital joint is an equal restriction of extension and lateral flexion. Rotation and flexion are not affected.[1]

INTERVERTEBRAL AND ZYGAPOPHYSIAL JOINTS C2 TO C7

STRUCTURE

The intervertebral joints are composed of the superior and inferior vertebral plateaus and adjacent intervertebral discs. The joints are reinforced anteriorly by the anterior longitudinal ligament, which limits extension, and posteriorly by the posterior longitudinal ligament, ligamentum nuchae, and ligamentum flavum, which help to limit flexion.

The zygapophysial joints are formed by the right and left superior articular processes (facets) of one vertebra and the right and left inferior articular processes of an adjacent superior vertebra. Each joint has its own capsule and capsular ligaments, which in the cervical region are lax and permit a relatively large ROM. The ligamentum flavum helps to reinforce the joint capsules.

OSTEOKINEMATICS AND ARTHROKINEMATICS

According to White and Punjabi,[2] one vertebra can move in relation to another adjacent vertebra in six different directions (three translations and three rotations) along and around three axes. The compound effects of sliding and tilting at a series of vertebrae produce a large ROM for the column as a whole, including flexion-extension, lateral flexion, and rotation. Some motions in the vertebral column are coupled with other motions; this coupling varies from region to region. A coupled motion is one in which one motion around one axis is consistently associated with another motion or motions around a different axis or axes. For example, left lateral flexion from C2 to C5 is accompanied by rotation to the left (spinous processes move to the right) and forward flexion. In the cervical region from C2 to C7, flexion and extension are the only motions that are not coupled.[2]

The intervertebral joints are cartilaginous joints of the symphysis type. These joints permit a small amount of sliding and tilting of one vertebra on another. In all of the motions at the intervertebral joints, the nucleus pulposus of the intervertebral disc acts as a pivot for the tilting and sliding motions of the vertebrae. Flexion is a result of anterior sliding and tilting of a superior vertebra on the interposed disc of an adjacent inferior vertebra. Extension is the result of posterior sliding and tilting.

The zygapophysial joints are synovial plane joints that permit small amounts of sliding of the right and left inferior facets on the right and left superior facets of an adjacent inferior vertebra. In the cervical region, the facets are oriented at 45 degrees to the transverse plane. The inferior facets of the superior vertebrae face anteriorly and inferiorly. The superior facets of the inferior vertebrae face posteriorly and superiorly. In flexion, the inferior facets of the superior vertebrae slide anteriorly and superiorly on the superior facets of the inferior vertebrae. In extension, the inferior facets of the superior vertebrae slide posteriorly and inferiorly on the superior facets of the inferior vertebrae. In lateral flexion and rotation, one inferior facet of the superior vertebra slides inferiorly and posteriorly on the superior facet of the inferior vertebra on the side to which the spine is laterally flexed. The opposite inferior facet of the superior vertebra slides superiorly and anteriorly on the superior facet of the adjacent inferior vertebra.

The orientation of the facets, which varies from region to region, determines the direction of the tilting and sliding of the vertebra, whereas the size of the disc determines the amount of motion. In addition, passive tension in a number of soft tissues and bony contacts controls and limits motions of the vertebral column. In general, although regional variations exist, the soft tissues that control and limit extremes of motion in forward flexion include the supraspinous and interspinous ligaments, zygapophysial joint capsules, ligamentum flavum, posterior longitudinal ligament, posterior fibers of the annulus fibrosus of the intervertebral disc, and back extensors.

Extension is limited by bony contact of the spinous processes and by passive tension in the zygapophysial joint capsules, anterior fibers of the annulus fibrosus, anterior longitudinal ligament, and anterior trunk muscles. Lateral flexion is limited by the intertransverse ligaments and by passive tension in the annulus fibrosus on the side opposite the motion on the convexity of the curve.

CAPSULAR PATTERN

The capsular pattern for C2 to C7 is recognizable by pain and equal limitation of all motions except flexion, which is usually barely restricted. The capsular pattern for unilateral facet involvement is a greater restriction of movement in lateral flexion to the opposite side and in rotation to the same side. For example, if the right facet joint capsule is involved, lateral flexion to the left and rotation to the right are the motions most restricted.[1]

RANGE OF MOTION

Table 10–1 provides cervical spine ROM values from selected sources. The measurements cited in the study by Capuano-Pucci et al.[6] were obtained using the cervical ROM (CROM) device, an instrument specifically designed to measure motion of the cervical spine. The instrument consists of two gravity goniometers, a compass, and a shoulder-mounted magnetic yoke. The goniometers and compass are attached to a frame mounted over the bridge of a subject's nose and ears. Measurements were obtained from 20 volunteer subjects (16 females and four males) with no history of cervical problems. The mean age of the subjects was 23.5 years, with a standard deviation of 3 years.

The values presented in Tables 10–2 to 10–7 should be used for reference *only* if examiners are using a CROM device for their measuring instrument. Ideally, the examiner should use norms that are appropriate to the method of measurement and the age and gender of the individuals being examined.

EFFECTS OF AGE AND GENDER

Tables 10–2 through 10–7 show the effects of age and gender on cervical spine ROM. The values presented in Tables 10–2 to 10–7 were obtained from 337 healthy volunteers (171 females and 166 males) ranging from 11 to 97 years of age. These subjects had no current neck or shoulder pain and no previous history of neck trauma or treatment, and were not receiving any pain medications. The subjects were measured by five full-time physical therapy faculty members.

In Tables 10–2 and 10–3, the mean values for active neck flexion in the two oldest groups of males and females are considerably less than the mean values obtained in the youngest group. Eighty-year-old subjects show about 20 degrees less motion than 20-year-old subjects. A comparison between the neck extension mean values for males

Table 10–1 **CERVICAL SPINE MOTION: MEAN VALUES IN DEGREES FROM SELECTED SOURCES**

Motion	AMERICAN ACADEMY OF ORTHOPAEDIC SURGEONS[4]*	AMERICAN MEDICAL ASSOCIATION[5]†	CAPUANO-PUCCI ET AL.[6]‡ (N = 20)	
			Mean	Standard Deviation
Flexion	45	60	50.9	9
Extension	45	75	69.5	9.1
Left lateral flexion	45	45	43.7	8.3
Right lateral flexion	45	45		
Left rotation	60	80	70.8	5.3
Right rotation	60	80		

*Values were obtained using a universal goniometer.
†Values obtained using an inclinometer.
‡Values obtained using the CROM.

Table 10–2 **EFFECTS OF AGE ON ACTIVE FLEXION OF THE CERVICAL SPINE: MEAN VALUES IN DEGREES FOR MALES AND FEMALES AGE 11–59 YR***

Motion	11–19 YR (N = 40)		20–29 YR (N = 42)		30–39 YR (N = 41)		40–49 YR (N = 42)		50–59 YR (N = 40)	
	Mean	Standard Deviation	Mean	Standard Deviation	Mean	Standard Deviation	Mean	Standard Deviation	Mean	Standard Deviation
Flexion	64.0	8.6	54.3	8.8	47.3	9.5	49.5	11.4	45.5	9.1

Adapted from Youdas, et al.[7] Reprinted from Physical Therapy with the permission of the American Physical Therapy Association.
*Measurements were obtained using a CROM instrument.

Table 10–3 **EFFECTS OF AGE ON ACTIVE FLEXION OF THE CERVICAL SPINE: MEAN VALUES IN DEGREES FOR MALES AND FEMALES AGE 60–97 YR***

Motion	60–69 YR (N = 40)		70–79 YR (N = 40)		80–89 YR (N = 38)		90–97 YR (N = 14)	
	Mean	Standard Deviation	Mean	Standard Deviation	Mean	Standard Deviation	Mean	Standard Deviation
Flexion	41.0	8.4	39.2	8.8	40.4	8.7	36.4	9.8

Adapted from Youdas, et al.[7] Reprinted from Physical Therapy with the permission of the American Physical Therapy Association.
*Measurements were obtained using a CROM instrument.

Table 10 – 4 **EFFECTS OF AGE AND GENDER ON ACTIVE CERVICAL SPINE MOTION: MEAN VALUES IN DEGREES FOR MALES AND FEMALES AGE 11 – 29 YR***

| | 11 – 19 YR | | | | 20 – 29 YR | | | |
| | MALES (N = 20) | | FEMALES (N = 20) | | MALES (N = 20) | | FEMALES (N = 20) | |
Motion	Mean	Standard Deviation	Mean	Standard Deviation	Mean	Standard Deviation	Mean	Standard Deviation
Extension	85.6	11.5	84.0	14.9	76.7	12.8	85.6	10.6
Left lateral flexion	46.3	6.7	46.6	7.3	41.4	7.1	42.8	4.6
Right lateral flexion	44.8	7.7	48.9	7.1	44.9	7.2	46.2	6.7
Left rotation	72.3	7.0	70.5	9.8	69.2	7.0	71.6	5.7
Right rotation	74.1	7.6	74.9	9.8	69.6	6.0	74.6	5.9

Adapted from Youdas, et al.[7] Reprinted from Physical Therapy with the permission of the American Physical Therapy Association.

*Measurements were obtained using a CROM instrument.

found in Table 10 – 4 with extension values for males found in Table 10 – 5 shows that the younger group's extension ROM is more than one standard deviation greater than the older group's ROM.

An examination of Tables 10 – 5 to 10 – 7 shows that females in almost all age groups over 30 years of age generally appear to have greater mean values for active cervical motion than males for the majority of motions measured. Furthermore, the oldest age groups in both genders have less active motion than the youngest group. Youdas et al.[7] concluded that each gender loses about 5 degrees of active extension, and 3 degrees of active lateral flexion and rotation, with each 10-year increase in age. Accordingly, one can expect to find approximately 15 to 20 degrees less active neck extension in a healthy 60-year-old compared with a healthy 20-year-old of the same gender.

O'Driscoll and Tomenson[8] also studied cervical ROM across age groups. These investigators used a spirit inclinometer (a hydrogoniometer that works on a pendulum principle) for their measurements. They measured 79 females and 80 males ranging in age from 0 to 79 years. ROM decreased with increasing age, and differences existed between males and females. A regression analysis showed that only age explained a significant amount of the variation. Regression lines for males and females were significantly different. However, the values obtained by these authors cannot be compared with the values in Tables 10 – 2 to 10 – 7 because the authors presented total ranges such as flexion-extension, rather than individual motions such as flexion.

Keske et al.[9] used an electromagnetic ROM (ENROM) system to compare cervical ROM in males and females age 21 to 29 years with a group of elderly females age 66 to 85 years. These authors also found age-related changes. The

Table 10 – 5 **EFFECTS OF AGE AND GENDER ON ACTIVE CERVICAL SPINE MOTION: MEAN VALUES IN DEGREES FOR MALES AND FEMALES AGE 30 – 49 YR***

| | 30 – 39 YR | | | | 40 – 49 YR | | | |
| | MALES (N = 20) | | FEMALES (N = 21) | | MALES (N = 20) | | FEMALES (N = 22) | |
Motion	Mean	Standard Deviation	Mean	Standard Deviation	Mean	Standard Deviation	Mean	Standard Deviation
Extension	68.2	12.8	78.0	13.8	62.5	12.2	77.5	13.2
Left lateral flexion	41.2	10.3	43.6	7.9	35.6	8	40.8	9.3
Right lateral flexion	42.9	8.5	46.5	8.4	38.0	10.9	42.5	9.2
Left rotation	65.4	9.1	65.9	8.1	62.0	7.6	64.0	7.9
Right rotation	67.1	7.4	71.7	5.7	64.6	9.6	70.2	6.6

Adapted from Youdas, et al.[7] Reprinted from Physical Therapy with the permission of the American Physical Therapy Association.

*Measurements were obtained using a CROM instrument.

Table 10–6 **EFFECTS OF AGE AND GENDER ON ACTIVE CERVICAL SPINE MOTION: MEAN VALUES IN DEGREES FOR MALES AND FEMALES AGE 50–69 YR***

| | 50–59 YR | | | | 60–69 YR | | | |
| | MALES (N = 20) | | FEMALES (N = 20) | | MALES (N = 20) | | FEMALES (N = 20) | |
Motion	Mean	Standard Deviation	Mean	Standard Deviation	Mean	Standard Deviation	Mean	Standard Deviation
Extension	59.9	10.4	65.3	16	57.4	10.5	65.2	13.3
Left lateral flexion	34.9	6.6	35.1	6	30.4	4.7	34.4	8.1
Right lateral flexion	35.6	5.4	37.3	6.8	29.8	5.4	32.7	9.6
Left rotation	58	8.8	62.8	8.4	56.6	6.7	59.7	9.1
Right rotation	61	7.7	61.2	8.6	53.6	7.4	65.2	9.7

Adapted from Youdas, et al.[7] Reprinted from Physical Therapy with the permission of the American Physical Therapy Association.

*Measurements were obtained using a CROM instrument.

means of lateral flexion, extension, and rotation were less in the sample of 11 elderly females than in the 20 males and females in the youngest group.

RELIABILITY AND VALIDITY

Many different methods and instruments have been employed to assess motion of the head and neck. However, the majority of the studies have focused on reliability rather than validity. Some of the studies that have been conducted to assess the reliability or validity, or both, of the various instruments and methods are reviewed in the following section. Goniometric instruments that have been studied include the universal goniometer,[10,11] CROM device,[6,7,11,12] pendulum goniometer,[13,14] gravity goniometer,[15] and electrogoniometer.[9] Nongoniometric methods that have been

studied include the tape measure,[15] visual estimation,[11,16] flexible ruler,[17] and radiograph.[14]

Universal Goniometer, Gravity Goniometer, Cervical Range of Motion Device, and Visual Estimation

Two of the most relevant studies for users of this manual are by Tucci et al.[10] and Youdas et al.[11] Tucci et al. compared the intratester and intertester reliability of cervical spine motions measured with a universal goniometer and a gravity goniometer. ICCs for intertester reliability ranged from −0.084 for flexion to 0.82 for extension, for measurements taken with the universal goniometer by two experienced testers on 10 volunteer subjects. ICCs for intertester reliability ranged from 0.80 for right rotation to 0.91 for left rotation, for measurements using the gravity gonio-

Table 10–7 **EFFECTS OF AGE AND GENDER ON ACTIVE CERVICAL SPINE MOTION: MEAN VALUES IN DEGREES FOR MALES AND FEMALES AGE 70–89 YR***

| | 70–79 YR | | | | 80–89 Yr | | | |
| | MALES (N = 20) | | FEMALES (N = 20) | | MALES (N = 20) | | FEMALES (N = 18) | |
Motion	Mean	Standard Deviation	Mean	Standard Deviation	Mean	Standard Deviation	Mean	Standard Deviation
Extension	53.7	14.4	54.8	10.2	49.4	11.5	50.3	14.5
Left lateral flexion	25	8.4	26.9	6.7	23.5	6.8	22.6	7.1
Right lateral flexion	25.8	7.3	27.7	7.3	23.8	6.2	26.3	5.7
Left rotation	49.7	8.8	50.1	7.9	46.8	9.2	50.5	10.7
Right rotation	50	10.2	53.4	8.8	46.4	8.2	52.6	10.5

Adapted from Youdas, et al.[7] Reprinted from Physical Therapy with the permission of the American Physical Therapy Association.

*Measurements were obtained using a CROM instrument.

meter by one experienced and one novice tester on 11 different volunteers. The authors concluded that the gravity goniometer that they had developed had good intertester reliability and was an accurate and reliable instrument.

In the study by Youdas et al.,[11] 11 physical therapists used the following three methods to determine active cervical ROM: visual estimation, a universal goniometer, and the CROM device. The physical therapists measured cervical ROM on 60 patients with orthopedic disorders (39 females and 21 males whose ages ranged from 21 to 84 years). Prior to testing, the therapists had 1 hour of instruction and practice on standardized measurement procedures for each instrument. Intratester and intertester reliability varied among the motions tested, but generally the intratester reliability for goniometric measurements using either the universal goniometer or the CROM device were good (ICCs above 0.80). Intertester reliability for the CROM device also was good. The ICCs for intertester reliability for both the universal goniometer and visual estimates were less than 0.80. The ICCs were poor to fair for interdevice comparisons among the three methods (visual estimation, the universal goniometer, and the CROM device) for all cervical motions. Intertester ICCs for visual estimation were lower than for the universal goniometer for all motions except rotation. The authors concluded that, because of poor interdevice reliability, the three methods should not be used interchangeably. The fact that intertester reliability was higher when using the CROM device than when using the universal goniometer suggests that use of the CROM device for measuring cervical ROM is preferable to either the universal goniometer or visual estimation when different therapists take measurements on a particular patient.

Garrett et al.[12] used the CROM device in a study to determine the intratester and intertester reliability of measurements of forward head posture in 40 patients with orthopedic disorders of the cervical spine. Intratester reliability was high (ICC = 0.93), and intertester reliability among seven different therapists was good (ICC = 0.83).

Capuano-Pucci et al.[6] also studied intratester and intertester reliability using the CROM device. Measurements of CROM were taken by two examiners on four males and 16 females with a mean age of 23.5 years. These authors concluded that the CROM device had acceptable reliability. Intertester reliability was slightly higher than intratester reliability, a finding attributed to the fact that the time interval between testers was only minutes, whereas the time interval between the first and second trials by one tester was 2 days.

Youdas et al.[7] employed five full-time physical therapy faculty members to determine intratester reliability of cervical ROM measurements during repeated testing on six healthy subjects. The testers followed a written protocol and were given a 30-minute training session using the CROM device prior to testing. Intertester reliability was determined on measurements of 20 healthy volunteers (11 females and 9 males) between 22 and 50 years of age. Each

subject's active ROM in six cervical motions was measured independently by three testers within moments of each other. The ICCs differed with the motions being measured. Median ICCs demonstrated that intratester reliability was fair for measurements of neck flexion (ICC = 0.76); high for measurements of neck extension (ICC = 0.94); and good for measurements of neck left lateral flexion (ICC = 0.86), right lateral flexion (ICC = 0.85), left rotation (ICC = 0.84), and right rotation (ICC = 0.80). Intertester reliability was high for measurements of neck extension (ICC = 0.90) and good for neck flexion (ICC = 0.83), left lateral flexion (ICC = 0.89), right lateral flexion (ICC = 0.87), and right rotation (ICC = 0.82). However, intertester reliability for measurements of left rotation was poor (ICC = 0.66).

Pendulum Goniometer

Defibaugh[13] used a pendulum goniometer with a mouthpiece attached to measure cervical motion. The 30 male subjects in this study ranged in age from 20 to 40 years. The author found coefficients of 0.909 to 0.711 for intratester reliability and coefficients of correlations of 0.939 to 0.660 for intertester reliability. Unlike the majority of other researchers, the author found that intertester reliability was higher than intratester reliability for some motions. However, 1 to 7 days had elapsed between the first and second measurements by the same tester, whereas only 2 hours had elapsed between one tester's and another tester's measurements. The higher intertester reliability was attributed to the short time between measurements.

Herrmann[14] took radiographic measurements of passive ROM of neck flexion-extension on 16 individuals 2 to 68 years of age. The radiographic measurements were compared with measurements obtained with a pendulum goniometer. ICCs of 0.98 indicated a good agreement between the two methods.

Gravity Goniometer and Tape Measure

Balogun et al.,[15] in a study that employed three testers and 21 healthy subjects, compared the reliability of measurements obtained with a Myrin Gravity-Reference Goniometer (OB Rehab AB, Soina, Sweden) with measurements taken by a tape measure. Intratester reliability coefficients for both the goniometer and the tape measure were moderately high, with the exception of those for flexion ROM. Intertester reliability was slightly higher for the tape measure method than for the goniometric method. However, intertester reliability of flexion measurements was poor for both methods.

Visual Estimation

The reliability of visual estimates has been studied by Viikari-Juntura[16] in a neurological patient population and by Youdas et al.[11] in an orthopedic patient population. In the study by Viikari-Juntura, the subjects were 52 male and female neurological patients ranging in age from 13 to 66 years who had been referred for cervical myelography. Intertester reliability between two testers of visual estimates of cervical ROM was determined to be fair.

In the study by Youdas et al.,[11] the subjects were 60 orthopedic patients ranging in age from 21 to 84 years. Intertester reliability for visual estimates of both active flexion and extension was poor (ICC = 0.42). Intertester reliability for visual estimates of active neck lateral flexion ROM was fair. The ICC for left lateral flexion was 0.63; for right lateral flexion it was 0.70. The intertester reliability for visual estimates of rotation was poor for left rotation (ICC = 0.69) and good for right rotation (ICC = 0.82).

Flexible Ruler

Rheault et al.[17] found that the intertester reliability was good (r = 0.80) for obtaining measurements of the neutral cervical spine position, and high (r = 0.90) for obtaining measurements of cervical spine flexion, using a flexible ruler. Measurements were taken on 20 healthy subjects (14 women and six men).

Summary

Each of the techniques for measuring cervical ROM discussed above has certain advantages and disadvantages.

The universal goniometer, tape measure, and flexible ruler are the most inexpensive and easy to obtain, transport, and use. Reliability tends to be motion specific, and generally, intratester reliability is better than intertester reliability. Therefore, if these methods are used to determine a patient's progress, measurements should be taken by a single therapist. The low reliability of visual estimation found in the studies militates against its use.

The advantages of the CROM device, gravity goniometer, and pendulum goniometer are that for some motions, intertester reliability is higher than for measurements obtained with the universal goniometer, tape measure, or flexible ruler. Also, Herrmann[14] has shown some evidence of the validity of measurements taken with a pendulum goniometer. The major disadvantages of these instruments are that they are expensive, may involve additional instruction and practice to use properly, and may not be readily available.

In consideration of the cost and availability of the various instruments for measuring cervical ROM, and the fact that the intratester reliability of the universal goniometer and tape measure appears comparable to that of measurements taken with other instruments, we decided to retain the universal goniometer and tape measure methods in this edition.

TESTING PROCEDURES

FLEXION

Motion occurs in the sagittal plane around a medial-lateral axis.

Recommended Testing Position

Position the subject sitting, with the thoracic and lumbar spine well supported by the back of a chair. The cervical spine is positioned in 0 degrees of rotation and lateral flexion. A tongue depressor can be held between the teeth for reference.

Stabilization

The shoulder girdle is stabilized to prevent flexion of the thoracic and lumbar spine. Usually the stabilization is achieved through the cooperation of the patient and support from the back of the chair (Fig. 10–1).

Goniometer Alignment

See Figures 10–2 and 10–3.

1. Center the fulcrum of the goniometer over the external auditory meatus.
2. Align the proximal arm so that it is either perpendicular or parallel to the ground.
3. Align the distal arm with the base of the nares. If a tongue depressor is used, align the arm of the goniometer parallel to the longitudinal axis of the tongue depressor.

Tape Measure Alternative Measurement Method

A tape measure can be used to measure the distance between the tip of the chin and the sternal notch. Make sure that the subject's mouth remains closed (Fig. 10–4).

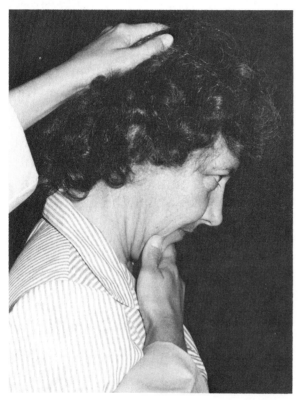

FIGURE 10–1. This photograph shows the end of the cervical flexion ROM. The examiner's left hand pushes gently on the posterior aspect of the subject's head to maintain cervical flexion. At the same time, the examiner's right hand pulls the subject's chin toward her chest. The examiner places her right arm across the subject's chest to prevent thoracic and lumbar spine flexion.

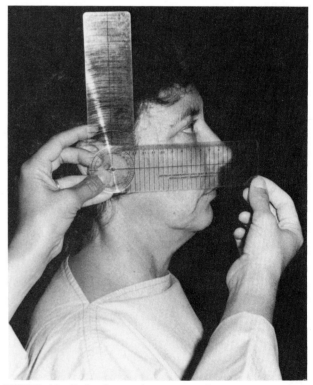

FIGURE 10–2. In the starting position for measuring cervical flexion ROM, the examiner aligns the proximal goniometer arm so that it is perpendicular to the floor. The goniometer body is centered over the subject's external auditory meatus. The examiner aligns the distal arm with the base of the nares. The goniometer will read 90 degrees in the zero starting position. This goniometer reading should be transposed and recorded as 0 degrees.

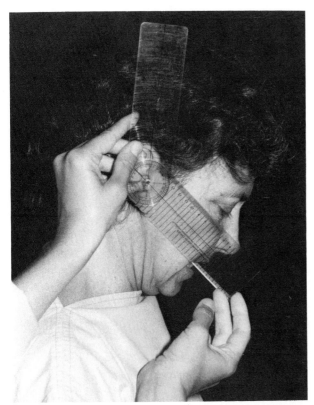

FIGURE 10-3. At the end of the ROM, the examiner's left hand aligns the proximal goniometer arm. The examiner uses her right hand to maintain alignment of the distal arm with the base of the nares. In this photograph, the goniometer reads 130 degrees at the end of the ROM. The cervical flexion ROM should be recorded as 0 to 40 degrees because the goniometer reads 90 degrees in the zero starting position. Alternatively, the examiner can align the distal arm parallel to the tongue depressor that the subject is holding between her teeth.

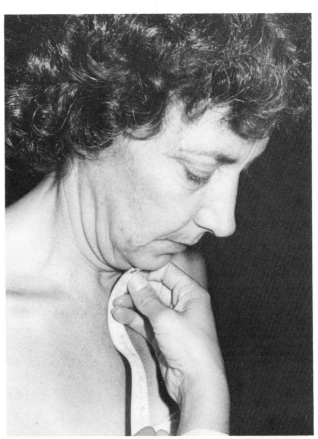

FIGURE 10-4. In the alternative method for measuring cervical flexion, the examiner uses a tape measure to determine the distance from the tip of the chin to the sternal notch.

EXTENSION

Motion occurs in the sagittal plane around a medial-lateral axis.

Recommended Testing Position, Stabilization, and Goniometer Alignment

The testing position, stabilization, and alignment are the same as for measuring cervical flexion (Figs. 10–5 to 10–7).

Tape Measure Alternative Measurement Method

A tape measure can be used to measure the distance between the tip of the chin and the sternal notch. Be sure that the subject's mouth remains closed (Fig. 10–8).

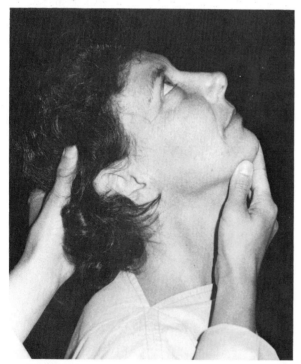

FIGURE 10–5. This photograph shows the end of the cervical extension ROM. The examiner prevents both cervical rotation and lateral flexion by holding the subject's chin with her right hand and the subject's posterior head with her left hand. The back of the chair (not visible) helps to prevent thoracic and lumbar extension.

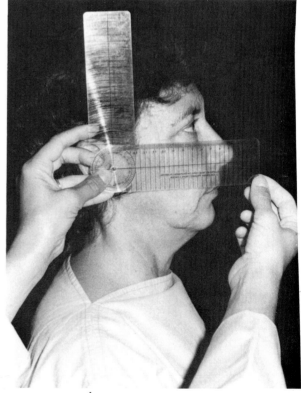

FIGURE 10–6. In the starting position for measuring cervical extension ROM, goniometer alignment is the same as for measuring cervical flexion ROM.

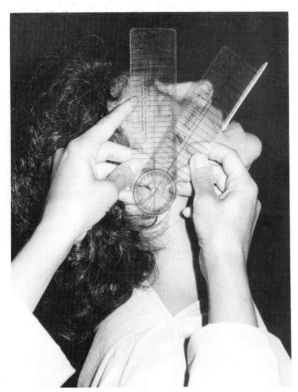

FIGURE 10-7. At the end of cervical extension, the examiner maintains the perpendicular alignment of the proximal goniometer arm with her left hand. With her right hand she aligns the distal arm with the base of the nares. The tongue depressor between the subject's teeth also can be used to align the distal arm.

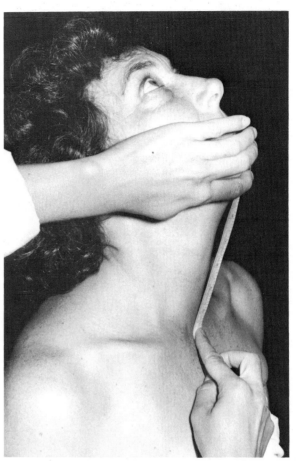

FIGURE 10-8. In the alternative method for measuring cervical extension, one end of the tape measure is placed on the tip of the subject's chin; the other end is placed at the subject's sternal notch. The distance between the two points of reference is recorded in inches or centimeters. The examiner measures the distance between the two reference points in the starting position first and then at the end of the ROM; the examiner records both beginning and ending measurements. The difference between the two measurements is the ROM. For example: Starting position: 2 inches; end ROM: 5 inches; ROM: 3 inches.

LATERAL FLEXION

Motion occurs in the frontal plane around an anterior-posterior axis.

Recommended Testing Position

Position the subject sitting, with the thoracic and lumbar spine well supported by the back of a chair. The cervical spine is positioned in 0 degrees of flexion, extension, and rotation.

Stabilization

Stabilize the shoulder girdle to prevent lateral flexion of the thoracic and lumbar spine (Fig. 10–9).

Goniometer Alignment

See Figures 10–10 and 10–11.

1. Center the fulcrum of the goniometer over the spinous process of the C7 vertebra.
2. Align the proximal arm with the spinous processes of the thoracic vertebrae so that the arm is perpendicular to the ground.
3. Align the distal arm with the dorsal midline of the head, using the occipital protuberance for reference.

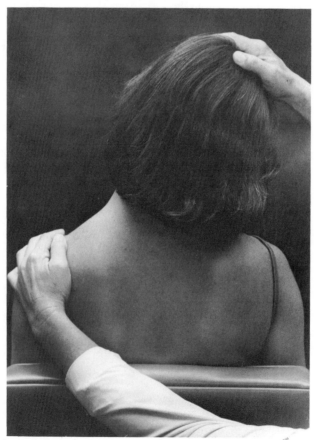

FIGURE 10–9. This photograph shows the end of the cervical lateral flexion ROM. The examiner's left hand holds the subject's left shoulder to prevent lateral flexion of the thoracic and lumbar spine. The examiner's right hand maintains cervical lateral flexion by pulling the subject's head laterally.

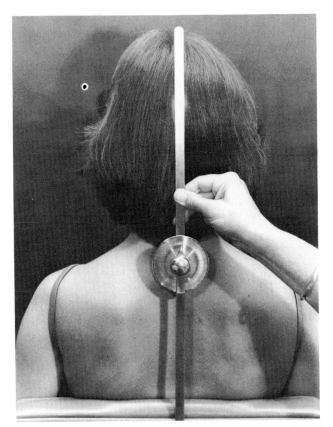

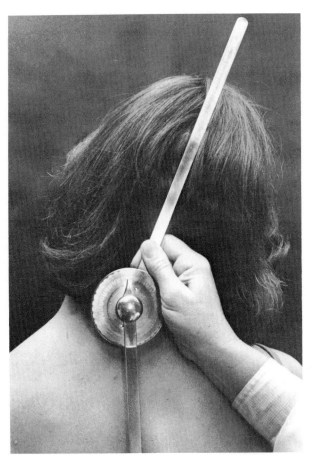

FIGURE 10–10. In the starting position for measuring lateral flexion ROM, the examiner centers the body of the goniometer over the subject's seventh cervical vertebra. The freely movable proximal goniometer arm hangs so that it is perpendicular to the floor.

FIGURE 10–11. At the end of the lateral flexion ROM, the examiner maintains alignment of the proximal goniometer arm with her right hand. In practice, the examiner would have one hand on the subject's head to maintain lateral flexion; for this photograph, the examiner is using only one hand so that the goniometer alignment is visible.

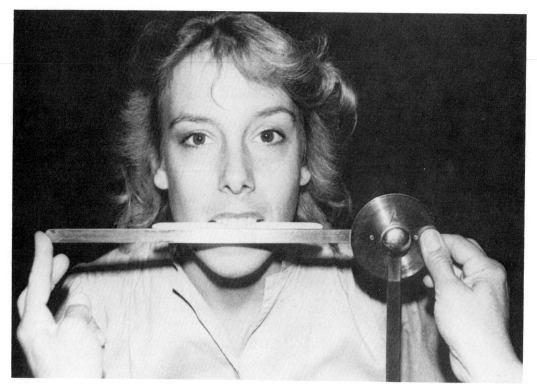

FIGURE 10–12. In the alternative method for measuring cervical lateral flexion, the subject holds a tongue depressor between her teeth (in this photograph the tongue depressor is almost completely hidden by the goniometer arm). The examiner aligns the distal goniometer arm parallel to the longitudinal axis of the tongue depressor. The proximal arm hangs so that it is perpendicular to the floor.

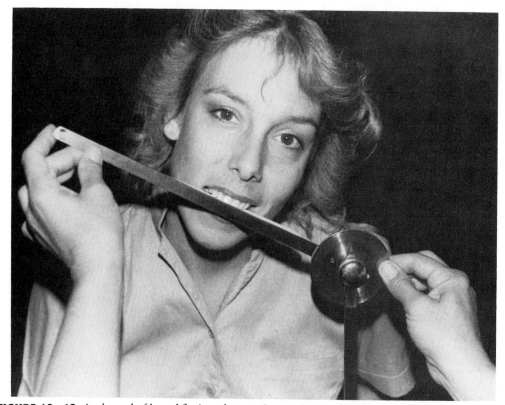

FIGURE 10–13. At the end of lateral flexion, the examiner maintains alignment of the distal goniometer arm with her left hand while holding the fulcrum of the instrument with her right hand.

Alternative Goniometer Alignment

A tongue depressor is held between the upper and lower teeth of both sides of the mouth (Figs. 10–12 and 10–13).

1. Center the fulcrum of the goniometer near one end of the tongue depressor.
2. Align the proximal arm so that it is either perpendicular or parallel to the ground.

3. Align the distal arm with the longitudinal axis of the tongue depressor.

Tape Measure Alternative Measurement Method

A tape measure can be used to measure the distance between the mastoid process and the acromial process (Fig. 10–14).

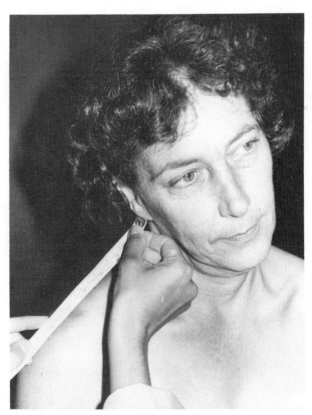

FIGURE 10–14. The distance between the subject's mastoid process and acromion process also can be used as a measurement of cervical lateral flexion ROM. The examiner measures the distance between the two reference points both in the starting position and at the end of the ROM. Both measurements are recorded, as well as the difference between them, which constitutes the ROM (the same method as described in Fig. 10–8). In this photograph, the subject is shown at the end of cervical lateral flexion ROM.

ROTATION

Motion occurs in the transverse plane around a vertical axis.

Recommended Testing Position

Position the subject sitting, with the thoracic and lumbar spine well supported by the back of the chair. The cervical spine is positioned in 0 degrees of flexion, extension, and lateral flexion. A tongue depressor can be held between the front teeth for reference.

Stabilization

Stabilize the shoulder girdle to prevent rotation of the thoracic and lumbar spine (Fig. 10–15).

Goniometer Alignment

See Figures 10–16 and 10–17.

1. Center the fulcrum of the goniometer over the center of the cranial aspect of the head.
2. Align the proximal arm parallel to an imaginary line between the two acromial processes.
3. Align the distal arm with the tip of the nose. If a tongue depressor is used, align the arm of the goniometer parallel to the longitudinal axis of the tongue depressor.

Tape Measure Alternative Measurement Method

A tape measure can be used to measure the distance between the tip of the chin and the acromial process (Fig. 10–18).

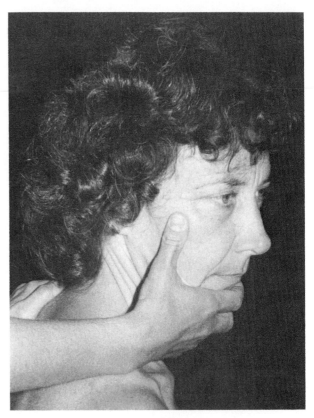

FIGURE 10–15. This photograph shows the end of the cervical rotation ROM. The examiner's right hand maintains rotation and prevents cervical flexion and extension. The examiner's left hand is placed on the subject's left shoulder to prevent rotation of the thoracic and lumbar spine.

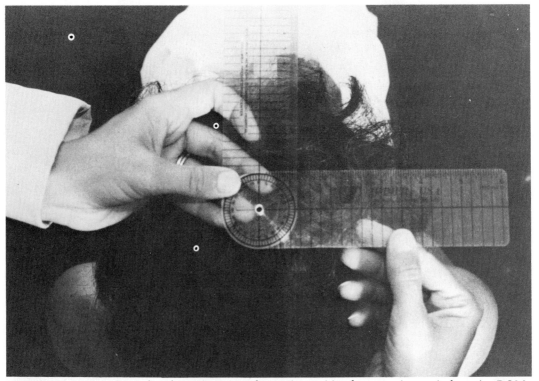

FIGURE 10–16. In order to align the goniometer at the starting position for measuring cervical rotation ROM, the examiner stands in back of the subject, who is seated in a low chair. The examiner centers the goniometer fulcrum on top of the subject's head and aligns the proximal goniometer arm parallel to an imaginary line between the subject's acromion processes. The examiner uses her left hand to align the distal goniometer arm with either the tip of the subject's nose or the tip of the tongue depressor.

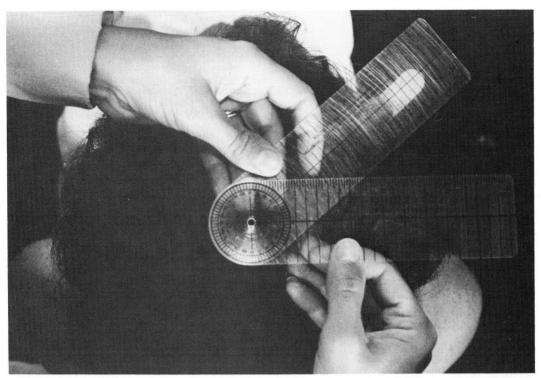

FIGURE 10–17. At the end of the range of right cervical rotation, the examiner's left hand maintains alignment of the distal goniometer arm with the tip of the subject's nose and with the tip of the tongue depressor. The examiner's right hand keeps the proximal arm aligned parallel to the imaginary line between the acromion processes.

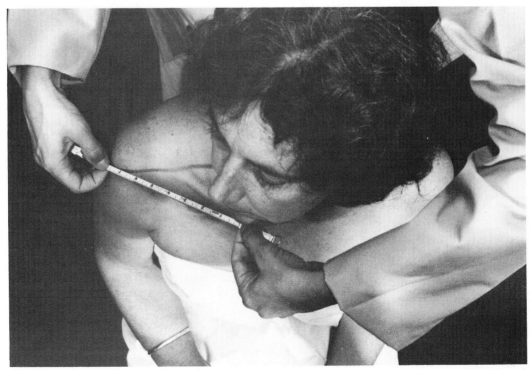

FIGURE 10–18. At the end of the right cervical ROM, the examiner is using a tape measure to determine the distance between the tip of the subject's chin and her right acromion process. The difference between the measurement taken in the starting position and the measurement at the end of the ROM provides information about the subject's right cervical rotation ROM.

REFERENCES

1. Hertling, D and Kessler, RM: Management of Common Musculo-skeletal Disorders, ed 2. JB Lippincott, Philadelphia, 1990.
2. White, AA and Punjabi, MM: Clinical Biomechanics of the Spine, ed 2. JB Lippincott, Philadelphia, 1990.
3. Norkin, CC and Levangie, PK: Joint Structure and Function: A Comprehensive Analysis, ed 2. FA Davis, Philadelphia, 1992.
4. American Academy of Orthopaedic Surgeons: Joint Motion: Method of Measuring and Recording. AAOS, Chicago, 1965.
5. American Medical Association: Guides to the Evaluation of Permanent Impairment, ed 3. AMA, Chicago, 1988.
6. Capuano-Pucci, D et al: Intratester and intertester reliability of the cervical range of motion. Arch Phys Med Rehabil 72:338, 1991.
7. Youdas, JW, et al: Normal range of motion of the cervical spine: An initial goniometric study. Phys Ther 72:770, 1992.
8. O'Driscoll, SL and Tomenson, J: The cervical spine. Clinics in Rheumatic Disease 8:617, 1982.
9. Keske, J, Johnson, G, and Ellingham, C: A reliability study of cervical range of motion of young and elderly subjects using an electromagnetic range of motion system (ENROM) [Abstract]. Phys Ther 71:S94, 1991.
10. Tucci, SM et al: Cervical motion assessment: A new, simple and accurate method. Arch Phys Med Rehabil 67:225, 1986.
11. Youdas, JW, Carey, JR, and Garrett, TR: Reliability of measurements of cervical spine range of motion: Comparison of three methods. Phys Ther 71:2, 1991.
12. Garrett, TR, Youdas, JW, and Madson, TJ: Reliability of measuring the forward head posture in patients [Abstract]. Phys Ther 71:S54, 1991.
13. Defibaugh, JJ: Measurement of head motion. Part II: An experimental study of head motion in adult males. Phys Ther 44:163, 1964.
14. Herrmann, DB: Validity study of head and neck flexion-extension motion comparing measurements of a pendulum goniometer and roentgenograms. Journal of Orthopaedic and Sports Physical Therapy 11:414, 1990.
15. Balogun, JA, et al: Inter- and intratester reliability of measuring neck motions with tape measure and Myrin Gravity-Reference Goniometer. Journal of Orthopaedic and Sports Physical Therapy: Jan:248, 1989.
16. Viikari-Juntura, E: Interexaminer reliability of observations in physical examination of the neck. Phys Ther 67:1526, 1987.
17. Rheault, W, et al: Intertester reliability of the flexible ruler for the cervical spine. Journal of Orthopaedic and Sports Physical Therapy Jan:254, 1989.

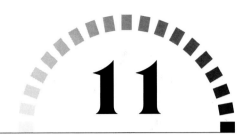

11

The Thoracic and Lumbar Spine

THORACIC SPINE: INTERVERTEBRAL, ZYGAPOPHYSIAL, COSTOVERTEBRAL, AND COSTOTRANSVERSE JOINTS

STRUCTURE

The intervertebral and zygapophysial joints have essentially the same structure as described for the cervical region, except that the superior zygapophysial facets face posteriorly and slightly laterally and cranially. The superior facet surfaces are slightly convex, whereas the inferior facet surfaces are slightly concave. The inferior facets face anteriorly and slightly medially and caudally. In addition, the joint capsules are tighter than in the cervical region and the spinous processes overlap each other.

The costovertebral joints are formed by a slightly convex costal facet on the head of a rib. From T2 to T8 they articulate with two concave demifacets on the inferior body of one vertebra and the superior aspect of the adjacent inferior vertebral body. Some of the costal facets also articulate with the interposed intervertebral disc, whereas the first, 11th, and 12th ribs articulate with only one vertebra. The costovertebral joints are surrounded by a thin fibrous capsule, which is strengthened by radial ligaments and the posterior longitudinal ligament. An intra-articular ligament lies within the capsule and holds the head of the rib to the annulus pulposus.

The costotransverse joints are formed by the concave costal tubercle and a convex costal facet on the transverse processes of T1 to T10. Costotransverse joints are not present in the last two or three ribs. The costotransverse joint capsules are strengthened by the medial, lateral, and superior costotransverse ligaments.

OSTEOKINEMATICS

The zygapophysial facets lie in the frontal plane from T1 to T6 and therefore limit flexion and extension in this region. The ribs and costal joints restrict lateral flexion. The facets in the lower thoracic region are oriented more in the sagittal plane and thus permit somewhat more flexion and extension. The thoracic region is, in general, less flexible than the cervical spine because of the limitations on movement imposed by the overlapping spinous processes, the tighter joint capsules, and the rib cage.

CAPSULAR PATTERN

The capsular pattern for the thoracic spine is a greater limitation of extension, lateral flexion, and rotation than of forward flexion.

LUMBAR SPINE: INTERVERTEBRAL AND ZYGAPOPHYSIAL JOINTS

STRUCTURE

The bodies of the five lumbar vertebrae are more massive than those in the other regions of the spine. The spinous processes are broad and thick and extend horizontally. The surfaces of the superior facets at the zygapophysial joints are concave and face medially and posteriorly. The inferior facet surfaces are convex and face laterally and anteriorly. The facets lie primarily in the sagittal plane, which favors flexion and extension and limits lateral flexion and rotation. The fifth lumbar vertebra differs from the other four vertebrae in having a wedge-shaped body, with the anterior height greater than the posterior height. The inferior facets of the fifth vertebra are widely spaced for articulation with the sacrum.

The joint capsules are strong. The ligaments of the region are essentially the same as for the thoracic region, except for the addition of the iliolumbar and thoracolumbar fascia. The iliolumbar ligament helps to stabilize the lumbosacral joint and prevent anterior displacement. The intertransverse ligament is well developed in the lumbar area and helps to limit lateral flexion. The posterior longitudinal ligament is not well developed in the lumbar area, but the anterior longitudinal ligament is strongest in this area.

OSTEOKINEMATICS

The zygapophysial facets of L1 to L4 lie primarily in the sagittal plane, which favors flexion and extension and limits lateral flexion and rotation. Flexion of the lumbar spine is more limited than extension. The greatest amount of flexion takes place at the lumbosacral joint. Lateral flexion and rotation are greatest in the upper lumbar region. Little or no lateral flexion is present at the lumbosacral joint because of the orientation of the facets.

CAPSULAR PATTERN

The capsular pattern for the lumbar spine is a marked and equal restriction of lateral flexion followed by restriction of flexion and extension.[1]

RANGE OF MOTION

Table 11–1 shows thoracolumbar spine ROM values from the AAOS and AMA.

EFFECTS OF AGE AND GENDER

Tables 11–2 and 11–3 show the effects of age and gender on thoracolumbar ROM as reported by Moll and Wright.[4] The measurement values in Tables 11–2 and 11–3 were obtained from a sampling of clinically and radiologically normal relatives of patients with psoriatic arthritis. The total number of subjects who participated in the study was 237 (118 females and 119 males) between 15 and 90 years of age. The method used to determine flexion ROM was the modified Schober technique as described by Macrae and Wright[5] in 1969. Lateral flexion was measured using a tape measure placed between the highest point on the iliac crest and the intersection of a horizontal line through the xiphisternum with a vertical line. Extension was measured using a plumb line and the same landmarks as for lateral flexion. They found that male ROM exceeded female ROM in forward flexion and extension, but that female ROM exceeded male ROM in lateral flexion. An initial increase in mean mobility occurred between 15 and 24 years of age, followed by a progressive decrease in succeeding decades. These authors suggested that age alone may decrease spinal mobility by as much as 23 percent to 52 percent.

Table 11–4 shows the results of a study by Fitzgerald et al.[6] on the effect of age on thoracolumbar ROM. The subjects who were measured to obtain the values presented in

Table 11–1 **THORACIC AND LUMBAR SPINE MOTION: MEAN VALUES IN DEGREES FROM SELECTED SOURCES**

Motion	AMERICAN ACADEMY OF ORTHOPAEDIC SURGEONS[2]*	AMERICAN MEDICAL ASSOCIATION[3]†
Flexion	80 (4 in)	60
Extension	20–30	25
Right lateral flexion	35	25
Left lateral flexion	35	25
Right rotation	45	30
Left rotation	45	30

*Values represent thoracolumbar motion. Flexion measurement in inches was obtained with a tape measure using the spinous processes of C7 and S1 as reference points.

†Lumbosacral motion was measured from midsacrum to T12 using a two-inclinometer method.

Table 11 – 2 **EFFECTS OF AGE AND GENDER ON THORACOLUMBAR MOTION IN INDIVIDUALS AGE 15 – 44 YR: MEAN VALUES IN CENTIMETERS**

| | 15 – 24 YR | | | | 25 – 34 YR | | | | 35 – 44 YR | | | |
| | MALE (N = 21) | | FEMALE (N = 10) | | MALE (N = 13) | | FEMALE (N = 16) | | MALE (N = 14) | | FEMALE (N = 18) | |
Motion	Mean	Standard Deviation	Mean	Standard Deviation	Mean	Standard Deviation	Mean	Standard Deviation	Mean	Standard Deviation	Mean	Standard Deviation
Flexion	7.23	0.92	6.66	1.03	7.48	0.82	6.69	1.09	6.88	0.88	6.29	1.04
Extension	4.21	1.64	4.34	1.52	5.05	1.41	4.76	1.53	3.73	1.47	3.09	1.31
Right lateral flexion	5.43	1.30	6.85	1.46	5.34	1.06	6.32	1.93	4.83	1.34	5.30	1.61
Left lateral flexion	5.06	1.40	7.20	1.66	5.93	1.07	6.13	1.42	4.83	0.99	5.48	1.30

Adapted from Moll and Wright.[4]

Table 11 – 3 **EFFECTS OF AGE AND GENDER ON THORACOLUMBAR MOTION IN INDIVIDUALS AGE 45 – 74 YR: MEAN VALUES IN CENTIMETERS**

| | 45 – 54 YR | | | | 55 – 64 YR | | | | 65 – 74 YR | | | |
| | MALE (N = 19) | | FEMALE (N = 23) | | MALE (N = 34) | | FEMALE (N = 30) | | MALE (N = 14) | | FEMALE (N = 14) | |
Motion	Mean	Standard Deviation	Mean	Standard Deviation	Mean	Standard Deviation	Mean	Standard Deviation	Mean	Standard Deviation	Mean	Standard Deviation
Flexion	7.17	1.20	6.02	1.32	6.87	0.89	6.08	1.32	5.67	1.31	4.93	0.90
Extension	3.88	1.19	3.12	1.36	3.56	1.28	3.57	1.32	3.41	1.56	2.72	0.95
Right lateral flexion	4.71	1.35	5.37	1.54	5.05	1.30	5.10	1.85	4.44	1.03	5.56	2.04
Left lateral flexion	4.55	0.94	5.14	1.54	4.94	1.22	4.88	1.61	4.38	0.98	5.55	2.16

Adapted from Moll and Wright.[4]

Table 11 – 4 **EFFECTS OF AGE ON LUMBAR SPINE MOTION: MEAN VALUES IN DEGREES**

| | 20 – 29 YR (N = 31) | | 30 – 39 YR (N = 42) | | 40 – 49 YR (N = 16) | | 50 – 59 YR (N = 43) | | 60 – 69 YR (N = 26) | | 70 – 79 YR (N = 9) | |
Motion	Mean	Standard Deviation	Mean	Standard Deviation	Mean	Standard Deviation	Mean	Standard Deviation	Mean	Standard Deviation	Mean	Standard Deviation
Flexion*	3.7	0.7	3.9	1.0	3.1	0.8	3.0	1.1	2.4	0.7	2.2	0.6
Extension	41.2	9.6	40.0	8.8	31.1	8.9	27.4	8.0	17.4	7.5	16.6	8.8
Right lateral flexion	37.6	5.8	35.3	6.5	27.1	6.5	25.3	6.2	20.2	4.8	18.0	4.7
Left lateral flexion	38.7	5.7	36.5	6.0	28.5	5.2	26.8	6.4	20.3	5.3	18.9	6.0

Adapted from Fitzgerald et al.[6] with the permission of the American Physical Therapy Association.
*Measurements obtained using the Schober method and reported in centimeters. All other measurements were obtained using a universal goniometer and are reported in degrees.

Table 11–4 were 172 patient volunteers (four females and 168 males). None of the patients had current back pain. The authors used the Schober technique to measure flexion and the universal goniometer to measure extension and lateral flexion. A review of the values in Table 11–4 shows that the oldest group had considerably less motion than the youngest group. The difference in values is greater than two standard deviations for all motions. The coefficients of variation indicated that a greater amount of variability exists in the ROM in the oldest groups.

The following authors, among others, also have contributed to our understanding of the effects of age and gender on ROM and the difficulties encountered in obtaining accurate and valid information: Macrae and Wright,[5] Moll and Wright,[4] Loebl,[7] Moll et al.,[8] Hart et al.,[9] Anderson and Sweetman,[10] Sughara et al.,[11] and Bookstein, et al.[12]

As with the cervical spine, a wide range of instruments and methods has been used to determine the range of thoracic, thoracolumbar, and lumbar motion. Therefore comparisons between studies are difficult. As is true for other regions of the body, conflicting evidence exists regarding the effects of age and gender on ROM. However, most studies indicate that age- and gender-related changes in the ROM occur and that these changes may affect certain motions more than other motions at the same joint or region.

In one of the earlier studies, Loebl[7] used an inclinometer to measure the active ROM of the thoracic and lumbar spine of 126 males and females between 15 and 84 years of age. He found no significant gender differences between males and females for measurements of lumbar flexion and extension. However, he found age-related effects for both males and females, and concluded that both genders should expect a loss of about 8 degrees of spinal ROM per decade with increases in age.

Macrae and Wright[5] used a modification of the Schober technique to measure forward flexion in 195 females and 147 males age 18 to 71 years. In the original Schober method, the subject was positioned in normal standing posture, and the examiner made two marks on the subject's back. The first mark was made on the spine at the lumbosacral junction. The second mark was made on the spine 10 cm superior to the first mark. A tape measure was held directly over the spine between the two marks. When the subject bent forward, the increase in the distance between the two marks was measured as the ROM in flexion.

Macrae's and Wright's[5] modification of the original Schober technique included a third mark made 5 cm below the lumbosacral junction mark. The inferior mark instead of the lumbosacral junction mark was used for the inferior placement of the tape measure. Therefore the measurement began with a 15-cm difference between the inferior and superior marks. Macrae and Wright decided on the modification because they found that the skin over the lumbosacral junction moved upward in relation to the spinous processes of both the inferior and superior marks in the original method. These authors believed that the skin

was more firmly attached 5 cm lower. Using the modified technique, Macrae and Wright found that active ROM decreased with age and that females had significantly less forward flexion than males across all age groups.

Moll et al.[8] used skin markings and a plumb line to measure the range of lumbar extension in a study involving 237 subjects (119 males and 118 females) age 20 to 90 years. In contrast to the findings of Loebl,[7] these authors found differences between males and females in different age groups. However, they also found a wide variation in normal values. They detected a gradual decrease in mobility from 35 to 90 years of age and determined that male mobility in extension significantly exceeded female mobility by 7 percent.

Hart et al.[9] used a spondylometer to measure ROM in 24 male and three female subjects who were observed for 10 to 26 years. These authors found no decreases in ROM that could be attributed to age.

Anderson and Sweetman[10] employed a device that combined a flexible rule and a hydrogoniometer to measure the ROM of 432 working males age 20 to 59 years. Increasing age was associated with a lower total lumbar spine ROM (flexion and extension). Of a total of 74 males who had less than 50 degrees combined flexion-extension, 32 were in the 50 to 59-year-old category, compared with 9 in the 20- to 29-year-old group. Of the 162 men who had more than 60 degrees total ROM, 22 were in the 50- to 59-year-old group and 60 were in the 20- to 29-year-old category. These authors also measured the angle of sacral tilt and found no age-related changes in the angle.

Sughara et al.,[11] using a device called a spinometer, studied age- and occupation-related changes in thoracolumbar active ROM in 1071 males and 1243 females ages 20 to 60 years. The subjects were selected from three occupational groups: fishermen, farmers, and industrial workers. These authors found that although both flexion and extension decreased with increasing age, decreases in the extension ROM were greater than decreases in flexion. Decreases in the extension active ROM were less in the group of fishermen and their wives than in the farmer and industrial worker groups and their wives. The authors concluded that because the fishermen's wives, like the fishermen, had more extension than other groups, variables other than the physical demands of fishing were affecting the maintenance of extension ROM in the fisherman group. The authors related decreases in body height and extension ROM as being indicators of senility.

Bookstein et al.[12] used a tape measure to measure the lumbar extension ROM in 75 elementary school children 6 to 11 years of age. No differences were found for age or gender, but a significant difference was found for age-gender interaction in the 6-year-old group. Girls aged 6 had a mean range of extension of 4.1 cm in contrast to the 6-year-old boys, who had a mean range of extension of 2.1 cm.

Although comparisons between the studies are not possible because of differences in measurement methods, the preponderance of evidence appears to indicate that age and gender affect active ROM in the thoracolumbar spine and that these changes are motion specific. The fact that ROM appears to decrease with age is consistent with the literature on age-related changes in the intervertebral discs, which would produce decreases in the ROM as well as decreases in height.

RELIABILITY AND VALIDITY

The following section on reliability and validity has been divided according to the instruments and procedures used to obtain the measurements. Some overlap occurs between the divisions because several investigators have compared different methods and instruments.

Inclinometer

Loebl[7] has stated that the only reliable method of measuring lumbar spine motion is radiography. However, radiography is not only expensive but poses a risk to the subject. Therefore, researchers have used many different instruments and methods in a search for reliable and valid measures of lumbar spine motion. Loebl used an inclinometer to measure flexion and extension in nine subjects. He found that the active ROM among the five measurements that he performed varied by 5 degrees in the most consistent subject and by 23 degrees in the most inconsistent subject. Variability decreased when measurements were taken on an hourly rather than on a daily basis. Patel,[13] who used the double inclinometer method to measure lumbar flexion on 25 subjects age 21 to 37 years, found intratester reliability to be high ($r = 0.91$) but intertester reliability to be only moderate ($r = 0.68$).

The AMA *Guides to the Evaluation of Permanent Impairment*[3] states that "measurement techniques using inclinometers are necessary to obtain reliable spinal mobility measurements." However, in a recent study by Williams et al.[14] comparing the inclinometer with the tape measure, the authors found that the double inclinometer technique had questionable reliability. ICCs for intertester reliability for measurements with the inclinometer were 0.60 for flexion and 0.48 for extension, in comparison with measurements with the tape measure, which had ICCs of 0.72 for flexion and 0.76 for extension.

Schober Technique, Inclinometer, Spondylometer, Gravity Goniometer, Universal Goniometer, and Fingertip-to-Floor Method

Macrae and Wright,[5] using both the original two-mark Schober technique and a three-mark modification of the Schober technique, found a linear relationship between these methods and radiography. The correlation coefficient was 0.90 between the Schober technique and radiographs with a standard error of 6.2 degrees. The correlation coefficient was 0.97 between the modified Schober method and radiographs, with a standard error of 3.25 degrees. Clinical identification of the lumbosacral junction was not easy, and faulty placement of skin marks seriously impaired the accuracy of the unmodified technique. Placement of marks 2 cm too low led to an overestimate of 14 degrees. Marks placed 2 cm too high led to an underestimate of 15 degrees. In the modified Schober technique, the same errors in placement led to overestimates and underestimates of 5 and 3 degrees, respectively.

Moll and Wright,[4] using a plumb line and skin marks to measure spinal extension in 14 subjects, found a positive correlation ($r = 0.75$) between displacement of lateral trunk skin marks and the true angle of thoracolumbar spinal extension as measured by radiography. These authors cited this finding as evidence of the validity of using lateral skin marks as an index of thoracolumbar extension.

Reynolds[15] compared intratester and intertester reliability using a spondylometer, a plumb line and skin distraction, and an inclinometer. Intertester error was calculated by comparing the results of two testers taking 10 repeated measurements of lumbar flexion, extension, and lateral flexion on 30 volunteers with a mean age of 38.1 years. Highly significant positive correlations were found between flexion-extension ROM measured with the inclinometer and the spondylometer. Lumbar flexion measurements correlated well with skin distraction and the inclinometer. Both the spondylometer and the inclinometer had acceptable intertester reliability. The skin distraction method had acceptable intertester reliability only for extension. The highest intratester reliability was found for lateral flexion to the right using the inclinometer and the spondylometer.

Miller et al.[16] compared the following four methods for measuring thoracolumbar mobility: the fingertip-to-floor method, the modified Schober technique, the OB Myrin gravity goniometer (LIC Rehab, Sweden), and a skin contraction 10-cm-segment method using a tape measure. Four testers measured four subjects (one healthy subject and three patients with ankylosing spondylitis) using all four methods. Intertester error was not found to be a significant source of variation. The 10-cm-segment method was found to be the most sensitive in detecting a loss of spinal mobility in the upper and middle 10-cm segments. The fingertip-to-floor method was the next sensitive, followed by the 10-cm-segment technique for the lower 10-cm segment, and the modified Schober technique. The least sensitive was the OB Myrin goniometric measurement. The testers rated the fingertip-to-floor method as the most convenient, followed by the modified Schober technique, the 10-cm-segment method, and the OB Myrin goniometer.

Portek et al.[17] studied 11 normal males between 25 and 36 years of age and 14 patients (nine males 16 to 58 years of age and five females 18 to 69 years of age). These authors found little correlation either among measurements obtained by two testers using three clinical techniques or among the three clinical techniques and radiographs. The clinical measures used were an inclinometer technique described by Loebl,[7] a plumb line method for measuring extension, and a skin distraction technique for measuring flexion. The inclinometer provided reproducible results, but only with careful monitoring. The coefficient of variation (CV) for flexion for the inclinometer was 16.4%. The intertester error for the skin distraction method for flexion showed significant differences between testers, according to paired t-tests. However, intertester error was calculated between 10 measurements on 10 different days, and the authors attributed the error to difficulties in reestablishing a neutral starting position and mobility of the skin over the landmarks.

Gill et al.[18] compared the reliability of four methods of measurement including fingertip-to-floor distance, the modified Schober technique, the two-inclinometer method, and a photometric technique. The subjects of the study were 10 volunteers (five males and five females) 24 to 34 years of age. Repeatability of the fingertip-to-floor method was poor (CV = 14.1%). Repeatability of the inclinometer for the measurement of full flexion was also poor (CV = 33.9%). However, the modified Schober technique yielded a CV of 0.9% for full flexion and a CV of 2.8 for extension.

Fitzgerald et al.[11] used the Schober technique to measure forward thoracolumbar flexion and the universal goniometer to measure lateral flexion and extension. Intertester reliability was calculated from measurements taken by two testers on 17 physical therapy student volunteers. Pearson reliability coefficients were calculated on paired results of the two testers. Intertester reliability for the Schober test for flexion was 1.0. Intertester reliability for the goniometric measurements were 0.88 for extension, 0.76 for right lateral flexion, and 0.91 for left lateral flexion.

Williams et al.[14] measured flexion and extension on 15 patient volunteers (eight females and seven males) with a mean age of 35.7 years with chronic low back pain. They used a modified–modified Schober technique (MMS), and the double-inclinometer method. The MMS uses two marks—one over the spine on a line connecting the two posterior superior iliac spines (PSIS) and one over the spine 15 cm superior to the first mark. This technique was developed to eliminate errors in identification of the lumbosacral junction. Intertester ICCs between the three physical therapist testers were 0.72 for flexion and 0.765 for extension using the MMS. Intertester ICCs for the double inclinometers were 0.60 for flexion and 0.48 for extension. The therapists underwent training in the use of standardized procedures for each method prior to testing. According to the testers, the Schober method was easier and quicker to use than the double-inclinometer method.

Flexible Ruler

Reliability and validity of measurements of lumbar spine motion and position have been conducted using the flexible ruler by Lindahl,[19] Bryan et al.,[20] and Lovell et al.[21]

Lindahl[19] evaluated five methods of measuring lumbar spine motion, including the fingertips-to-floor method and the flexible ruler. In the fingertip-to-floor method, the authors found that values in maximum flexion ranged from −10 to 50 cm and included hip joint motion, whereas the flexible ruler provided a fairly accurate record of range of spinal mobility in maximum extension and flexion.

Bryan et al.[20] used the flexible ruler to measure lumbar lordosis in 45 adult females (21 blacks and 24 whites) between 18 and 40 years of age. The authors found poor correlation between the measurements obtained with the flexible ruler and the radiograph. Because of the poor criterion validity of the flexible ruler, the authors suggested that its use be discontinued.

Lovell et al.[21] examined the intratester and intertester reliability of lumbar lordosis measurements taken with the flexible ruler on 80 subjects (40 with low back pain and 40 without low back pain). Intratester reliability ranged from 0.73 to 0.94, but intertester reliability was poor.

Automated Video System

Robinson et al.[22] used Spinetrak (Motion Analysis Corp., Santa Rosa, CA), an automated video motion analysis system, to obtain ROM and velocity measurements on a clinical population consisting of 33 men and nine women with a mean age of 38.5 years. All subjects had complained of back pain for more than 6 months and were being evaluated for a back rehabilitation program. Correlation coefficients ranged from 0.77 for thoracolumbar flexion to 0.95 for thoracolumbopelvic flexion. The authors concluded that intrasubject reliability had been established through their study.

Summary

The sampling of studies reviewed above reflects the amount of effort that has been directed toward finding a reliable and valid method for measuring spinal motion. Each method reviewed has advantages and disadvantages, and clinicians should select a method that appears to be appropriate for their particular clinical situation and then determine its reliability. The advantages of using a tape measure technique for measuring spinal ROM are that the tape measure is easy to obtain, inexpensive, and quick and easy to use. As with other methods, intertester reliability is motion specific and is lower than intratester reliability. However, in at least one study, the tape measure was found to have higher intertester reliability than the double-inclinometer method.

The Schober technique is reported to be easier to use than the double-inclinometer method and has been found to have good reliability and validity. This method is slightly more difficult to use than the simple tape measure method but is inexpensive and can be performed quickly. The major disadvantage of this technique is difficulty in locating the lumbosacral junction, which can lead to errors in measurement.

According to Fitzgerald et al.,[11] intertester reliability was good for measurements of extension and left lateral flexion using the universal goniometer. The advantages of the universal goniometer are that it is readily available, inexpensive, and easy to use. The disadvantage is that it is difficult to align for flexion and extension.

The advantage of the double-inclinometer method is that it is the method mandated by the AMA for disability evaluations of the spine. The disadvantages of this method are that the inclinometers are relatively expensive and difficult to manipulate, and errors in locating landmarks and placing the instrument are problematic. Therefore, to master the technique and obtain accurate measurements, a considerable amount of practice time and careful monitoring is necessary. Because intratester reliability of the inclinometer method has been found to be only moderate, and because intertester reliability ranges between poor and high in different studies, the double-inclinometer method does not appear to be superior to the tape measure and Schober techniques. An examiner who must use the double-inclinometer method to evaluate spinal ROM for a disability determination should follow the instructions in the AMA *Guides to the Evaluation of Permanent Impairment.*[3]

The flexible ruler has been reported by Bryan et al.[20] to have low criterion validity and therefore is not recommended.

TESTING PROCEDURES

The testing procedures that are discussed in the following section include the universal goniometer, the simple tape measure method, and the modified Schober technique as described by Macrae and Wright.[4] These methods were selected because they are inexpensive, relatively easy to use, and have comparable reliability and validity with other methods. We hope that by the time the next edition of this textbook is being prepared, conclusive evidence regarding the reliability and validity of some of the newer methods of measuring spinal ROM will be available.

FLEXION

Motion occurs in the sagittal plane around a medial-lateral axis.

Recommended Testing Position

Position the subject standing with the cervical, thoracic, and lumbar spine in 0 degrees of lateral flexion and rotation.

Stabilization

Stabilize the pelvis to prevent anterior tilting (Fig. 11 – 1).

Measurement

One method for determining the range of thoracic and lumbar flexion is to measure the distance between the spinous processes of C7 and S1 with a tape measure. The initial measurement is made with the subject in the upright zero starting position, and the final measurement is made at the end of the ROM (Figs. 11 – 2 and 11 – 3). The difference between these two measurements indicates the amount of

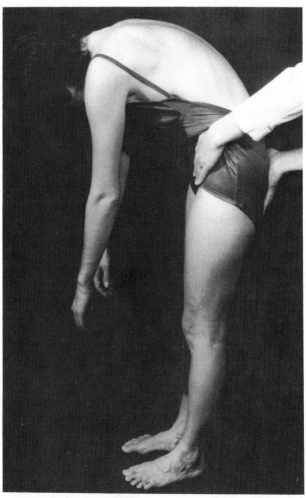

FIGURE 11 – 1. This photograph shows the end of thoracic and lumbar flexion ROM. The examiner stabilizes the subject to prevent anterior pelvic tilting while the subject bends forward.

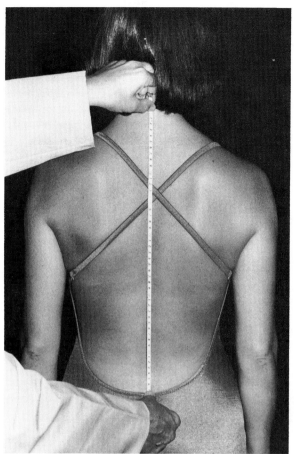

FIGURE 11–2. In the starting position for measuring thoracic and lumbar flexion ROM, the examiner positions one end of the tape measure at the subject's seventh cervical vertebra and the other end over the first sacral vertebra.

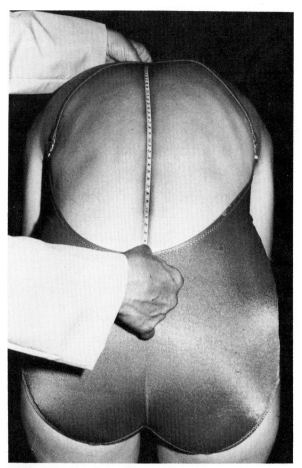

FIGURE 11–3. At the end of the ROM, the examiner is maintaining the cervical end of the tape measure over the spinous process of the subject's seventh cervical vertebra. The sacral end of the tape measure is allowed to unwind and accommodate the spinal movement. The metal tape measure case (not visible in the photo) is in the examiner's right hand.

thoracic and lumbar flexion that is present. Magee[23] states that a 10-cm difference in tape measure length is normal for this measurement. The AAOS[2] states that 4 inches is an average measurement for healthy adults.

Another method used by some examiners assesses thoracic and lumbar flexion by measuring, at the end of the ROM, the distance between the tip of the subject's middle finger and the floor. This fingertip-to-floor, or forward bending, test combines spinal flexion and hip flexion, making it difficult to isolate and measure spinal flexion. Therefore, this test is not recommended for measuring thoracic and lumbar flexion but can be used to assess general body flexibility.[24–26]

Alternative Measurement Method: Modified Schober Technique

The subject stands with the feet about 15 cm apart. The examiner stands behind the subject and makes the following three marks:

1. One mark on the lumbosacral junction
2. A second mark on a spinous process 10 cm above the first mark (measure to the nearest millimeter)
3. A third mark 5 cm below the first mark

Align the tape measure between the most superior and most inferior marks, with 0 at the inferior mark. Ask the subject to bend forward as far as possible while keeping the knees straight. Maintain the tape measure against the subject's back during the movement and record the distance between the most superior and inferior marks at the end of the ROM. The ROM is the difference between the 15 cm and the length measured at the end of the motion.

Tables 11–2 and 11–3 may also be used as references for this measurement.

EXTENSION

Motion occurs in the sagittal plane around a medial-lateral axis.

Recommended Testing Position, Stabilization, and Measurement

The testing position, stabilization, and measurement are the same as for thoracic and lumbar flexion (Figs. 11–4 to 11–6).

Alternate Measurement Method: Modified Schober Technique

The testing position and tape measure alignment are the same as those used in the modified Schober technique of measuring flexion. However, the examiner should ask the patient to put his hands on his buttocks and to bend backward as far as possible. The ROM is the difference between the initial length of 15 cm and the length obtained at the end of the ROM.

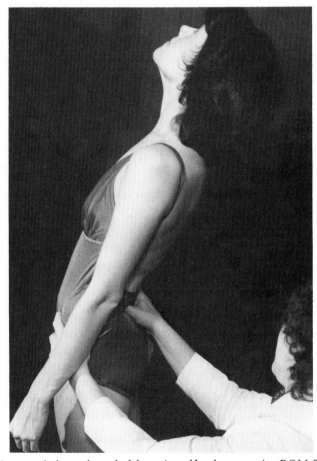

FIGURE 11–4. This photograph shows the end of thoracic and lumbar extension ROM. The examiner uses her left hand on the subject's anterior pelvis and her right hand on the posterior pelvis to prevent posterior pelvic tilting. If the subject has balance problems or muscle weakness in the lower extremities, the measurement can be taken in either the prone or side-lying position.

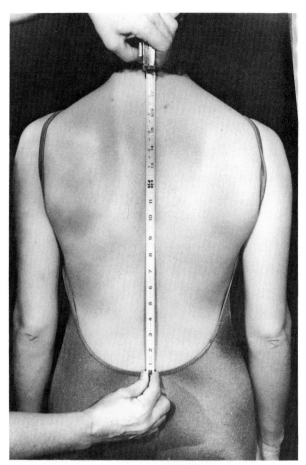

FIGURE 11-5. The positioning of the tape measure for measuring thoracic and lumbar extension ROM is the same as that for measuring thoracic and lumbar flexion ROM. In this photograph, the tape measure case is in the examiner's left hand. When the subject moves into extension, the tape slides into the case.

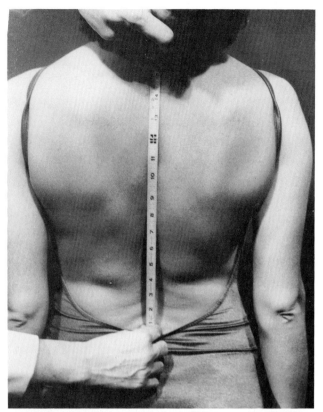

FIGURE 11-6. At the end of thoracic and lumbar extension ROM, the distance between the two reference points is less than that in the starting position. The difference between the measurement taken in the starting position and that at the end of the ROM constitutes the total ROM. The starting measurement, the end measurement, and the difference between these measurements are recorded in either inches or centimeters.

LATERAL FLEXION

Motion occurs in the frontal plane around an anterior-posterior axis.

Recommended Testing Position

Position the subject standing, with the cervical, thoracic, and lumbar spine in 0 degrees of flexion, extension, and rotation.

Stabilization

Stabilize the pelvis to prevent lateral tilting (Fig. 11–7).

Goniometer Alignment

See Figures 11–8 and 11–9.

1. Center the fulcrum of the goniometer over the posterior aspect of the spinous process of S1.
2. Align the proximal arm so that it is perpendicular to the ground.
3. Align the distal arm with the posterior aspect of the spinous process of C7.

Tables 11–1 and 11–4 can be used as references for normal ROM values.

Alternative Measurement Method

To measure the distance between the tip of the middle finger and the floor, both feet must be flat on the ground and the knees extended (Fig. 11–10).

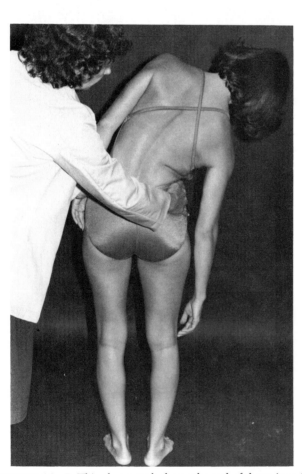

FIGURE 11–7. This photograph shows the end of thoracic and lumbar lateral flexion ROM. The examiner places both hands on the subject's pelvis to prevent lateral pelvic tilting.

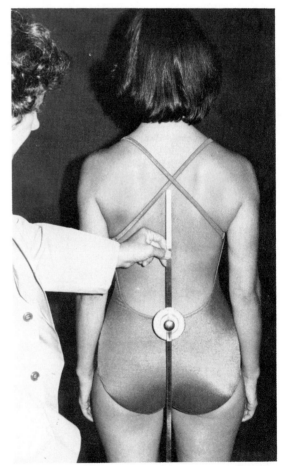

FIGURE 11–8. In the starting position for measuring thoracic and lumbar lateral flexion, the examiner centers the fulcrum of the goniometer over the spinous process of the subject's first sacral vertebra; the freely movable proximal goniometer arm hangs so that it is perpendicular to the floor. The examiner aligns the distal goniometer arm with the spinous process of the subject's seventh cervical vertebra.

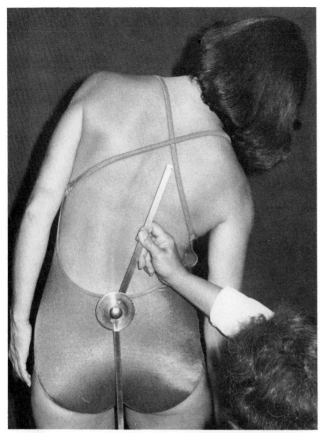

FIGURE 11–9. At the end of thoracic and lumbar lateral flexion, the examiner keeps the distal goniometer arm aligned with the subject's seventh cervical vertebra. The examiner makes no attempt to align the distal arm with the subject's vertebral column. As can be seen in the photograph, the lower thoracic and upper lumbar spine become convex to the left during right lateral flexion.

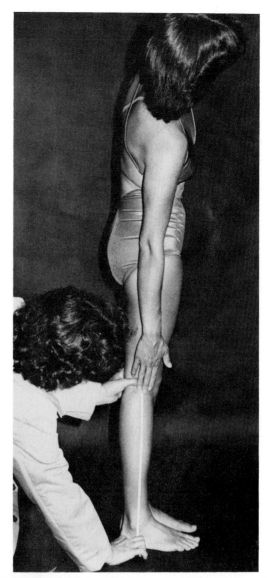

FIGURE 11–10. At the end of thoracic and lumbar lateral flexion ROM, the examiner is using a tape measure to determine the distance from the tip of the subject's third finger to the floor. Lateral pelvic tilting should be avoided.

ROTATION

Motion occurs in the transverse plane around a vertical axis.

Recommended Testing Position

Position the subject sitting, with the feet on the floor to help stabilize the pelvis. A seat without a back support is preferred so that rotation of the spine can occur freely. The cervical, thoracic, and lumbar spine are in 0 degrees of flexion, extension, and lateral flexion.

Stabilization

Stabilize the pelvis to prevent rotation (Fig. 11–11). Avoid flexion, extension, and lateral flexion of the spine.

Goniometer Alignment

See Figures 11–12 and 11–13.

1. Center the fulcrum of the goniometer over the center of the cranial aspect of the head.
2. Align the proximal arm parallel to an imaginary line between the two prominent tubercles on the iliac crests.
3. Align the distal arm with an imaginary line between the two acromial processes.

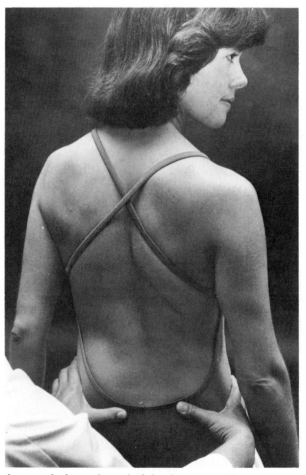

FIGURE 11–11. This photograph shows the end of the thoracic and lumbar rotation ROM. The subject is seated on a low stool without a back rest, so that spinal movement can occur without interference. The examiner positions her hands on the subject's iliac crests to prevent pelvic rotation.

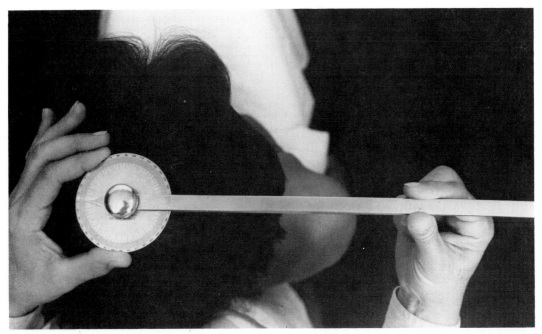

FIGURE 11-12. In the starting position for measuring rotation ROM, the examiner stands behind the seated subject. The examiner positions the fulcrum of the goniometer on the superior aspect of the subject's head. The examiner's right hand is holding both arms of the goniometer aligned with the subject's acromion processes. The subject should be positioned so that the acromion processes are aligned directly over the iliac tubercles.

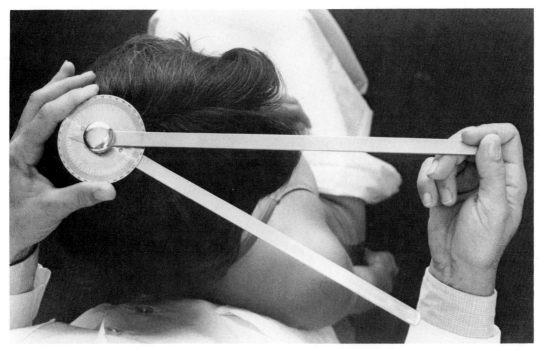

FIGURE 11-13. At the end of rotation, the examiner's right hand keeps the proximal goniometer arm aligned with the subject's iliac tubercles while keeping the distal goniometer arm aligned with the subject's right acromion process.

REFERENCES

1. Cyriax, JH and Cyriax, P: Illustrated Manual of Orthopaedic Medicine. Butterworths, London, 1983.
2. American Academy of Orthopaedic Surgeons: Joint Motion: Method of Measuring and Recording. AAOS, Chicago, 1965.
3. American Medical Association: Guides to the Evaluation of Permanent Impairment, ed 3. AMA, Chicago, 1988.
4. Moll, JMH and Wright, V: Normal range of spinal mobility: An objective clinical study. Ann Rheum Dis 30:381, 1971.
5. Macrae, IF and Wright, V: Measurement of back movement. Ann Rheum Dis 28:584, 1969.
6. Fitzgerald, GK et al: Objective assessment with establishment of normal values for lumbar spine range of motion. Phys Ther 63:1776, 1983.
7. Loebl, WY: Measurement of spinal posture and range of spinal movement. Annals of Physical Medicine 9:103, 1967.
8. Moll, JMH, Liyange, SP, and Wright, V: An objective method to measure lateral spinal flexion. Rheumatology and Physical Medicine 11:225, 1972.
9. Hart, FD, Strickland, D, and Cliffe, P: Measurement of spinal mobility. Ann Rheum Dis 33:136, 1974.
10. Anderson, JAD and Sweetman, BJ: A combined flexi-rule hydrogoniometer for measurement of lumbar spine and its sagittal movement. Rheumatology and Rehabilitation 14:173, 1975.
11. Sughara, M et al: Epidemiological study on the change of mobility of the thoraco-lumbar spine and body height with age as indices for senility. J Hum Ergol (Tokyo) 10:49, 1981.
12. Bookstein, NA et al: Lumbar extension range of motion in elementary school children [abstract]. Abstracts in Physical Therapy 72:S35, 1992.
13. Patel, RS: Intratester and intertester reliability of the inclinometer in measuring lumbar flexion [abstract]. Abstracts in Physical Therapy 72:S44, 1992.
14. Williams, R et al: Reliability of the modified–modified Schober and double inclinometer methods for measuring lumbar flexion and extension. Phys Ther 73:26, 1993.
15. Reynolds, PMG: Measurement of spinal mobility: A comparison of three methods. Rheumatology and Rehabilitation 14:180, 1975.
16. Miller, MH et al: Measurement of spinal mobility in the sagittal plane: New skin distraction technique compared with established methods. J Rheumatol 11:4, 1984.
17. Portek, I et al: Correlation between radiographic and clinical measurement of lumbar spine movement. Br J Rheumatol 22:197, 1983.
18. Gill, K et al: Repeatability of four clinical methods for assessment of lumbar spinal motion. Spine 13:50, 1988.
19. Lindahl, O: Determination of the sagittal mobility of the lumbar spine. Acta Orthop Scand 37:241, 1966.
20. Bryan, JM et al: Investigation of the flexible ruler as a noninvasive measure of lumbar lordosis in black and white adult female sample populations. Journal of Orthopaedic and Sports Physical Therapy 11:3, 1989.
21. Lovell, FW, Rothstein, JM, and Personius, WJ: Reliability of clinical measurements of lumbar lordosis taken with a flexible rule. Phys Ther 69:96, 1989.
22. Robinson, ME et al: Intrasubject reliability of spinal range of motion and velocity determined by video motion analysis. Phys Ther 73:626, 1993.
23. Magee, DJ: Orthopedic Physical Assessment. WB Saunders, Philadelphia, 1987.
24. Kraus, H and Hirschland, RP: Minimum muscular fitness tests in school children. Res Q Exerc Sport 25:178, 1954.
25. Nicholas, JA: Risk factors, sports medicine and the orthopedic system: An overview. J Sports Med 3:243, 1975.
26. Brodie, DA, Bird, HA, and Wright, V: Joint laxity in selected athletic populations. Med Sci Sports Exerc 14:190, 1982.

12

The Temporomandibular Joint

STRUCTURE

The temporomandibular joint (TMJ) is the articulation between the mandible, the articular disc, and the temporal bone. The disc divides the joint into two distinct joints, which are referred to as the upper and lower joints. The upper joint consists of the convex articular eminence of the temporal bone and the concave superior surface of the disc. The lower joint consists of the anterior convex surface of the mandibular condyle and the concave inferior surface of the disc.[1]

The joint is enclosed in a joint capsule, which is thin and loose above the disc, but tight in the lower joint anteriorly, medially, and posteriorly. The lateral aspect of the capsule is thick and strong because it is reinforced by the temporomandibular ligament. This ligament limits downward and posterior motions of the mandible and lateral displacement of the condyle.

OSTEOKINEMATICS AND ARTHROKINEMATICS

The upper joint is an amphiarthrodial gliding joint. The lower joint is a hinge joint. The TMJ as a whole allows motions in three planes around three axes. The functional motions permitted are mandibular elevation and depression, protrusion and retrusion, and lateral deviation.

Mandibular depression (mouth opening) in the sagittal plane is accomplished by rotation of the condyles on the disc around a medial-lateral axis combined with anterior and inferior sliding of the condyles with the disc on the articular eminence. Mandibular elevation (mouth closing) is accomplished by rotation of the mandibular condyles on the disc and sliding of the disc with the condyles posteriorly and superiorly on the articular eminence.

In protrusion, the condyles and disc move anteriorly and inferiorly on the articular eminence. In lateral deviation, one condyle and disc slide inferiorly, anteriorly, and medially along the articular eminence. The other condyle rotates about a vertical axis and slides medially within the fossa. For example, in left lateral deviation the left condyle spins and the right slides anteriorly.

CAPSULAR PATTERN

In the capsular pattern, mouth opening is limited to 1 cm and is accompanied by deviation.

RANGE OF MOTION

The normal, or average, ROM for mouth opening is considered to be a distance sufficient for the subject to place two or three flexed PIP joints within the opening. That distance may range from 35 to 50 mm. The average ROM for protrusion (jutting out of the jaw) is 5 mm, and the normal ROM for retrusion is 3 to 4 mm. The normal ROM for lateral deviation is 10 to 12 mm.[2]

EFFECTS OF AGE AND GENDER

We are not aware of any studies that have been conducted to determine the effects of age or gender on the ROM of the TMJ. However, TMJ dysfunction, a common disorder that affects more women than men, initially causes hypermobility of the joint but later may cause limitation of motion.[3]

RELIABILITY AND VALIDITY

We are not aware of any reliability or validity studies that have been conducted on ROM measurements of the TMJ.

TESTING PROCEDURES

DEPRESSION OF THE LOWER JAW (OPENING MOUTH)

Motion occurs in sagittal plane around a medial-lateral axis.

Recommended Testing Position

Position the subject sitting, with the cervical spine in 0 degrees of flexion, extension, lateral flexion, and rotation.

Stabilization

Stabilize the posterior aspect of the head and neck to prevent flexion, extension, lateral flexion, and rotation of the cervical spine (Fig. 12–1).

Normal End-Feel

The end-feel is firm because of tension in the temporomandibular, sphenomandibular, and stylomandibular ligaments.

Measurement

Measure the distance between the upper and lower central incisor teeth with a tape measure or ruler (Fig. 12–2). Normally the lower jaw is reported to depress approximately 35 to 50 mm, so that the subject's three fingers[3] or two knuckles can be placed between the upper and lower central incisor teeth. In normal active movement, no lateral deviation occurs during depression. If lateral deviation does occur, it may take the form of either a C- or an S-shaped curve. In a C curve, the deviation is to one side and should be noted on the recording form. In an S curve, the deviation occurs first to one side and is followed by deviation to the opposite side.[2] A description of the deviations should be included on the recording form (Fig. 12–3).

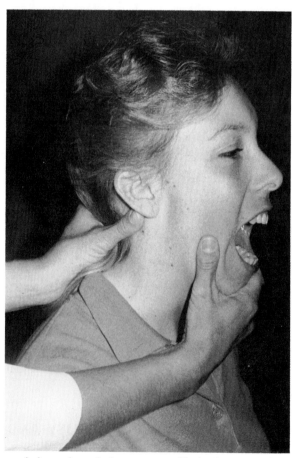

FIGURE 12–1. This photograph shows the end of temporomandibular depression ROM. The examiner's right hand maintains depression by pulling the lower jaw inferiorly. The examiner's left hand holds the back of the subject's head to prevent cervical motion.

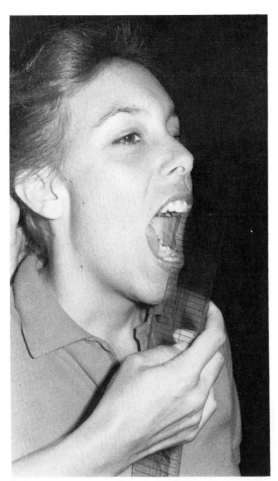

FIGURE 12-2. At the end of depression, the examiner uses an arm of a plastic goniometer to measure the distance between the subject's upper and lower central incisors.

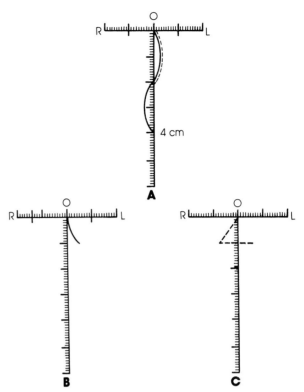

FIGURE 12-3. Examples of recording deviations in temporomandibular motions. (*A*) Deviation R and L on opening; maximum opening, 4 cm; lateral deviation equal (1 cm each direction); protrusion on functional opening (*dashed lines*). (*B*) Capsule-ligamentous pattern: opening limited to 1 cm; lateral deviation greater to R than to L; deviation to L on opening. (*C*) Protrusion is 1 cm; lateral deviation to R on protrusion (indicates weak lateral pterygoid on opposite side). (From Magee, DJ: Orthopedic Physical Assessment, ed 2. WB Saunders, Philadelphia, 1992, p. 81, with permission.)

ANTERIOR PROTRUSION OF THE LOWER JAW

Translatory motion occurs in the transverse plane.

Recommended Testing Position

Position the subject sitting, with the cervical spine in 0 degrees of flexion, extension, lateral flexion, and rotation. The TMJ is opened slightly.

Stabilization

Stabilize the posterior aspect of the head and neck to prevent flexion, extension, lateral flexion, and rotation of the cervical spine (Fig. 12–4).

Measurement

Measure the distance between the lower central incisor teeth and the upper central incisor teeth with a tape measure or ruler (Fig. 12–5). Normally, the lower central incisor teeth are able to protrude beyond the upper central incisor teeth 6 to 9 mm.[4,5]

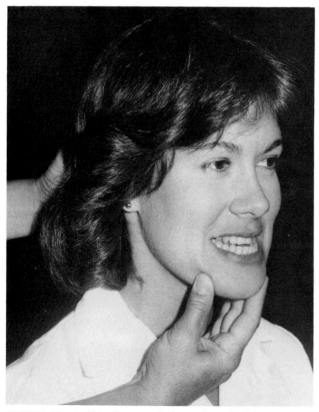

FIGURE 12–4. This photograph shows the end of the temporomandibular anterior protrusion ROM. The examiner's left hand stabilizes the posterior aspect of the subject's head to prevent cervical motion, while her right hand maintains anterior protrusion.

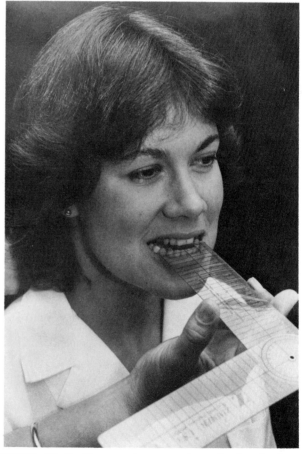

FIGURE 12–5. The examiner uses the end of a plastic goniometer to measure the distance between the subject's upper and lower central incisors. The subject maintains the position.

LATERAL DEVIATION OF THE LOWER JAW

Translatory motion occurs in the transverse plane.

Recommended Testing Position and Stabilization

The testing position and stabilization are the same as for anterior protrusion of the lower jaw (Fig. 12–6).

Measurement

Measure the distance between the most lateral points of the lower and upper cuspid teeth or first bicuspid teeth with a tape measure or ruler (Fig. 12–7). The amount of lateral movement to the right and left sides should be similar, between 10 and 12 mm.[2]

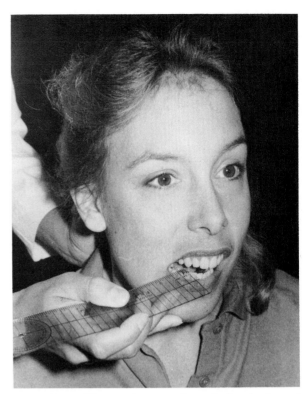

FIGURE 12–7. The examiner uses the end of a plastic goniometer to measure the distance between the upper and lower cuspids. The examiner maintains her grasp on the subject's head during the measurement.

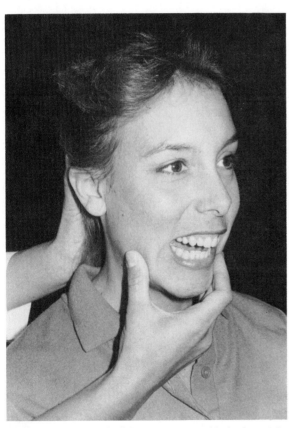

FIGURE 12–6. The end of the temporomandibular lateral deviation ROM. The examiner places her left hand at the back of the subject's head to prevent cervical motion while using her right hand to pull the lower jaw laterally to maintain lateral deviation to the right. The examiner avoids pulling the lower jaw into depression.

REFERENCES

1. Norkin, CC and Levangie, PK: Joint Structure and Function: A Comprehensive Analysis, ed 2. FA Davis, Philadelphia, 1992.
2. Magee, DJ: Orthopedic Physical Assessment, ed 2. WB Saunders, Philadelphia, 1992.
3. Hertling, D and Kessler, RM: Management of Musculoskeletal Disorders, ed 2. JB Lippincott, Philadelphia, 1990.
4. Hoppenfeld, S: Physical Examination of the Spine and Extremities. Appleton Century-Crofts, New York, 1976.
5. Friedman, MH and Weisberg, J: Application of orthopedic principles in evaluation of the temporomandibular joint. Phys Ther 62:597, 1982.

APPENDIX A: Average Ranges of Motion

**AVERAGE RANGES OF MOTION FOR THE UPPER EXTREMITIES
IN DEGREES FROM SELECTED SOURCES**

Joint	Motion	American Academy of Orthopaedic Surgeons[1]	Kendall and McCreary[2]	Hoppenfeld[3]	American Medical Association[4]
Shoulder	Flexion	0–180	0–180	0–90	0–150
	Extension	0–60	0–45	0–45	0–50
	Abduction	0–180	0–180	0–180	0–180
	Medial rotation	0–70	0–70	0–55	0–90
	Lateral rotation	0–90	0–90	0–45	0–90
Elbow	Flexion	0–150	0–145	0–150	0–140
Forearm	Pronation	0–80	0–90	0–90	0–80
	Supination	0–80	0–90	0–90	0–80
Wrist	Extension	0–70	0–70	0–70	0–60
	Flexion	0–80	0–80	0–80	0–60
	Radial deviation	0–20	0–20	0–20	0–20
	Ulnar deviation	0–30	0–35	0–30	0–30
Thumb					
CMC	Abduction	0–70	0–80	0–70	0–8 cm
	Flexion	0–15	0–45		
	Extension	0–20	0		
	Opposition	Tip of thumb to base or tip of fifth digit	Pad of thumb to pad of fifth digit	Tip of thumb to tip of fingers	
MCP	Flexion	0–50	0–60	0–50	0–60
IP	Flexion	0–80	0–80	0–90	0–80
Digits Second– Fifth					
MCP	Flexion	0–90	0–90		
	Hyperextension	0–45		0–90	0–90
	Abduction			0–45	0–20
				0–20	
PIP	Flexion	0–100		0–100	0–100
DIP	Flexion	0–90		0–90	0–70
	Hypertension	0–10		0–10	0–30

AVERAGE RANGES OF MOTION FOR THE LOWER EXTREMITIES
IN DEGREES FROM SELECTED SOURCES

Joint	Motion	American Academy of Orthopaedic Surgeons[1]	Kendall and McCreary[2]	Hoppenfeld[3]	American Medical Association[4]
Hip	Flexion	0–120	0–125	0–135	0–100
	Extension	0–30	0–10	0–30	0–30
	Abduction	0–45	0–45	0–50	0–40
	Adduction	0–30	0–10	0–30	0–20
	Lateral rotation	0–45	0–45	0–45	0–40
	Medial rotation	0–45	0–45	0–35	0–50
Knee	Flexion	0–135	0–140	0–135	0–150
Ankle	Dorsiflexion	0–20	0–20	0–20	0–20
	Plantar flexion	0–50	0–45	0–50	0–40
	Inversion	0–35	0–35		0–30
	Eversion	0–15	0–20		0–20
Subtalar	Inversion	0–5		0–5	
	Eversion	0–5		0–5	
Transverse tarsal	Inversion	0–20		0–20	
	Eversion	0–10		0–10	
Toes					
First MTP	Flexion	0–45		0–45	0–30
	Extension	0–70		0–90	0–50
First IP	Flexion	0–90			0–30
	Extension	0			0
Second–Fifth MTP	Flexion	0–40			
	Extension	0–40			
Second MTP	Flexion				0–30
	Extension				0–40
Third MTP	Flexion				0–20
	Extension				0–30
Fourth MTP	Flexion				0–10
	Extension				0–20
Fifth MTP	Flexion				0–10
	Extension				0–10
Second–Fifth PIP	Flexion	0–35			
Second–Fifth DIP	Flexion	0–60			

AVERAGE RANGES OF MOTION FOR THE SPINE AND THE TEMPOROMANDIBULAR IN DEGREES

Joint	Motion	American Academy of Orthopaedic Surgeons[1]	Kendall and McCreary[2]	Hoppenfeld[3]	American Medical Association[4]
Cervical spine	Flexion	0–45	0–45	Chin touches chest	0–60
	Extension	0–45	0–45		0–75
	Lateral flexion	0–45		Looking at ceiling	0–45
	Rotation	0–60		0–45	0–80
				Chin in line with shoulder	
Thoracic spine	Flexion				0–50
	Rotation				0–30
Thoracic and lumbar spine	Flexion	0–80 4 in			
	Extension	0–25			
	Lateral flexion	0–35			
	Rotation	0–45			
Lumbosacral spine	Extension				0–25
	Lateral flexion				0–25
Temporomandibular joint	Depression			Three finger widths	
	Anterior protrusion			Beyond upper teeth	
	Lateral deviation			Beyond upper teeth	

REFERENCES

1. American Academy of Orthopaedic Surgeons: Joint Motion: Method of Measuring and Recording. AAOS, Chicago, 1965.
2. Kendall, FP and McCreary, EK: Muscles: Testing and Function, ed 3. William & Wilkins, Baltimore, 1983.
3. Hoppenfeld, S: Physical Examination of the Spine and Extremities. Appleton Century-Crofts, New York, 1976.
4. American Medical Association: Guides to the Evaluation of Permanent Impairment. AMA, Chicago, 1988.

APPENDIX B: Joint Measurements by Body Position

	Prone	Supine	Sitting	Standing
Shoulder	Extension	Flexion Abduction Medial rotation Lateral rotation	(Abduction)	
Elbow		Flexion		
Forearm			Pronation Supination	
Wrist			Flexion Extension Radial deviation Ulnar deviation	
Hand			All motions	
Hip	Extension	Flexion Abduction Adduction	Medial rotation Lateral rotation	
Knee		Flexion		
Ankle and foot	Subtalar inversion Subtalar eversion	Dorsiflexion Plantar flexion Inversion Eversion Midtarsal inversion Midtarsal eversion	Dorsiflexion Plantar flexion Inversion Eversion Midtarsal inversion Midtarsal eversion	
Toes		All motions	All motions	
Cervical spine			Flexion Extension Lateral flexion Rotation	
Thoracolumbar spine			Rotation	Flexion Extension Lateral flexion
Temporomandibular joint			Depression Anterior protrusion Lateral deviation	

APPENDIX C: Sample Numerical Recording Form

RANGE OF MOTION RECORD

Name _____ Date of Birth _____

Diagnosis _____ Date of Onset _____

Recording:
1. Passive motion is recorded unless notation of active motion is made.
2. Space is left at the end of each section to record comments regarding type of goniometer used, patient positioning, pain, edema, crepitus, end-feel.

				Left / Right				
				Examiner				
				Date				
				Temporomandibular Joint Depression				
				Anterior Protrusion				
				Lateral Deviation				
				Comments:				
				Cervical Spine Flexion				
				Extension				
				Lateral Flexion				
				Rotation				
				Comments:				
				Thoracolumbar Spine Flexion				
				Extension				
				Lateral Flexion				
				Rotation				
				Comments:				

RANGE OF MOTION RECORD - UPPER EXTREMITY

NAME								
		Left				Right		
				Examiner				
				Date				
				Shoulder				
				Flexion				
				Extension				
				Abduction				
				Medial Rotation				
				Lateral Rotation				
				Comments:				
				Elbow and Forearm				
				Flexion				
				Supination				
				Pronation				
				Comments:				
				Wrist				
				Flexion				
				Extension				
				Ulnar Deviation				
				Radial Deviation				
				Comments:				

RANGE OF MOTION RECORD - UPPER EXTREMITY

				NAME				
			Left				Right	
				Examiner				
				Date				
				Thumb				
				CMC				
				Flexion				
				Extension				
				Abduction				
				Opposition				
				MCP				
				Flexion				
				DIP				
				Flexion				
				Extension				
				Comments:				
				Second Digit				
				MCP				
				Flexion				
				Extension				
				Abduction				
				Adduction				
				PIP				
				Flexion				
				DIP				
				Flexion				
				Comments:				

RANGE OF MOTION RECORD - UPPER EXTREMITY

NAME								
	Left						Right	
				Examiner				
				Date				
				Third Digit				
				MCP				
				Flexion				
				Extension				
				Abduction (Radial)				
				Abduction (Ulnar)				
				PIP				
				Flexion				
				DIP				
				Flexion				
				Comments:				
				Fourth Digit				
				MCP				
				Flexion				
				Extension				
				Abduction				
				Adduction				
				PIP				
				Flexion				
				DIP				
				Flexion				
				Comments:				

RANGE OF MOTION RECORD - UPPER EXTREMITY

				NAME				
		Left				Right		
				Examiner				
				Date				
				Fifth Digit MCP				
				Flexion				
				Extension				
				Abduction				
				Adduction				
				PIP				
				Flexion				
				DIP				
				Flexion				
				Comments:				

Summary:

RANGE OF MOTION RECORD - LOWER EXTREMITY

				NAME				
			Left				Right	
				Examiner				
				Date				
				Hip				
				Flexion				
				Extension				
				Abduction				
				Adduction				
				Medial Rotation				
				Lateral Rotation				
				Comments:				
				Knee				
				Flexion				
				Comments:				
				Ankle				
				Dorsiflexion				
				Plantar flexion				
				Inversion				
				Eversion				
				Comments:				

RANGE OF MOTION RECORD - LOWER EXTREMITY

				NAME				
		Left					Right	
				Examiner				
				Date				
				Great Toe				
				MTP				
				Flexion				
				Extension				
				Abduction				
				IP				
				Flexion				
				Comments:				
				Second Digit				
				MTP				
				Flexion				
				Extension				
				Abduction				
				PIP				
				Flexion				
				DIP				
				Flexion				
				Comments:				
				Third Digit				
				MTP				
				Flexion				
				Extension				
				Abduction				
				PIP				
				Flexion				
				DIP				
				Flexion				
				Comments:				

RANGE OF MOTION RECORD - LOWER EXTREMITY

NAME									
		Left						Right	
				Examiner					
				Date					
				Fourth Digit					
				MTP					
				Flexion					
				Extension					
				Abduction					
				PIP					
				Flexion					
				DIP					
				Flexion					
				Comments:					
				Fifth Digit					
				MTP					
				Flexion					
				Extension					
				Abduction					
				PIP					
				Flexion					
				DIP					
				Flexion					
				Comments:					

Index

An "f" following a page number indicates a figure; a "t" following a page number indicates a table.

Abduction
  carpometacarpal joint, 108, 108f, 109f
  hip, 128, 128f, 129f
  metacarpophalangeal joint, 98, 99f
  metatarsophalangeal joint, 174, 174f,
    175f
  shoulder, 58, 58f, 59f, 60f, 61, 61f
Acromioclavicular joint(s), 50
Active range of motion (AROM), 8
Activities of daily living. See Functional
    range of motion
Adduction
  carpometacarpal joint, 108
  hip, 130, 130f, 131f
  metacarpophalangeal joints, 98
  metatarsophalangeal joints, 174
  shoulder, 61
Adhesions, joint capsule, 10
Age and range of motion
  ankle and foot, 150–151, 151t,
    152t
  cervical spine, 182–185, 183t, 184t,
    185t
  elbow and forearm, 70, 70t, 71t
  hip, 121, 122t, 123
  knee, 139t, 139–140, 140t
  metacarpophalangeal joints, 93
  shoulder, 50–52, 51t, 52t
  studies of, 7
  thoracic spine, 200–203, 201t
  wrist and hand, 81–82, 81t
Alignment, goniometer arms, 22f,
    22–25, 23f, 24f, 25
American Medical Association (AMA),
    30, 203, 205
Anatomical landmarks, 22
Anatomical position, 6f

Angles, measurement of. See
    Goniometry
Ankle and foot
  dorsiflexion, 15
  functional range of motion, 149
  interphalangeal joints, 149
  metatarsophalangeal joints, 149
  midtarsal joint, 148
  range of motion, 149–151, 150t
  reliability/validity, ROM
    measurements, 151–153
  subtalar joint, 148
  talocrural joint, 147–148
  tarsometatarsal joints, 148–149
  testing procedures, 154–177
  tibiofibular joints, proximal and
    distal, 147–148
  transverse tarsal joint, 148
Ankylosis, notation/charting, 30
Anterior-posterior axis, 4, 5f
Anterior protrusion, lower jaw, 218
Arthritis, capsular patterns and, 10
Arthrokinematics
  acromioclavicular joint, 50
  carpometacarpal joint, 102–103
  defined, 4
  glenohumeral joint, 49
  hip, 119
  humeroulnar and humeroradial
    joints, 67
  interphalangeal joints, foot, 149
  interphalangeal joints, hand, 92, 103
  intervertebral joints, C2 to C7,
    181–182
  knee, 138
  metacarpophalangeal joints, 92, 103
  metatarsophalangeal joints, 149

  midcarpal joint, 79
  midtarsal joint, 148
  radiocarpal joint, 79
  radioulnar joints, superior and
    inferior, 67–68
  scapulothoracic joint, 50
  sternoclavicular joint, 50
  subtalar joint, 148
  talocrural joint, 147–148
  tarsometatarsal joints, 149
  temporomandibular joint, 215
  tibiofibular joint, proximal and distal,
    147–148
  transverse tarsal joint, 148
  zygapophysial joints, C2 to C7,
    181–182
Atlanto-occipital joint(s), 181
Atlantoaxial joint(s), 181
Automated video system, 204
Axes, joint motion, 4f, 4–6, 5f

Biological variation
  defined, 37
  standard deviation indicating, 38–39
Body, universal goniometer, 16–17, 17f
Body positioning. See Positioning, for
    goniometry procedures
Bubble goniometer(s), 20

Calcaneus. See Subtalar joint(s)
Capsular fibrosis, 10
Capsular patterns
  atlanto-occipital and atlantoaxial
    joints, 181
  carpometacarpal joint, 103
  defined, 10

237

Capsular patterns—*Continued*
  glenohumeral joint, 49
  hip, 119
  humeroulnar and humeroradial
      joints, 67
  interphalangeal joints, hand, 92, 103
  intervertebral joints, C2 to C7,
      181–182
  knee, 138
  lumbar spine, 200
  metacarpophalangeal joints, 92, 103
  metatarsophalangeal joints, 149
  midcarpal joint, 79
  noncapsular patterns, 10
  radiocarpal joint, 79
  radioulnar joints, superior and
      inferior, 68
  subtalar joint, 148
  talocrural joint, 148
  temporomandibular joint, 215
  thoracic spine, 199
  tibiofibular joint, 148
  zygapophysial joints, C2 to C7,
      181–182
Carpometacarpal joint(s)
  abduction, 108, 108f, 109f
  adduction, 108
  arthrokinematics, 102–103
  capsular pattern, 103
  extension, 106, 106f, 107f
  flexion, 104, 104f, 105f
  opposition, 110f, 110–111, 111f
  osteokinematics, 102
  range of motion, 103
  structure, 102
  testing procedures, 104–111
"Carrying angle," humerus and
    forearm, 67
Cervical spine
  atlanto-occipital joint, 181
  atlantoaxial joint, 181
  extension, 190, 190f, 191f
  flexion, 188, 188f, 189f
  intervertebral joints, C2 to C7,
      181–182
  lateral flexion, 192, 192f, 193f, 194f,
      195f
  range of motion, 182–185, 183t,
      184t, 185t, 223t
  reliability/validity, ROM
      measurements, 185–187
  rotation, 196, 196f, 197f
  testing procedures, 188–197
  zygapophysial joints, C2 to C7,
      181–182
Clavicle. *See* Acromioclavicular joint(s);
    Sternoclavicular joint(s)
Coefficient of variation, evaluating
    reliability, 39–40
Content validity, 35
Correlation coefficients, evaluating
    reliability, 40t, 40–41
Costotransverse joint(s), thoracic spine,
    199
Costovertebral joint(s), thoracic spine,
    199
Coxa. *See* Hip

Criterion-related validity, 35
"cubitus valgus," 67

Depression of lower jaw (opening
    mouth), 216–217
DIPs. *See* Distal interphalangeal joints
    (DIPs)
Distal arm, goniometer, 23
Distal interphalangeal joints (DIPs)
  foot, 176–177
  hand, 92–93, 102
Distal tibiofibular joint(s), 147–148
Dorsiflexion
  ankle, 15
  talocrural joint, 154, 154f, 155f
  wrist and hand, 86, 86f, 87f

Elbow and forearm
  extension, 16, 72, 73f
  flexion, 15, 23f, 24f, 25, 32, 72, 72f,
      73f
  functional range of motion, 69, 69t
  humeroradial joint, 67
  humeroulnar joint, 67
  pronation, 74, 74f, 75f
  radioulnar joints, superior and
      inferior, 67–68
  range of motion, 68t, 68–70
  reliability/validity, ROM
      measurements, 70–71
  supination, 76, 76f, 77f
  testing procedures, 72–77
Electrogoniometer(s), 20–21
Empty end-feel, 9t
End-feel
  abnormal (pathological), 9t
  differentiating types of, 15–16
  normal (physiological), 9t
  range of motion and, 9–10
  soft/firm/hard, 9t
Errors. *See* Reliability; Validity
Eversion
  subtalar joint, 164, 164f, 165f
  tarsal joints, 160, 160f, 161f
  transverse tarsal joint, 168, 168f, 169f
Extension
  carpometacarpal joint, 106, 106f, 107f
  cervical spine, 190, 190f, 191f
  defined, 6
  distal interphalangeal joints, foot,
      177
  distal interphalangeal joints, hand,
      102
  elbow and forearm, 16, 72, 73f
  hip, 126, 126f, 127f
  interphalangeal joints, thumb, 116
  knee, 144
  lumbar spine, 208, 208f, 209f
  metacarpophalangeal joint, 96, 96f,
      97f, 112
  metatarsophalangeal joint, 172, 172f,
      173f
  proximal interphalangeal joints, foot,
      176

proximal interphalangeal joints,
    hand, 100–101
  shoulder, 7f, 56, 57f
  thoracic spine, 208, 208f, 209f
  wrist and hand, 86, 86f, 87f
External rotation. *See* Lateral (external)
    rotation

Fibula. *See* Talocrural joint(s);
    Tibiofibular joint(s), proximal
    and distal
Fingers. *See* Distal interphalangeal
    joints (DIPs);
    Metacarpophalangeal joint(s);
    Proximal interphalangeal
    joints (PIPs)
Fingertip-to-floor measurement
    method, 203–204
Firm end-feel, 9t, 15
Flexible rulers, 187
Flexion. *See also* Dorsiflexion; Palmar
    flexion
  carpometacarpal joint, 104, 104f, 105f
  cervical spine, 188, 188f, 189f
  distal interphalangeal joints, foot,
      176–177
  distal interphalangeal joints, hand, 102
  elbow and forearm, 15, 23f, 24f, 25,
      32, 72, 72f, 73f
  hip, 120t, 124, 124f, 125f
  interphalangeal joints, thumb, 114,
      115f
  knee, 142f, 142–144, 143f, 144f, 145f
  lumbar spine, 206f, 206–207, 207f
  metacarpophalangeal joint, fingers,
      94, 94f, 95f
  metacarpophalangeal joint, thumb,
      112, 112f, 113f
  metatarsophalangeal joint, 170, 170f,
      171f
  proximal interphalangeal joints, foot,
      176
  proximal interphalangeal joints,
      hand, 100–101
  shoulder, 7f, 54–55
  thoracic spine, 206f, 206–207, 207f
  wrist and hand, 84, 84f, 85f
Fluid (bubble) goniometer(s), 20
Foot. *See* Ankle and foot
Forearm. *See* Elbow and forearm
Frontal plane, 4, 5, 5f, 28–30
Fulcrum, goniometer alignment, 23, 25
Full-circle goniometer(s), 17f, 18f, 19f
Functional range of motion
  ankle and foot, 149, 151t
  elbow and forearm, 69, 69t
  hip, 120t, 120–121
  knee, 138–139, 139t
  metacarpophalangeal joints, 92–93
  shoulder, 50, 51t
  wrist and hand, 80–81, 81t

Gender and range of motion
  ankle and foot, 150–151
  cervical spine, 182–185, 183t, 184t,
      185t

elbow and forearm, 70
hip, 121, 123
knee, 139–140
metacarpophalangeal joints, 93
related studies, 7–8
shoulder, 50–52
thoracic spine, 200–203, 201t
wrist and hand, 81t, 81–82
Glenohumeral joint(s)
   abduction, 58f, 58–61
   adduction, 61
   extension, 56–57
   flexion, 54–55, 54f, 55f
   lateral rotation, 64–65
   structure/kinematics/capsule, 49
   testing procedure, 53
Glenoid fossa, 49
Goniometer(s)
   alignment of arms, 22f, 22–25, 23f,
      24f, 25
   cervical spine measurements,
      185–187
   electrogoniometers, 20–21
   explanation to subject, 30–31
   gravity-dependent, 18–20, 20f
   half- or full-circle, 17f, 18f, 19f
   selection, 19f
   universal, 16–18, 17f, 21
Goniometry
   applications/uses, 3–4
   basic concepts, 3–10
   defined, 3
   end-feel, 9–10
   joint motion, 4–6
   range of motion, 6–10
   visual estimation, 21
Goniometry testing procedures
   12-step sequence, 31–32
   ankle and foot, 154–177
   carpometacarpal joint, 104–111
   cervical spine, 188–197
   elbow and forearm, 72–77
   explanation to subject, 30–31
   hip, 124–135
   joint measurements by body
      position, 225t
   knee, 142–145
   lumbar spine, 206–213
   measurement instruments, 16–21
   positioning, 13–14
   recording measurements, 26–30, 27f
   shoulder, 53–65
   stabilization, 14f, 14–15
   temporomandibular joint, 216–219
   thoracic spine, 206–213
   validity/reliability, 35–45
   wrist and hand, 84–91, 94–116
Gout, 10
Gravity-dependent goniometer(s)
   cervical spine ROM, 185, 186
   features, 18–20, 20f
   thoracolumbar spine ROM, 203–204
Guides to the Evaluation of Permanent
      Impairment, 30, 203, 205

Half-circle goniometer(s), 17f, 18f, 19f
Hand. See Wrist and hand

Hard end-feel, 9t, 16
Hindfoot. See Subtalar joint(s)
Hip
   abduction, 128, 128f, 129f
   adduction, 130, 130f, 131f
   extension, 126, 126f, 127f
   flexion, 120t, 124, 124f, 125f
   functional range of motion, 120t,
      120–121
   lateral (external) rotation, 134, 134f,
      135f
   medial (internal) rotation, 132, 132f,
      133f
   range of motion, 119–123, 120t
   reliability/validity, ROM
      measurements, 123
   structure/kinematics/capsule, 119
   testing procedures, 124–135
Humeroradial joint(s), 67
Humeroulnar joint(s), 67
Humerus. See Glenohumeral joint(s)
Hyperextension, defined, 6
Hypermobile, defined, 26
Hypomobility
   defined, 26
   notation/charting, 29

Inclinometer, 20, 203–204
Inferior radioulnar joint(s), 68
Internal rotation. See Medial (internal)
      rotation
Interphalangeal joint(s). See also Distal
      interphalangeal
      joints (DIPs); Proximal
      interphalangeal joints (PIPs)
   toes, 149
   fingers, 103
   thumb, 114–116, 115f
Intertester reliability, 36–37, 42, 44, 45f
Intervertebral joint(s)
   lumbar spine, 200
   thoracic spine, 199
Intraclass correlation coefficient (ICC),
      41
Intratester reliability, 36–37, 41–42, 43f
Inversion
   subtalar joint, 162, 162f, 163f
   tarsal joints, 158, 158f, 159f
   transverse tarsal joint, 166, 166f, 167f

Jaw. See Temporomandibular joint
      (TMJ)
Joint capsules. See Capsular patterns
Joint effusion, 10
Joint measurements by body position,
      225t
Joint motion
   arthrokinematics, 4
   osteokinematics, 4
   planes and axes, 4f, 4–6, 5f

Knee
   arthrokinematics, 138
   extension, 144

flexion, 142f, 142–144, 143f, 144f,
      145f
functional range of motion, 138–
      139, 139t
osteokinematics, 137–138
range of motion, 138t, 138–140
reliability/validity, ROM
      measurements, 140–141
structure, 137
testing procedures, 142–145

Landmarks, anatomical, 22
Lateral deviation, lower jaw, 219, 219f
Lateral (external) rotation
   hip, 134, 134f, 135f
   shoulder, 63f, 64f, 64–65, 65f
Lateral flexion
   cervical spine, 192, 192f, 193f, 194f,
      195f
   lumbar spine, 210, 211f
   thoracic spine, 210, 211f
Ligament shortening, 10
Lower extremity(ies), 222t. See also
      Ankle and foot; Hip;
      Knee
Lumbar spine
   capsular pattern, 200
   extension, 208, 208f, 209f
   flexion, 206f, 206–207, 207f
   intervertebral joints, 200
   lateral flexion, 210, 211f
   osteokinematics, 200
   range of motion, 200t, 200–203,
      201t, 223t
   reliability/validity, ROM
      measurements, 203–205
   rotation, 212, 212f, 213f
   structure, 200
   testing procedures, 206–213
   zygapophysial joints, 200

Mandible. See Temporomandibular
      joint (TMJ)
Mean (statistical), 38
Measurement error
   defined, 37
   standard deviation indicating, 39
Measurements, goniometry
   body position for, 225t
   instruments for, 16–21
   recording, 26–30
   validity/reliability, 35–45
Medial (internal) rotation
   hip, 132, 132f, 133f
   shoulder, 62f, 62–63, 63f
Medial-lateral axis, 4, 4f
Metacarpophalangeal joint(s)
   abduction, 98, 99f
   adduction, 98
   arthrokinematics, 103
   capsular pattern, 103
   extension, 96, 96f, 97f, 112
   flexion, 94, 94f, 95f, 112, 112f, 113f
   functional range of motion, 92–93
   osteokinematics, 103

Metacarpophalangeal
        joint(s)—*Continued*
    range of motion, 92, 92t, 103
    reliability/validity, ROM
            measurements, 93
    structure, 103
    thumb, 112, 112f, 113f
Metatarsal. *See* Tarsometatarsal joint(s)
Metatarsophalangeal joint(s)
    abduction, 174, 174f, 175f
    adduction, 174
    extension, 172, 172f, 173f
    flexion, 170, 170f, 171f
    structure/kinematics/capsule, 149
Midcarpal joint(s), 79–90
Midtarsal joint(s), 148
Mouth. *See* Temporomandibular joint
        (TMJ)
Moving arm, goniometer
    alignment, 23
    defined, 18
Muscle contractures, 10
Muscle strains, 10

Noncapsular patterns, range of motion,
        10
Notation system, degrees of ROM, 6
Numerical tables, recording ROM
        measurements, 28, 28f,
        228f–235f

180- to 0-degree notation system, 6
Opposition, carpometacarpal joint,
        110f, 110–111, 111f
Osteokinematics
    acromioclavicular joint, 50
    atlanto-occipital and atlantoaxial
            joints, 181
    carpometacarpal joint, 102
    defined, 4
    glenohumeral joint, 49
    hip, 119
    humeroulnar and humeroradial
            joints, 67
    interphalangeal joints, foot, 149
    interphalangeal joints, hand, 92, 103
    intervertebral joints, C2 to C7,
            181–182
    knee, 137–138
    lumbar spine, 200
    metacarpophalangeal joints, 92, 103
    metatarsophalangeal joints, 149
    midcarpal joint, 79
    midtarsal joint, 148
    radiocarpal joint, 79
    radioulnar joints, superior and
            inferior, 68
    scapulothoracic joint, 50
    sternoclavicular joint, 50
    subtalar joint, 148
    talocrural joint, 147
    tarsometatarsal joints, 149
    temporomandibular joint, 215
    thoracic spine, 199
    tibiofibular joint, proximal and
            distal, 147

transverse tarsal joint, 148
zygapophysial joints, C2 to C7,
        181–182

Palmar flexion, 84f, 85f
Passive range of motion (PROM). *See
        also* Capsular patterns;
        End-feel
    defined, 8–9
    noncapsular patterns, 10
Pearson product moment correlation
        coefficient, 40–41
Pendulum goniometer(s), 186
Phalanges. *See* Distal interphalangeal
        joints (DIPs);
        Metacarpophalangeal joint(s);
        Metatarsophalangeal
        joint(s); Proximal interphalangeal
        joints (PIPs)
Pictorial charts, recording ROM
        measurements, 28, 29f
PIPs. *See* Proximal interphalangeal
        joints (PIPs)
Planes, joint motion, 4f, 4–6, 5f
Plantar flexion, talocrural joint, 156,
        156f, 157f
Positioning, for goniometry procedures,
        13–14, 225t
Pronation, elbow and forearm, 74, 74f,
        75f
Proximal arm, goniometer, 23
Proximal interphalangeal joints (PIPs)
    foot, 176
    hand, 92–93, 100–101
Proximal tibiofibular joint(s), 147–148

Radial deviation (radial flexion), 88,
        88f, 89f
Radiocarpal joint(s), 79–90
Radiography, validity and, 35–36
Radioulnar joint(s), superior and
        inferior, 67–68
Radius. *See* Humeroradial joint(s)
Range of motion (ROM)
    active, 8
    age and, 7
    ankle and foot, 149–151, 150t
    carpometacarpal joint, 103
    cervical spine, 182–185, 223t
    defined, 6
    determining end of, 15–16
    elbow and forearm, 23f, 24f, 68t,
            68–70, 69t
    end-feel, 9–10
    factors affecting, 6–8
    gender and, 7–8
    glenohumeral joint, 53t
    hip, 119–123, 120t
    interphalangeal joints, hand, 103
    knee, 138t, 138–140
    limitation, capsular/noncapsular
            patterns, 10
    lower extremities, 222t
    lumbar spine, 200–203, 201t, 223t

metacarpophalangeal joints, 92, 92t,
        103
    passive, 8–9
    shoulder, 7f, 50–52
    temporomandibular joint, 215, 223t
    thoracic spine, 200–203, 201t, 223t
    upper extremities, 221t
    wrist and hand, 80–82
Recommended testing positions. *See*
        Positioning, for
        goniometry procedures
Recording
    AMA *Guides to Evaluation of
        Permanent Impairment*, 30, 203,
        205
    goniometric measurements, 26–30,
            27f, 217f
    intertester reliability, 45f
    intratester reliability, 43f
    numerical tables, 28, 28f, 228f–235f
    pictorial charts, 28, 29f
    SFTR method, 28–30
Reliability, ROM measurements
    ankle and foot, 151–153
    cervical spine, 185–187
    defined, 36
    elbow and forearm, 70–71
    exercises to evaluate, 41–45
    hip, 123
    intertester, 44, 45f
    intratester, 42, 43f
    knee, 140–141
    lumbar spine, 203–205
    mathematical methods of evaluating,
            37–41
    metacarpophalangeal joint, 93
    shoulder, 52–53
    summary, research studies, 36–37
    temporomandibular joint, 215
    thoracic spine, 203–205
    wrist and hand, 82–83
Rheumatoid arthritis, 10
Rotation
    cervical spine, 196, 196f, 197f
    lumbar spine, 212, 212f, 213f
    thoracic spine, 212, 212f, 213f

Sagittal-frontal-transverse rotation
        (SFTR) recording
        method, 28–30
Sagittal plane, 4, 4f
Scapulothoracic joint(s), 50
Schober technique, 203–204, 207, 208
SFTR recording method, 28–30
Shoulder
    abduction, 58, 58f, 59f, 60f, 61, 61f
    acromioclavicular joint, 50
    adduction, 61
    extension, 7f, 56, 57f
    flexion, 7f, 54f, 54–55, 55f
    functional range of motion, 51t
    glenohumeral joint, 49
    lateral (external) rotation, 63f, 64f,
            64–65, 65f
    medial (internal) rotation, 62f,
            62–63, 63f
    range of motion, 50–52, 51t

reliability/validity, ROM measurements, 52–53
scapulothoracic joint, 50
sternoclavicular joint, 49–50
testing procedures, 53–65
Soft end-feel, 9t, 15
Spine. *See* Cervical spine; Lumbar spine; Thoracic spine
Spondylometer, 203–204
Stabilization, for goniometry procedures, 14f, 14–15
Standard deviation, evaluating reliability, 38t, 38–39, 39t
Standard error of measurement, evaluating reliability, 41
Stationary arm, goniometer
alignment, 22–23
defined, 18
Sternoclavicular joint(s), 49–50
Subtalar joint(s)
eversion, 164, 164f, 165f
inversion, 162, 162f, 163f
structure/kinematics/capsule, 148
Superior radioulnar joint(s), 67–68
Supination, elbow and forearm, 76, 76f, 77f
Synovial inflammation, 10

Talocrural joint(s)
dorsiflexion, 154, 154f, 155f
plantar flexion, 156, 156f, 157f
structure/kinematics/capsule, 147–148
Talus. *See* Subtalar joint(s)
Tarsal joint(s)
eversion, 160, 160f, 161f
inversion, 158, 158f, 159f
midtarsal, 148
transverse tarsal, 166–169
Tarsometatarsal joint(s), 148–149
Temporal variation, defined, 37
Temporomandibular joint (TMJ)
anterior protrusion, lower jaw, 218, 218f
arthrokinematics, 215
capsular pattern, 215
depression of lower jaw (opening mouth), 216, 216f, 217f
lateral deviation, lower jaw, 219, 219f
osteokinematics, 215

range of motion, 215, 223t
reliability/validity, ROM measurements, 215
structure, 215
testing procedures, 216–219
Thoracic spine
capsular pattern, 199
costotransverse joints, 199
costovertebral joints, 199
extension, 208, 208f, 209f
flexion, 206f, 206–207, 207f
intervertebral joints, 199
lateral flexion, 210, 211f
osteokinematics, 199
range of motion, 200t, 200–203, 201t, 223t
reliability/validity, ROM measurements, 203–205
rotation, 212, 212f, 213f
structure, 199
testing procedures, 206–213
zygapophysial joints, 199
Thumb. *See* Carpometacarpal joint(s); Interphalangeal joint(s); Metacarpophalangeal joint(s)
Tibia. *See* Talocrural joint(s)
Tibiofibular joint(s), 147–148
Tipping (tilting), scapula, 50
Toes. *See* Distal interphalangeal joints (DIPs); Metatarsophalangeal joint(s); Proximal interphalangeal joints (PIPs)
Transverse plane, 4, 5, 5f, 28–30
Transverse tarsal joint(s)
eversion, 168, 168f, 169f
inversion, 166, 166f, 167f
structure/kinematics/capsule, 148

Ulna. *See* Humeroulnar joint(s); Radioulnar joints
Ulnar deviation (ulnar flexion), 89f, 90, 90f, 91f
Universal goniometer(s), 16–18, 17f, 21, 185–186, 203–204
Upper extremity(ies), 221t. *See also* Elbow and forearm; Shoulder; Wrist and hand

Validity, ROM measurements
ankle and foot, 151–153
cervical spine, 185–187
defined, 35–36
elbow and forearm, 70–71
hip, 123
knee, 140–141
lumbar spine, 203–205
metacarpophalangeal joint, 93
shoulder, 52–53
temporomandibular joint, 215
thoracic spine, 203–205
wrist and hand, 82–83
Vertebrae. *See* Costovertebral joint(s); Intervertebral joint(s)
Vertical axis, 4, 5f
Video motion analysis system, 204
Visual estimation, joint position/movement, 21, 185, 186–187

"Window" of a goniometer, 17f
Winging (abduction), scapula, 50
Wrist and hand
arthrokinematics, 79
capsular pattern, 79
carpometacarpal joint, thumb, 102–103
extension (dorsiflexion), 86, 86f, 87f
flexion, 84, 84f, 85f
functional range of motion, 80–81, 81t
interphalangeal joints, proximal and distal, 92–93, 100–103
metacarpophalangeal joints, 92–98, 103
midcarpal joints, 79–90
osteokinematics, 79
radial deviation (radial flexion), 88, 88f, 89f
radiocarpal joints, 79–90
range of motion, 80t, 80–82
reliability/validity, ROM measurements, 82–83
structure, 79
testing procedures, 84–91, 94–116
ulnar deviation (ulnar flexion), 90, 91f

0- to 180-degree notation system, 6, 30
Zygapophysial joint(s)
lumbar spine, 200
thoracic spine, 199